Lasers and Related Technologies in Dermatology

Lasers and Related Technologies in Dermatology

Roy G. Geronemus, MD
Director
Laser & Skin Surgery Center of New York
Clinical Professor of Dermatology
New York University Medical Center
New York, New York

Leonard J. Bernstein, MD
Associate Clinical Professor of Dermatology
Weill Cornell School of Medicine, New York
Laser & Skin Surgery Center of New York
New York, New York

Julie K. Karen, MD
Clinical Assistant Professor of Dermatology
New York University Medical Center
Laser & Skin Surgery Center of New York
New York, New York

Elizabeth K. Hale, MD
Clinical Associate Professor of Dermatology
NYU Langone Medical Center
Laser & Skin Surgery Center of New York
New York, New York

Elliot T. Weiss, MD
Clinical Assistant Professor of Dermatology
Weill-Cornell Department of Dermatology
Laser & Skin Surgery Center of New York
New York, New York

Lori A. Brightman, MD
Faculty
Department of Dermatology
Mt. Sinai School of Medicine
Laser & Skin Surgery Center of New York
New York, New York

Robert T. Anolik, MD
Clinical Assistant Professor of Dermatology
New York University Medical Center
Clinical Assistant Professor of Dermatology
Weill Cornell Medical College
Laser & Skin Surgery Center of New York
New York, New York

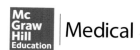 | Medical

New York   Chicago   San Francisco   Athens   London   Madrid
Mexico City   Milan   New Delhi   Singapore   Sydney   Toronto

LASERS AND RELATED TECHNOLOGIES IN DERMATOLOGY

1 2 3 4 5 6 7 8 9 0   CTP/CTP   18 17 16 15 14 13

BOOK ISBN: 978-0-07-174644-1
BOOK MHID: 0-07-174644-7

This book was set in Stempel Schneidler by Thomson Digital.
The editors were Anne Sydor and Regina Y. Brown.
The production supervisor was Sherri Souffrance.
Project management was provided by Sowmya Ramalingam, Thomson Digital.
China Translation & Printing Services, Ltd. was printer and binder.

This book is printed on acid-free paper.

Cataloging-in-Publication Data on file with the Library of Congress.

McGraw-Hill books are available at special quantity discounts to use as premiums and sales promotions, or for use in corporate training programs. To contact a representative please visit the Contact Us pages at www.mhprofessional.com.

Dedication

To my wife Gail, for her unwavering support over the years as I have built my career and channeled much of my energy into the evolving field of lasers and related technologies. Thank you for the encouragement to pursue my interests, *which*, *at* many times, *was* at the expense of our personal and family time.

To my sons Evan and Greg as well as their wonderful new brides Ashley and Katherine, for their significant interest in my clinical and academic life and providing me incredible joy and pride that I have witnessed in your personal and professional growth.

To my parents Terry and Al, and my sister Lynn, for making the sacrifices that were necessary for my education and for being my biggest fans for as long as I can remember.

To my co-authors Leon Bernstein, Lori Brightman, Liz Hale, Julie Karen, Elliot Weiss, and Rob Anolik, for their contribution not only to this book but also to making the Laser & Skin Surgery of New York a special place to work and advance the field in which we are immersed.

To Jeremy Brauer and Kavitha Reddy, fellows extraordinaire, for their tireless efforts in preparing many of the chapters and also for their major contributions to the field in such a short period of time.

To Joan Agnetti and Allison McDonough as well as the staff at the Laser & Skin Surgery of New York for helping me build a dynamic and exciting clinical and research practice that has allowed our physicians to provide state-of-the-art quality care to our patients.

To the 25 fellows who have shared my vision and enthusiasm for the extraordinary opportunities placed before us.

Roy G. Geronemus, MD

Contents

Contributors

Robert T. Anolik, MD
Clinical Assistant Professor of Dermatology
New York University Medical Center
Clinical Assistant Professor of Dermatology
Weill Cornell Medical College
Laser & Skin Surgery Center of New York
New York, New York
Chapters 5, 6, and 8

Leonard J. Bernstein, MD
Associate Clinical Professor of Dermatology
Weill Cornell School of Medicine, New York
Laser & Skin Surgery Center of New York
New York, New York
Chapter 4

Jeremy A. Brauer, MD
Clinical & Research Associate
Laser & Skin Surgery Center of New York
New York, New York
Chapters 3, 5, 9, and 11

Lori A. Brightman, MD
Faculty
Department of Dermatology
Mt. Sinai School of Medicine
Laser & Skin Surgery Center of New York
New York, New York
Chapters 5 and 6

Roy G. Geronemus, MD
Director
Laser & Skin Surgery Center of New York
Clinical Professor of Dermatology
New York University Medical Center
New York, New York
Chapters 2 and 10

Elizabeth K. Hale, MD
Clinical Associate Professor of Dermatology
NYU Langone Medical Center
Laser & Skin Surgery Center of New York
New York, New York
Chapters 3 and 7

Julie K. Karen, MD
Clinical Assistant Professor of Dermatology
New York University Medical Center
Laser & Skin Surgery Center of New York
New York, New York
Chapters 7 and 11

Christine A. Liang, MD
Associate Physician and Instructor in Dermatology
Department of Dermatology
Brigham and Women's Hospital
Harvard Medical School
Boston, Massachusetts
Chapter 7

Kira Minkis, MD, PhD
Clinical Associate in Dermatology
Weill Cornell School of Medicine
New York Presbyterian Hospital
New York, New York
Chapter 4

Tracey Newlove, MD
Department of Dermatology
New York University School of Medicine
New York, New York
Chapter 8

Kavitha K. Reddy, MD
Fellow, Procedural Dermatology
Laser & Skin Surgery Center of New York
New York, New York
Chapters 2, 5, 6, and 10

Melanie A. Warycha, MD
Faculty
Department of Dermatology
Mount Kisco Medical Group
Mount Kisco, New York
Chapter 3

Elliot T. Weiss, MD
Clinical Assistant Professor of Dermatology
Weill-Cornell Department of Dermatology
Laser & Skin Surgery Center of New York
New York, New York
Chapters 1 and 9

Preface

This book represents the collective experience of the Laser & Skin Surgery Center of New York, arguably one of the largest and most comprehensive private laser and technology centers in the world. Our physicians as the primary authors of each chapter are all fellowship trained in procedural dermatology and have been active in the clinical development of many of the devices you will be reading about in this book. It is my hope that this experience will help the reader understand the science and the rationale for the clinical use of each of the devices and the conditions for which their use is indicated.

My interest in lasers began as a senior resident in dermatology at the New York University Medical Center Skin & Cancer Unit in 1983. At that point I established the Department of Dermatology's laser program. I began with 2 lasers that are now essentially defunct, the argon and continuous-wave carbon dioxide lasers. By today's standards our results from those lasers were marginal and grossly inferior to what can be achieved with current technologies.

The field of lasers was transformed in 1994 with the introduction of the theory of selective photothermolysis allowing for the selective destruction of a vascular target in the skin (Chapter 1). I was fortunate to have been involved in the clinical trials of the first of the lasers (pulsed dye) that was developed in accordance with the selective photothermolysis theory. As the forerunner of the long and growing list of lasers capable of selective injury, the pulsed dye laser was initially designed and developed for the safe treatment of port-wine stains and has subsequently been utilized as an effective treatment for many additional vascular conditions, scars, and numerous inflammatory conditions (Chapter 2). In 1990 and 1991 selective photothermolysis of pigment including tattoo pigment was introduced with the Q-switched ruby and Nd:YAG lasers and subsequently with the Q-switched alexandrite lasers (Chapter 3). The ability to safely and effectively remove tattoos and many types of epidermal and dermal pigmentation helped the concept of laser technology gain broader acceptance in the dermatologic community. These lasers were further modified in the later part of the 1990s with longer pulse widths for the removal of hair, which has experienced worldwide popularity (Chapter 4). Rejuvenation of the skin and the removal of neoplasms were promulgated in the mid-1990s with the use of sophisticated scanning and delivery systems for the ablative carbon dioxide laser. While in theory the SP concept would apply to the absorption of water allowing for precise thermal injury of the skin, extraordinary results were by thermal side effects with higher than expected incidence of depigmentation and scarring allowing this resurfacing procedure to lose popularity.

Fortunately, in the early 2000s the concept of fractional resurfacing was introduced, addressing many of the concerns of prolonged healing and untoward side effects. Initially as a nonablative procedure and subsequently as an ablative rejuvenation technique, effective and safe resurfacing has become a viable option for a broad segment of the public (Chapter 5). The first decade of this century also brought about the introduction of non-laser technologies including monopolar and bipolar radio frequency, focused ultrasound, low-level light, and the use of cold for therapeutic purposes. This broad range of energy devices has further expanded the options for resurfacing and has provided unique nonablative options for skin tightening and body contouring (Chapter 6). The past decade or so has also seen the modification of wavelengths and techniques to allow for the safe and effective treatment of the skin of color as well as the treatment of inflammatory diseases such as acne (Chapter 7) and precancerous lesions in combination with light or lasers (Chapter 8). The use of laser technology for traumatic, surgical, and acne scars has been well accepted by a population of patients with limited therapeutic options (Chapter 9).

The future of lasers and light sources may well be exemplified by the introduction of home-based devices for hair removal, acne, and rejuvenation (Chapter 10).

This book was intended to give a broad overview and update on the range of technologies offered as of 2013. While this didactic review is intended to provide physicians and their professional staff the background required to appreciate the use of technology for the skin, it will not replace the need for an understanding of skin biology and hands-on training and experience.

The enclosed DVD should embellish the didactic content of what has been written.

This book and the accompanying DVD should be considered part of an ongoing learning experience as this is a rapidly changing field that will continue to evolve at a rapid pace with increasing importance in field of dermatologic care.

Lasers and Related Technologies in Dermatology

CHAPTER 1

Fundamentals of Lasers and Related Technology

Elliot T. Weiss

The field of laser-, light-, and energy-based technology has grown tremendously since the introduction of the first medical laser. These technologies continue to benefit from ongoing research and technical advancements, and the practicing surgeon must continuously learn and adapt to new and changing devices. The purpose of this book is to provide the laser surgeon with an updated comprehensive clinical guide to laser-, light-, and energy-based devices used in dermatology and dermatologic surgery. While a detailed overview of the physics of laser- and energy-based devices is beyond the scope of this book, a brief summary of the fundamentals of lasers and related technologies is included for general review. These concepts should help guide practitioners as they learn and modify techniques in response to new and changing technology.

■ OVERVIEW

The term *laser* stands for *l*ight *a*mplification by *s*timulated *e*mission of *r*adiation. While differing laser designs exist, the basic components are similar. Energy or light passes through a gain medium where an amplified beam of light is generated through stimulated emission. The gain medium may consist of a gas, liquid, plasma, or solid, and the medium's electrons absorb external energy (often from a light source or electrical field) and enter an excited quantum state. The electrons' eventual transition back to a relaxed state from the excited state results in a predictable emission of radiation. Various design techniques exist to create a stimulated emission of radiation at a desired wavelength. Differing designs and gain mediums have enabled the production of lasers at many different desired wavelengths.

Emitted laser light is classically characterized as exhibiting temporal and spatial coherence. Temporal coherence implies polarized light waves of a single frequency moving in phase, troughs aligned with troughs and peaks aligned with peaks. Spatial coherence, on the other hand, describes a narrow beam of light with minimal diffraction or divergence. These characteristics of laser emissions distinguish them from other high-energy emissions of light. Laser emissions can be precisely measured, and several terms are commonly used to describe the energy output of a laser device. Fluence is the term used to describe the quantity of laser energy delivered to a given area (fluence = Joules/[centimeter]^2). Pulse energy describes the quantity of energy delivered with each individual pulse of laser light. Power is a term used to describe the rate at which energy is transferred, and it is expressed in watts (1 W = 1 J/s).

Laser devices can deliver energy continuously over time (continuous mode) or in short pulses separated by intervals of time (pulsed mode). Most medical lasers used in dermatology operate in pulsed mode, and, conceptually, devices can be divided into categories based on wavelength and pulse duration. Wavelengths utilized in medical lasers include those in the ultraviolet, visible, and infrared spectra (see Table 1-1). Extremely short pulse durations, in the nanosecond and picosecond range, can be generated through engineered design features known as quality-switching (Q-switching) and mode-locking. These features allow the laser to generate large quantities of energy that are released in nanosecond or picosecond pulses, and these ultrashort pulses of laser light are capable of generating photoaccoustic effects on target tissues.[1] Current medical lasers used in dermatology offer pulse durations ranging from the picosecond to continuous wave, and many devices are capable of adjusting pulse durations to meet the needs of the operator.

The principle of selective photothermolysis governs the selection of a laser wavelength to match a peak in the absorption spectrum of the targeted chromophore. A chromophore is a material that absorbs specific wavelengths of light and transmits others. An absorption spectrum describes the degree at which a chromophore absorbs incident radiation over a range of frequencies.

TABLE 1-1
Commercial Medical Lasers Available According to Wavelength

Name	Wavelength (nm)	Photon Emitting Medium	Substrate	Type	Typical Mode Pulse Duration
Excimer laser	308	Excited dimer molecules (Xe-Cl)	Different gases	Gas	Pulsed µs–ms
"KTP" laser (Nd:YAG laser) frequency doubled) with KTP crystal)	532	Nd^{3+}	Crystal: Yttrium-aluminum Garnet ($Y_3Al_5O_{12}$)	Solid state	Pulsed ms–ns
Dye laser	585–600	Dyes, eg, Rhodamines	Organic solvents	Liquid	Pulsed ms
Ruby laser	694	Cr^{3+}	Al_2O_3	Solid state	Pulsed ms–ns
Alexandrite laser	755	Cr^{3+}	Chrysoberyl ($BeAl_2O_4$)	Solid state	Pulsed ms–ns
Diode laser	Different wavelengths (eg, 810, 940)	InGaAs AlGaAs	Semiconductor material	Solid state	Pulsed ms
Nd:YAG laser	1,064	Nd^{3+}	Crystal: Yttrium-aluminum Garnet ($Y_3Al_5O_{12}$)	Solid state	cw, pulsed ms–ns
Er:YAG laser	2,940	Er^{3+}	Crystal: Yttrium-Aluminum Garnet ($Y_3Al_5O_{12}$)	Solid state	Pulsed ms
CO_2 laser	10,600	CO_2	Different gases	Gas	cw, pulsed ms

The absorption spectra of each of the skin's major chromophores, melanin, water, and oxyhemoglobin, have been well characterized, and the wavelengths of most available medical lasers correspond to peaks in these absorption spectra (see Figure 1-1). Each chromophore has multiple absorption peaks, and the relative absorption of one chromophore versus another for a particular wavelength changes as one moves across the visible light and infrared spectrum. When treating the skin, the laser operator must account for the fact that all 3 major chromophores are always present to some degree and will absorb laser energy according to their respective absorption spectrum.

The first step in selecting the appropriate laser device entails identifying the target chromophore to be treated (melanin, exogenous pigment, water, oxyhemoglobin). Once identified, the surgeon can select a laser with an emission spectrum that corresponds to a peak in the target's absorption spectrum. The depth of the target chromophore must also be taken into account, and longer wavelengths are selected, when possible, for treating more deeply located targets. The presence of competing chromophores must always be considered when selecting a wavelength and treatment parameters.

Selective photothermolysis is based on the concept of delivering sufficient energy to heat and destroy a target before it can cool by dissipating thermal energy to surrounding tissue, causing nonselective heating and tissue damage. This principle allows for laser energy to be deposited specifically at a target chromophore in such a manner that the tissue effect or thermal injury is spatially confined to the target chromophore. The laser pulse duration (Tp) thus largely controls the spatial confinement of the laser energy. The thermal relaxation time describes the rate at which a material dissipates absorbed thermal energy. The thermal relaxation time (Tr) is a function of the square of the target diameter (d) and is inversely related to the thermal diffusivity of the target, as expressed in the following formula: Tr = $d^2/16X$. Selecting a pulse duration equal to or less than the thermal relaxation time of the target is necessary to selectively heat the chromophore while avoiding collateral tissue damage. This delivery of laser energy using a specific wavelength and pulse duration to selectively create a spatially confined thermal injury is the operating principle for aesthetic lasers used for treating vascular lesions, pigmentation, tattoos, and hair.

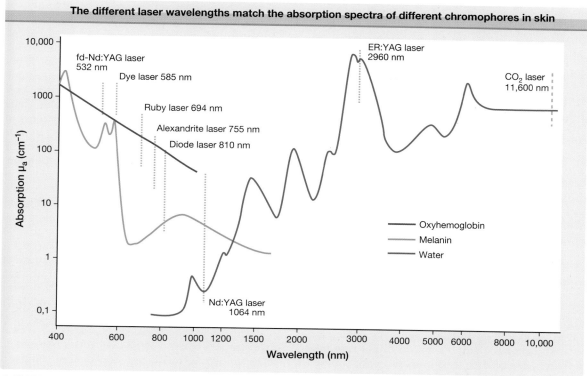

▲ FIGURE 1-1 The different laser wavelengths match the absorption spectra of different chromophores in skin.

Many of the tissue targets treated with laser therapy are located underneath the melanin-containing epidermis. While treating these dermal or subcutaneous targets with high fluences, epidermal cooling mechanisms must be employed to prevent thermal injury to the overlying epidermis resulting from melanin's absorption of laser energy. Various technologies have been developed to cool the epidermis during laser- and energy-based device treatment. One of the first technologies to be developed that is still in use is the dynamic cooling device (DCD). This technology utilizes a cryogen spray that is delivered to the skin in adjustable amounts. The cryogen spray rapidly evaporates on the surface of the skin and cools the skin in preparation for the laser pulse. Care must be taken to use the appropriate amount of cryogen cooling to avoid overheating the epidermis during treatment, but excessive cryogen cooling can result in a cold-induced injury to the epidermis (cryogen burn). Forced-air cooling is another method of protecting the epidermis. With this technique, chilled air is blown from a hose onto the treatment area to cool it in preparation for the energy pulse. Another very common method of epidermal cooling is contact cooling. With this technology, a chilled tip on the device handpiece is held in contact with the skin to be treated. Typically, the chilled tip consists of a transparent crystal (often sapphire) that is maintained at low temperature. When the tip is in contact with the treatment area, it absorbs the heat and cools the surface before the pulse of energy is delivered.

In recent decades, a non-laser, light-based technology known as intense pulsed light (IPL) has become increasingly popular in aesthetic medicine. These devices use various lamp designs to generate intense pulses of incoherent, polychromatic light, instead of coherent laser light, that can be delivered over short pulse durations to achieve the desired clinical effect. The principle of selective photothermolysis still governs the use of this technology in medicine. IPL devices utilize various filters that remove unwanted wavelengths of light and shape the emission spectrum to match the absorption spectrum of the targeted chromophores. Different filters are used when targeting pigmentation and hair (melanin) versus vascular lesions (oxyhemoglobin), and, similar to laser devices, pulse durations are modified based on the thermal relaxation time of the targeted chromophore. In order to avoid thermal injury to the epidermis, IPL also utilizes integrated epidermal cooling mechanisms, most commonly a chilled crystal which contacts the skin.

In addition to light- and laser-based devices, recent technological advancements have allowed the safe utilization of radio frequency (RF) and ultrasound energy (US) in aesthetic medicine. RF energy consists of electrical currents that oscillate at the rate of 3 kHz to 300 GHz. RF energy (MHz range) is used in dermatology to deliver heat to and to tighten deeper tissue layers in the skin. RF can be delivered into the skin via several methods, all of which rely on tissue resistance to transform delivered RF energy into thermal energy. RF is capable of penetrating deep into tissue and is not affected by epidermal melanin, making it safe for all skin types. Monopolar RF devices utilize a single RF electrode placed on the skin and a grounding pad located at a distant location. Bipolar RF devices utilize 2 electrodes placed on the skin and do not require a grounding electrode. Below the treatment electrodes, an oscillating electrical field passes through the tissue and is converted to thermal energy. The shape, size, and orientation of RF electrodes determine the depth and degree of volumetric tissue heating. Several new devices utilize fractional RF to generate dermal and subcutaneous heating. Fractional RF is designed to heat only a fraction of dermal and subcutaneous tissue while sparing the remaining tissue. Similar to fractionated laser treatment, this method is thought to enhance treatment effect while minimizing side effects and recovery. Fractional RF can be delivered via several methods. With one method, a handpiece consisting of numerous RF electrodes (contact points) is placed into contact with the skin. The RF energy passes selectively underneath and between adjacent RF contact points. The end result is a latticework of intersecting arcs of RF-treated tissue under the skin with only a fraction of the dermis treated with RF energy while the other portion is left untreated. Another method utilizes rows of RF electrodes that are inserted superficially into the skin. The RF energy selectively travels between adjacent pins and delivers spatially confined thermal injury to a portion of treated tissue. Similarly, the end result is a latticework of RF-treated tissue between the RF electrodes.

Focused ultrasound is the newest energy form to be utilized in aesthetic medicine for therapeutic purposes. US consists of high-frequency acoustic waves that can deeply penetrate human tissue. As US passes through tissue, some energy is transmitted and some is converted to heat. Ultrasound waves can be focused and thus concentrated at specific depths below the skin's surface to treat dermal and subcutaneous tissue. These focused waves can create spatially confined zones of thermal injury at various depths below the surface without injuring the overlying tissue. Treatment of the dermis and connective tissue results in thermal injury and subsequent neocollagenesis. Treatment of subcutaneous adipose tissue results in thermal injury and death of adipocytes in the treatment zones. Similar to RF, US is not absorbed by melanin and therefore may be safely used on all skin types.

A critically important principle of laser surgery is related to variability both in the tissue response of each individual and in the performance of each device. The skin's response to laser treatment is dynamic and varies with depth, breadth, degree, or density of laser injury. Essential to successful laser treatment of any dermatologic condition is a clear understanding of the desired clinical end point to be obtained during treatment. Experienced surgeons use the tissue response as a guide to ensure appropriate treatment parameters and desired end points. Energy settings for different devices of the same class are not always interchangeable and device performance varies from manufacturer to manufacturer. This concept cannot be overemphasized. Depending on the treatment delivered, varying degrees of purpura, vessel blanching, erythema, edema, or epidermal whitening may be desired.

EQUIPMENT

Common available vascular lasers and devices, including the long pulse 532, 595, 755, and 1064 nm, and IPL, all target the chromophore hemoglobin/oxyhemoglobin within dermal and subcutaneous vasculature. Due to the presence of epidermal melanin, which acts as a competing chromophore for the laser energy, vascular-specific devices must provide some form of epidermal cooling to prevent injury to the epidermis. Epidermal whitening during vascular treatment indicates excessive superficial energy deposition and/or inadequate epidermal cooling. Depending on the clinical scenario, appropriate treatment of vascular lesions is evident by transient or fixed purpura, erythema, or temporary vessel blanching without epidermal whitening. As will be discussed in later chapters, deeper or thicker vascular lesions may best respond to longer wavelengths that penetrate deeper into treated tissue or longer pulse durations that target larger-caliber vessels.

Epidermal and dermal melanin and exogenous pigments possess multiple absorption peaks within the visible light spectrum. As a result, multiple laser wavelengths are available for pigmented lesion treatment, including 532, 694, 755, and 1064 nm, and IPL. Targeted melanosomes or pigment particles measure in the micrometer range, and therefore nanosecond or picosecond pulse durations are required for the most selective destruction. Q-switched and mode-locked lasers generate picosecond- and nanosecond-range laser pulses best suited for selective destruction of melanosomes or tattoo pigment. Epidermal whitening occurs transiently during Q-switched laser treatment and often represents the desired clinical end point. In general, a clinical end point of uniform whitening without epidermal disruption is desired during Q-switched laser treatment or picosecond-laser treatment of epidermal pigmentation and tattoos. When treating darker skin types, care must be taken to avoid excessive whitening that may lead to hypopigmentation or even postinflammatory hyperpigmentation.

Laser hair removal targets melanin within the hair bulb and follicular unit located in the dermis. The most commonly used systems include the 755 nm alexandrite, 800 nm diode, the 1064 nm Nd:YAG, and appropriately filtered IPL. Laser hair removal targets the concentrated melanin found within the follicular bulb and matrix, and it requires epidermal cooling to protect the melanin-containing epidermis that functions as a competing chromophore for the laser energy. The clinical end point of therapy is typically follicular erythema without epidermal whitening or graying.

Numerous lasers are currently available for skin rejuvenation and resurfacing. These devices all target the chromophore water and rely on thermal injury to stimulate dermal remodeling and neocollagenesis. This category can be divided into ablative and nonablative and subdivided into fractionated and nonfractionated. The carbon dioxide (10,600 nm) and the erbium:YAG (2940 nm) lasers are the most commonly used ablative lasers. These wavelengths are highly absorbed by water, and thus delivery of short pulses of energy results in precise zones of tissue ablation and thermal injury. Nonablative lasers consist of infrared wavelengths with a relatively lower absorption by water, and therefore these lasers penetrate through

tissue and result in thermal coagulation, rather than ablation.

The introduction of the fractionated laser beam allowed users to generate deep columns of ablation or thermal injury extending into the dermis while avoiding confluent epidermal injury and subsequent scarring or pigmentary alteration. Fractional treatment results in a grid-like distribution of microscopic treatment zones (MTZ). With fractional ablative lasers, the pulse duration of each micropulse determines the ratio of ablation to thermal coagulation present at each MTZ. Ultrashort pulses, at one extreme, create ablative zones with very narrow zones of thermal coagulation at the periphery. Longer pulse durations result in ablation zones surrounded by wider zones of thermal coagulation that extend deeper and wider than the ablative zone. Each ablative device creates a different combination of ablation and thermal coagulation, and the surgeon must be aware of the characteristics of the device in use in order to avoid excessive injury to the skin. With nonablative fractional lasers, the wavelength and size of each microbeam determine the pattern and extent of tissue injury. Commonly used wavelengths for nonablative fractional resurfacing are 1410, 1440, 1540, 1550, and 1927 nm. With the exception of 1927 nm, the mid-infrared wavelengths are only moderately absorbed by water and therefore are capable of penetrating deeply into the dermis to generate thermal coagulation. The 1927 nm wavelength is more highly absorbed by water, and, therefore, this wavelength creates superficial, spatially confined thermal injury best suited to treat epidermal disorders.

Various ablative and nonablative fractional devices are available, and each device varies in its method of delivering the fractionated beam to the treatment area. One method entails a rolling handpiece that delivers fractionated laser treatment to the skin as the handpiece is continuously moved across the surface. Another method, known as stamping, utilizes a lens array inside the handpiece to fractionate the laser beam each time the laser is activated. The handpiece must be moved from area to area in a stamping movement to evenly deliver treatment to the skin. Some devices utilize a scanning handpiece to fractionate the beam. With this method, the handpiece is held over each area to be treated and an optical scanner generates a fractionated pattern within the treatment area each time the laser is activated.

Fractionated lasers allow the treatment of a percentage of the skin's surface, and, as a result, a fraction of epidermal and dermal tissue units in treated areas are

TABLE 1-2
Thermal Relaxation Times for Common Laser Targets in Skin

Target	Mean Diameter	Thermal Relaxation Time
Pigment (melanosome)	~0,1 μm	5 ns
Small vessel (eg, port-wine stain)	~50 μm	1.1 ms
Hair follicle	~0,2 mm	18 ms
Large vessel (eg, leg veins)	~1,5 mm	1,023 ms

uninjured and available to rapidly regenerate and repair zones of thermal injury (Table 1-2). This technology mitigates many of the risks and side effects associated with nonfractionated resurfacing or rejuvenation procedures.

MEDICOLEGAL ISSUES

Laser surgery, like any procedure, inherently entails some risk to the patient. From a medicolegal standpoint, an adequately documented discussion of the risks, benefits, and alternatives to treatment must occur before every treatment. While the most common risks should be clearly stated in the consent form, the physician should review the expected risks and outcomes prior to the patient signing the informed consent form. Furthermore, all safety precautions and laser parameters should be documented clearly in the patient record, and posttreatment skin care should also be reviewed with the patient and documented in the medical record.

As will be discussed in the following section, proper training and experience allows the operator to recognize the desired clinical end point during treatment and to ensure a safe outcome. The delegation of laser procedures to nonphysicians is a growing and concerning trend, and the level of training and experience achieved by nonphysician operators varies greatly. The likelihood of injury resulting from inappropriate treatment is thus higher with delegated procedures, and the liability risk to the supervising physician is subsequently elevated. When a physician is not directly performing or supervising a procedure, he or she assumes liability for any error that the lesser-trained operator may make.

Another important medicolegal issue involves wound care and follow-up. Documentation of patient education regarding wound care is essential. Additionally, the physician should establish follow-up visits, as appropriate, to ensure proper wound healing following laser treatment. This is particularly critical following ablative procedures. Failure to reasonably recognize and treat any deviation in the normal healing process may result in patient harm and subsequent liability risk to the physician.

PEARS AND PITFALLS

While laser surgery has the potential for serious side effects, most operator-dependent errors can be avoided when the surgeon has a clear understanding of laser–tissue interactions and desired clinical end points. For most available lasers, there exist multiple manufacturers offering similar products. Laser devices are not created equal, and laser parameters that are appropriate for one manufacturer may not be appropriate when applied to another manufacturer's device. Additionally, the laser output of a device may vary slightly over time and with extended use, and periodic servicing or preventive maintenance can result in minor differences in laser performance. These above-mentioned variables are easily detected and accounted for when surgeons use the real-time tissue reaction to guide therapy. While specific energy and treatment parameters must be noted and recorded, experienced practitioners continuously monitor the reaction of the skin to the laser energy and use this end point to guide therapy. This method allows the practitioner to immediately detect any unexpected tissue responses and to modify treatment parameters as needed. Failure to recognize appropriate and inappropriate tissue responses causes the practitioner to rely solely on numerical treatment parameters as guides, and in this circumstance, obvious undertreatment or overtreatment may occur and remain undetected during the treatment. Most treatment failures or side effects can be prevented altogether when this principle is followed.

This concept becomes particularly relevant when laser procedures are delegated to less experienced users who may not recognize the proper or improper tissue response. In these situations, the risk of injury to the patient is significantly increased.

The laser surgeon must carefully balance the potential risks of a procedure with the likelihood of achieving a successful outcome. Additionally, the degree of medical necessity or the severity of the condition being treated influences the level of risk that both the physician and patient are willing to tolerate. The treating physician and patient should discuss these factors prior to initiating treatment.

Finally, a satisfied patient is generally one whose expectations are met, and, therefore, properly managing patient expectations is essential to running a successful laser practice. The first step in this process is an accurate assessment of the wishes and desires of the patient. Carefully listening to patient concerns and clarifying the specific needs during the consultation allows the physician to identify the particular goal(s) of treatment. Once identified, the physician should confirm these goals with the patient and begin to establish reasonable expectations for the treatment. Specifically, the physician should carefully convey the likelihood of treatment success, the expected degree of improvement, and the predicted range of treatment sessions required. Patients should be made aware of the fact that treatment outcomes vary slightly from person to person, and exact percentages of improvement are often impossible to guarantee. The physician's word choice is very important, and simply stating "get rid of" rather than "improve significantly" may unknowingly create unreasonable expectations and ultimately a dissatisfied patient. Generally speaking, the goal is to create expectations that can always be met or exceeded by treatment, and this generates satisfied patients and a successful practice.

REFERENCE

1. Brauer J, Reddy K, Anolik R, et al. Successful and rapid treatment of blue and green tattoo pigment with a novel picosecond laser. *Arch Dermatol*. 2012;148(7):820–823.

CHAPTER 2

Laser Treatment of Cutaneous Vascular Lesions

Kavitha K. Reddy and Roy G. Geronemus

INTRODUCTION

Destruction of vascular lesions by laser treatment represents one of the earliest applications of selective photothermolysis, a principle elucidated by Anderson and Parrish.[1] The first reports of successful clinical laser treatment of vascular lesions were made by Goldman and colleagues in 1968.[2] Laser treatment of vascular lesions is accomplished most often using the principle of selective photothermolysis, using nonablative vascular-selective lasers that target hemoglobin in the vessel. Alternative choices such as ablative lasers or photodynamic therapy have also been used to destroy vessels. When the appropriate laser and settings are selected and applied, lasers demonstrate success in safely destroying cutaneous vessels of various types, sizes, and depths.

SELECTIVE PHOTOTHERMOLYSIS OF VESSELS

Vascular lesions are composed of endothelial cell–lined vessels containing colorless lymphatic fluid, blood colored by hemoglobin, or both. Vessels vary in diameter, thickness, and depth. Hemoglobin present may be in varying states of oxygenation, including deoxyhemoglobin, oxyhemoglobin, methemoglobin, or any combination of these forms. Selective photothermolysis (Figure 2-1) employs the observation that preferential absorption of a laser pulse by certain pigmented chromophores causes their heating and subsequent thermal destruction, with relative sparing of surrounding structures. Excess thermal energy absorbed by the pigmented target diffuses to surrounding targets in a process termed thermal relaxation. In order to selectively destroy vessels, the laser wavelength should be preferentially absorbed by the chromophore present in the vessel, which in the case of blood-filled lesions is hemoglobin in varying forms. The wavelength must also be sufficiently long to reach the targeted vessel depth. The pulse duration should be equal to or less than the vessel thermal relaxation time (τ_r) to avoid heat damage to the surrounding structures (for cylindrical vessels, $\tau_r = d^2/16\kappa$; $\kappa = 1.3 \times 10^{-3}$ cm²/s).[1] The energy delivered, or fluence, should be sufficient to damage the vessel(s) while also conservative enough to limit injury of surrounding tissue.

MECHANISM OF VASCULAR INJURY

The ultimate target is the vascular endothelium. Selective photothermolysis indirectly injures the endothelium by heating the chromophore hemoglobin

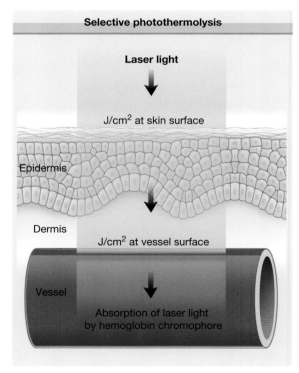

▲ **FIGURE 2-1** Selective photothermolysis of vascular lesions.

within the vessel, leading to formation of an occlusive mass of photocoagulated erythrocytes, with subsequent heat transfer to the endothelium and endothelial cell destruction by coagulation necrosis (achieved at a critical temperature of >70°C for thermal denaturation).[3] Photomechanical effects including cavitation (water vaporization with steam bubble expansion and collapse) may also damage endothelial cells.

Histologic evaluation after selective photothermolysis of cutaneous vessels (Figure 2-2) demonstrates immediate brown discoloration of the blood with a viscous decrease in flow, hemostasis, and formation of a coagulated erythrocyte mass. Vessel rupture with hemorrhage may be observed at purpuric settings.[1] By 24 hours, vasculitis-like changes of neutrophilic and lymphocytic perivascular infiltrate with karyorrhexis are seen.[1] Vascular remodeling is hypothesized to occur in many cases, replacing damaged vessels with normal ones.[4] At 1 month after effective treatment, reduction in the number and/or diameter of the targeted vessel(s) is seen.

■ EVALUATION OF THE PATIENT

History

Clinical evaluation of the patient is an essential first step in selection of the most effective and safe treatment. A thorough history with particular attention to historical elements that aid in accurate diagnosis and treatment of vascular lesions includes the following:

1. Time of onset: present at birth (congenital), or acquired
2. Changes in appearance over time
3. Growth in width and/or thickness, rate of growth
4. Associated tissue hypertrophy
5. Associated systemic disease
6. Associated bleeding or bruising
7. History of imaging or other studies
8. History of chemotherapy or radiation treatment
9. Medication list with particular attention to anticoagulants
10. History of isotretinoin use in the past 6 to 12 months
11. Skin phototype and tendency toward postinflammatory hyperpigmentation

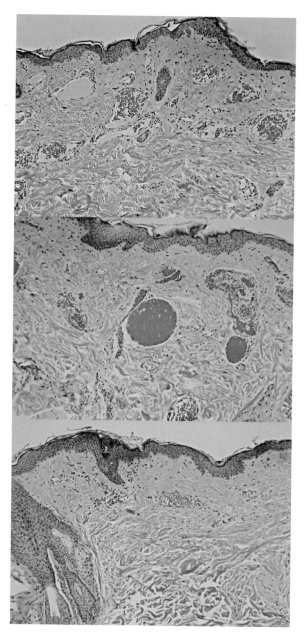

▲ **FIGURE 2-2** Histologic effects of laser treatment of cutaneous vessels. Port-wine stain capillaries before treatment, immediately after KTP laser treatment showing platelet thrombi and homogenized erythrocytes, and 1 month after laser treatment showing reduced vessel number and size.

Physical Examination

Close physical examination aids in diagnosis and selection of appropriate treatment parameters. The following may be estimated most often from the physical examination:

1. Type of vessel(s) present (lymphatic, arterial, venous, mixed, capillary). The color(s) of the lesion is helpful in determining the type and density of vessels present.
2. Thickness of the vessels.
3. Density of vessels.
4. Blood quantity in the vessel.
5. Blood quality in the vessel (type of hemoglobin present, oxyhemoglobin, deoxyhemoglobin, and/or methemoglobin).
6. Depth(s) of vessels.
7. Overall size of the lesion.
8. Diameter of vessels (small, medium, large).
9. Skin color (type and amount of epidermal melanin).
10. Hair follicle presence and type in affected area.

Consultation with a dermatologist, vascular specialist, or other physician as needed to determine the appropriate diagnosis and medical care may be considered. Other testing or imaging studies are sometimes required for accurate diagnosis or evaluation.

During and after each laser treatment, close physical examination should continue. Vascular lesions are dynamic and change is often visible during and after treatments. During treatment, the desired clinical end point should be monitored, and the treatment adjusted to safe and effective achievement of the end point. This includes observing for changes in the targeted vessel(s), and simultaneously observing the integrity and color of the epidermis. In general, clinical end points are transient purpura, persistent purpura, or disappearance of the vessel along with avoidance of graying, moderate to severe whitening, or blistering of the epidermis.[5] Multiple treatments are often required and treatment expectations of both physician and patient should be reasonable. A particular vascular lesion may contain vessels with varying characteristics, and may require multiple treatment modalities and/or continued evolution in choice of laser and settings at subsequent treatments. Clinically observed factors such as blanching, whitening, purpura, erythema, edema, pigmentary changes, scarring, or severe pain should be closely observed

and continually evaluated to guide optimal and safe treatment.

PARAMETER SELECTION

Wavelength

The first parameter selected is generally wavelength. Wavelength should be selected to achieve 3 goals: (1) strong and preferential absorption by the target chromophore (hemoglobin), as determined by published absorption spectra (Figure 2-3), (2) absorption to the least extent possible by competing chromophores (eg, melanin), and (3) sufficient depth to target the vessel(s).

The chromophore in blood-filled vascular lesions (arteries, veins, and capillaries) is hemoglobin, the red-colored oxygen carrier in erythrocytes. Hemoglobin may exist in varying states of oxygenation, including deoxyhemoglobin, oxyhemoglobin, and/or methemoglobin. Hemoglobin shows strong absorption at 400 to 600 nm (blue, green, yellow) and some absorption at 700 to 1100 nm (near-infrared) (Figure 2-3). Melanin absorbs wavelengths up to more than 1000 nm, with decreasing absorption as the wavelength increases. Therefore, when treating darker skin types (generally skin types III and higher, or tanned type II skin), longer wavelengths will provide greater safety and reduced risks of pigmentary changes, with 1064 nm Nd:YAG lasers frequently being the wavelength of choice in darker skin types.

Pulse Duration

The ideal pulse duration should be equal to or slightly less than the target's thermal relaxation time, or time for the central temperature to cool by 50%. A pulse duration long enough to deliver sufficient heat to the target vessel, while also short enough to limit transfer of damaging heat to surrounding structures, is desirable. Very short pulse durations far less than the thermal relaxation time rapidly deliver high energies, resulting in target rupture, shock wave propagation, and in some cases nonselective damage.[6] Pulse widths should be varied to match the appropriate vessel size.

Fluence

To determine the appropriate fluence, test spots are often helpful, beginning with a conservative fluence and gradually increased as necessary for the achievement of the goal response. The optimal fluence permits

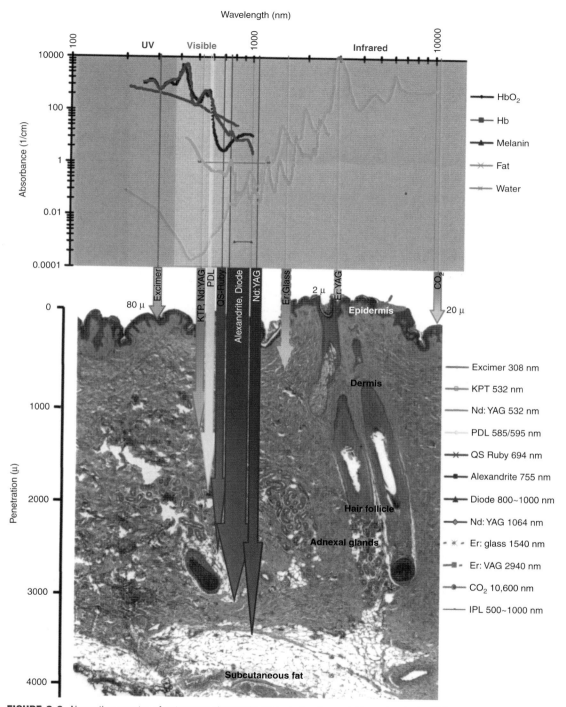

▲ **FIGURE 2-3** Absorption spectra of cutaneous chromophores including hemoglobin and melanin. Light absorption by skin chromophores as a function of wavelength, with the approximate 50 percent optical penetration depth. Erbium (Er), hemoglobin (Hb), oxygenated hemoglobin (HbO_2), potassium-titanyl-phosphate (KTP), intense pulsed light (source) (IPL), neodymium (Nd), yttrium-aluminum-garnet (YAG), pulsed dye laser (PDL), Q-switched (QS), ultraviolet (UV). (Created with permission from data of Drs. Scott Prahl, Thomas Flotte, and Dieter Manstein.)

vascular destruction while avoiding nonspecific thermal damage that may lead to immediate or delayed pigmentary change or scarring. The goal clinical response during treatment varies according to the lesion treated.[5] Blanching or disappearance of the vessel may be seen. Transient purpura indicates intravascular coagulation.[6] Vessel rupture and erythrocyte extravasation results in persistent purpura lasting several days.[6] In addition to the immediate clinical response, the long-term response 2 to 4 weeks after treatment should be evaluated when selecting subsequent fluence settings.

Spot Size and Spacing

Spot size is selected based on lesion size and desired depth of penetration. Increasing spot sizes penetrate to increasing depths and allow more convenient and rapid coverage of the lesion. The choice of spot size is limited by the desired fluence and pulse duration and adjustments may be required depending on the capability of the laser being used. Spacing should be individualized based on desired treatment density, shape and size of spots, risk of bulk heating, and the beam energy distribution profile of the particular laser being used.

Passes

Multiple passes may in some circumstances improve overall treatment success due to repeated vessel injury. Methemoglobin may also be formed after the first pass and subsequently targeted during succeeding passes.[7] Periods of cooling between each pass are generally recommended to reduce the risk of bulk heating. Pulse stacking consists of multiple pulses in the same area without significant cooling intervals, a technique that increases risks of bulk heating and scarring. Therefore, pulse stacking is usually avoided, particularly in children, except in occasional circumstances where repeated injury is desirable.

Epidermal Protection and Cooling

Competing chromophores overlying the intended target influence treatment efficacy and safety. For vascular lesions, overlying chromophore is found in overlying vessels and in epidermal melanin.[8] Longer wavelengths have a greater depth of penetration, reduced melanin absorption, and reduced risk of hypopigmentation or hyperpigmentation. Longer pulse widths or, in the case of intense pulsed light (IPL), longer delay times between pulses also reduce the risk of pigmentary changes.

Epidermal cooling methods further aid in reducing damage, allowing higher fluences to be used that more effectively heat target vessels.[9–12] Common cooling methods are cryogen spray cooling (also called "dynamic" cooling, CSC, 1,1,1,2-tetrafluoroethane, and/or R134a), contact cooling (chilled quartz or sapphire window, chilled gel or ice), and cold air cooling. Cryogen spray cools epidermis and at spray durations of 100 to 300 milliseconds may affect superficial vessels in the papillary dermis.[13] CSC may provide more effective cooling than contact cooling.[14] Contact cooling is nonetheless also effective in many circumstances, although the pressure of the glass window may blanch fine superficial vessels making them more difficult to visualize.

PHYSIOLOGIC INFLUENCES

Overlying Vessels

Vessels between the target and the initial laser pulse partially shield the target, reducing the fluence reaching the target and decreasing efficacy.[15] Dense overlying vessels are generally treated first in order to improve subsequent targeting of deeper vessels.

Cutaneous Temperature, Vascular Dilation, and Blood Flow

Decreased cutaneous temperature requires a slightly increased fluence to achieve purpura.[16] Vascular dilation and blood flow, as affected by conditions of suction, pressure, epinephrine effects, or UVB erythema, do not appear to significantly influence purpura thresholds.[16] Nonetheless, conditions that increase cutaneous temperature, bring greater blood (chromophore) into the treatment area, or aid in photocoagulation are predicted to improve treatment efficacy.[8]

ADJUNCTIVE METHODS

Diascopy

Nodular, hypertrophic, or high-flow lesions (eg, spider angioma) or lesions with superficial vessels above the target may benefit from compression during laser treatment using a glass slide.

Dependence/Tourniquets

Venous lesions will often darken as a result of increased blood content when in a dependent position or when outflow is constricted with a tourniquet. These techniques may be utilized to improve chromophore content and treatment efficacy.[17]

IMAGING METHODS

Video microscopy, optical coherence tomography, and other imaging methods that determine depth and pattern of vascular abnormality may aid in optimal treatment selection.[18] Imaging aids are likely to improve efficacy as technology develops.

ALTERNATIVE AND COMBINATION TREATMENT METHODS

Laser treatment of vascular lesions represents an effective and safe modality for the vast majority of cutaneous vascular lesions limited to the upper 3 to 4 mm of the skin. For lesions with a deeper portion or connection, such as compound or deep infantile hemangiomas (IH) or arteriovenous malformations, laser treatment from the surface of the skin does not reach the deep component and an alternative or adjunctive treatment method should be considered. Alternative or adjunctive treatment methods for vascular lesions include endovenous ablation, sclerotherapy, photodynamic therapy, embolization, and cosmetic camouflage. Topical and systemic inhibitors of angiogenesis, such as rapamycin, or medical therapy such as propranolol for deep IH, represent another alternative or adjunctive option.[19]

SIDE EFFECTS, RISKS, AND COMPLICATIONS

Erythema and Edema

Erythema and edema are common, lasting from a few hours to weeks after laser treatment of vascular lesions. Both may be reduced by posttreatment application of ice or chilled gel pads.

Purpura

Transient or persistent purpura is a desired clinical end point. Persistent purpura occurs frequently with pulse durations less than 6 to 10 milliseconds. Purpura will fade in 7 to 14 days, though may leave residual hemosiderin pigmentation. Pulsed dye laser (PDL) treatment of purpura beginning 2 to 3 days after the bruise is noted speeds resolution.[20]

Alopecia

Vascular-specific lasers frequently target follicular melanin and may lead to alopecia in the treated areas. Physicians may choose to avoid areas where hair is desired or the patient should be informed of risks of alopecia.

Risks and Complications

PIGMENTARY CHANGES Pigmentary changes are the result of direct effects on melanosomes and/or postinflammatory changes. Strong photoprotection is critical to both prevention and treatment in the majority of cases. In darker skin types, wavelengths with minimal melanin absorption, longer pulse widths, use of conservative fluences, and appropriate epidermal cooling methods help to prevent unintended thermal damage. Further, prevention and prompt treatment of inflammation reduce risks of postinflammatory changes. Test spots evaluated immediately after treatment and at 2 to 4 weeks posttreatment are recommended to assess the response and side effects prior to treating a large area. Hyperpigmentation may sometimes but not always be improved with photoprotection, time, and/or appropriate use of hydroquinone or melanin-reducing agents. Hypopigmentation may respond to ultraviolet light treatment in the form of excimer laser or narrowband UVB treatment.[21]

SCARRING Scarring is a rare complication when appropriate settings are employed. However, its avoidance requires careful attention to settings and clinical end points. Particular anatomic locations such as the neck, chest, and periorbital skin are more likely to scar. Conservative fluences reduced by 10% to 20% are recommended in scar-prone areas, even with traditionally lower-risk lasers such as the PDL.[22–24] Lasers with a high risk of scarring are often avoided in these areas entirely. Postprocedure care and avoidance of trauma are also critical. If scarring has occurred, the choice of wavelength, fluence, pulse duration, and influence of patient factors such as skin type and physiologic variables must be considered carefully to determine the contributing factors. Persistent gray coloration, development of blistering, or scabbing may be warning signs of impending scar development. Scarring should be managed by close observation, appropriate wound care, and consideration of intervention using intralesional agents, silicone gel dressings, and/or laser treatments.

OCULAR AND RETINAL SAFETY Appropriate eye protection for all individuals in the treatment room should be utilized, along with precautions to reduce scatter and accidental exposures such as use of appropriate warning signs. Patients should wear appropriate protective goggles, or if a periorbital area is being treated, a stainless steel eye shield. In addition to adverse effects on multiple structures in the eye, laser and light exposures can destroy retinal melanin, potentially resulting in rapid and painless blindness.[25]

OPERATING ROOM SAFETY The vast majority of laser procedures may be performed safely under local anesthesia using topical anesthesia, intralesional injection, or local nerve blockade. Laser treatment may also be performed under general anesthesia, for example, when an uncooperative child is of sufficient size to warrant ocular or other safety concerns, or when there is patient preference to undergo general anesthesia to reduce anxiety and/or pain. In the operating room setting, the presence of high-concentration oxygen in the presence of laser radiation presents a fire hazard.[26] When supplemental oxygen is required, laryngeal mask airways with clear tubing are preferred due to a more optimal seal and minimal laser light absorption.[26] Nasal cannulas leak significant amounts of oxygen. Flammable substances should not be used to clean the laser handpiece, or when used must be allowed to dry completely and then preferably rinsed with water. Wet drapes should be placed around the oxygen tubing, and wet gauze, water, and a fire extinguisher should be readily available (Figure 2-4). In addition, use of nonflammable water-soluble lubricant on hair-bearing sites and use of intraocular eye shields all reduce potential fire hazards.[26]

LASERS AND LIGHT SOURCES WITH VASCULAR EFFECTS

Argon

The first widely used vascular-selective laser, the argon laser generates blue-green 488 to 514 nm light strongly absorbed by oxyhemoglobin, and reaches 1 to 2 mm depth. The small spot size (0.1–1 mm) limits penetration depth and makes operator use difficult. Because of the continuous wave property, the pulse duration frequently exceeds the target thermal relaxation time, leading to a high rate of pigmentary change and scarring. Melanin also absorbs argon wavelengths, further increasing risk of pigmentary change and epidermal damage. After PDLs were developed, the argon laser fell out of favor due to higher risks. A quasi-continuous wave 488 to 638 nm argon-pumped tunable dye laser (APTDL)

exists, although the rate of scarring still remains high when compared with the PDL. For these reasons, argon lasers have been almost completely replaced by use of the pulsed dye and other vascular lasers.

Copper

Copper vapor and copper bromide lasers produce 578 nm yellow quasi-continuous light. Thermal necrosis is a common reaction with blistering and crusting. Melanin is also absorbed, limiting use to skin types I to II. For these reasons, copper lasers are infrequently used.

Krypton

Krypton lasers produce 520 to 530 nm quasi-continuous wave green light and 568 nm yellow light. Although infrequently used, the most common use of krypton lasers is in the treatment of facial telangiectasia (often

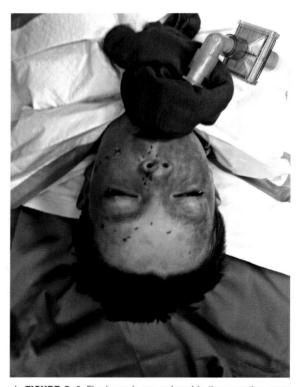

▲ **FIGURE 2-4** Fire hazards are reduced in the operating room with use of a laryngeal mask airway, wet towels around oxygen tubing, water-soluble lubricant over hair-bearing areas, and placement of intraocular eye shields. In addition, water, wet gauze, and a fire extinguisher are kept within reach.

at 568 nm, 1 mm spot size, 0.2 second pulse duration, power of 0.5–0.75 W, every 3–4 weeks).[27]

Potassium Titanyl Phosphate (KTP)

KTP lasers are 532 nm frequency-doubled Nd:YAG lasers. Most are quasi-continuous wave, although continuous wave KTP lasers have been developed. The laser has a short penetration depth and is absorbed by both melanin and oxyhemoglobin, limiting its use to superficial vascular lesions in skin types I to III. KTP lasers are most often used to treat telangiectasias, although a variety of applications exist.

Pulsed Dye Laser

First-generation PDLs produced 577 nm light, the wavelength of the third absorption peak of oxyhemoglobin. To increase penetration depth and improve dye efficiency, modern PDLs have been updated to produce 595 to 600 nm yellow light, although this does reduce absorption by hemoglobin. PDLs penetrate 2 mm into the skin and exhibit good absorption by oxyhemoglobin and deoxyhemoglobin, as well as some absorption by melanin. Pulse durations range from 0.45 to 40 milliseconds, allowing a variety of vessel types to be targeted. Spot sizes range from 2 to 12 mm, with circular and elliptical options. Modern PDLs with CSC have demonstrated an excellent safety profile when administered appropriately over many years.[28] As such, the PDL has become the standard of care for the majority of superficial vascular lesions in lighter skin types.

Alexandrite

Alexandrite lasers have a longer, near-infrared 755 nm wavelength best used to target deeper, larger vessels in the skin than those treated with the PDL or KTP lasers. In particular, the alexandrite laser is typically used for dark or resistant port-wine stains (PWS), and larger-caliber spider and reticular veins in the legs as an alternative to sclerotherapy.

Diode

Diode lasers (800–940 nm) are most commonly used to treat venous lakes[29] and to perform endovenous ablation of incompetent lower extremity veins[30] or other vessels.[31]

Nd:YAG

The 1064 nm Nd:YAG laser provides increased penetration depth, low epidermal melanin absorption, and good absorption by methemoglobin and deoxyhemoglobin. The Nd:YAG laser is therefore most commonly used for treatment of reticular veins and for vascular lesions in darker skin types. Reduced rates of purpura add to its value. Appropriate epidermal cooling is important given higher fluences are required to reach and heat deeper vessels. Crusting, scarring, and pigmentary change may occur due to high fluences. In high-risk sites such as inside the orbital rim, Nd:YAG treatment is generally avoided or performed with caution in the presence of an intraocular eye shield.

Intense Pulsed Light

IPL is noncoherent (non-laser) pulsed 500 to 1200 nm light most commonly produced by a xenon flashlamp. Filters can be used to select certain wavelengths (wavelengths below the filter level are eliminated; common filters are 420, 515, 550, 560, 570, 595, 610, 645, 695, and 755 nm). IPL may be given in 1, 2, or 3 pulses of 1.5 to 25 milliseconds each, with 2- to 500-millisecond intervals between each pulse and fluences of 3 to 90 J/cm². Spot sizes range from 8×15 to 15×35 mm, and can be reduced further by physically covering portions of the applicator with opaque paper. Cooling is most often through chilled gel or a chilled crystal. Despite its non-laser classification, IPL can result in pigmentary change and scarring when appropriate settings are not carefully selected and when clinical end points are not carefully evaluated before, during, and after treatment.

■ LASER TREATMENT OF SPECIFIC VASCULAR LESIONS

See Table 2-1.

Telangiectasia and Spider Angioma

Telangiectasias are small dilated superficial blood vessels (diameter 1–1.5 mm) that are most often macular and occasionally papular (spider angioma). They are most commonly acquired as a result of aging, genetics, and/or ultraviolet exposure. On sun-exposed areas of the neck and upper chest, they may be associated with poikiloderma (mottled pigmentation and telangiectasia). On the legs, venous stasis is a frequent cause. Occasionally, telangiectasia may develop as a result of prolonged or potent topical corticosteroid use, radiation dermatitis, or an underlying medical condition such as lupus erythematosus, hereditary hemorrhagic telangiectasia, systemic sclerosis/CREST (calcinosis, Raynaud

TABLE 2-1
Laser Treatment of Vascular Lesions[a]

Diagnosis	Clinical Appearance	Laser	Wavelength (nm)	Skin Phototypes	Settings	Clinical End Point	Treatment Interval	Treatment Expectations	Medical Considerations
Telangiectasia	0.1–1 mm diameter pink, red, or violaceous linear or arborizing macules or papules	KTP	532	I–III	7–16 J/cm², 3–7 mm, 10–30 ms; purpuric settings (<3–6 ms) improve efficacy; when nonpurpuric settings are chosen, pulse stacking at low fluences may improve efficacy	Blanching/disappearance of vessel	4–6 weeks	Individual lesions typically resolve in 1–2 treatments; perinasal vessels are often more resistant or may not resolve; new telangiectasias commonly appear over time	Hereditary hemorrhagic telangiectasia, lupus erythematosus, systemic sclerosis (CREST syndrome), rosacea, hyperestrogenic states, nevoid conditions, radiodermatitis, basal cell carcinoma, other conditions
Telangiectasia	0.1–1 mm diameter pink, red, or violaceous linear or arborizing macules or papules	PDL	585–595	I–III	5–8 J/cm², 10–12 mm, 0.45–6 ms (using Candela V Beam laser)	Blanching/disappearance of vessel	4–6 weeks	Individual lesions typically resolve in 1–2 treatments; perinasal vessels are often more resistant or may not resolve; new telangiectasias commonly appear over time	Hereditary hemorrhagic telangiectasia, lupus erythematosus, systemic sclerosis (CREST syndrome), rosacea, hyperestrogenic states, nevoid conditions, radiodermatitis, basal cell carcinoma, other conditions
Telangiectasia	0.1–1 mm diameter pink, red, or violaceous linear or arborizing macules or papules	IPL	500–1200	I–III, cautious use in type IV	550–570 nm filter in lighter skin types; 2.5–5 ms double pulse, 25–45 J/cm², 10–30 ms delay; may treat through hole in opaque white paper to target desired area	Little to no purpura	4–6 weeks	Gradual improvement over multiple sessions, new telangiectasias commonly appear over time	Hereditary hemorrhagic telangiectasia, lupus erythematosus, systemic sclerosis (CREST syndrome), rosacea, hyperestrogenic states, nevoid conditions, radiodermatitis, basal cell carcinoma, other conditions
Spider angioma	Pink to red blanching papule	PDL	585–595	I–III	6–8 J/cm²; 7–10 mm spot size, 1.5 ms pulse width; may treat center through glass slide or glass contact cooling window, followed by feeding vessels	Disappearance of the lesion or mild superficial whitening	4–6 weeks	Individual lesions typically resolve in 1–2 treatments	Hyperestrogenic states, pregnancy, children
Cherry angioma	Cherry-red dome-shaped papule	KTP	532	I–III	7–16 J/cm², 3–7 mm, 10–30 ms	Purpura	4–6 weeks	Individual lesions typically resolve in 1–2 treatments	Associated with chronologic aging

(continued)

TABLE 2-1

Laser Treatment of Vascular Lesions[a] *(Continued)*

Diagnosis	Clinical Appearance	Laser	Wavelength (nm)	Skin Phototypes	Settings	Clinical End Point	Treatment Interval	Treatment Expectations	Medical Considerations
Infantile hemangioma—superficial component	Pink patch to cherry-red plaque	PDL	585–595	I–IV	6–8 J/cm², 7–10 mm, 0.45–1.5 ms	Purpura	2–8 weeks depending on speed of proliferation	Slowed growth phase, reduced proliferation	Consider ophthalmologic referral if at or near orbit; large, extensive, or multiple lesions need medical evaluation
Infantile hemangioma—deep component	Skin colored to violaceous or blue nodule	Laser treatment ineffective, refer for medical or other procedural therapy	N/A	N/A	N/A	N/A	N/A	N/A	As above
Port-wine stain (capillary vascular malformation)—superficial	Pink to dusky pink patches	PDL	585–595	I–III	PDL: begin for infants at 8 J/cm², 10 mm, 1.5 ms; for children and adults at 8–8.5 J/cm², 10 mm, 1.5 ms; for darker skin types at 6.5 J/cm², 12 mm, 0.45–1.5 ms; may increase by 0.5 J/cm² per treatment only to desired clinical end point; cryogen spray cooling 30–50 ms spurt duration with 20–30 ms delay before pulse	Purpura	4–12 weeks	Gradual fading of color (10% per treatment); may reach treatment plateau	Consider glaucoma, Sturge-Weber syndrome, Klippel-Trenaunay, Cobb, or other associated syndrome
Port-wine stain	Pink to dusky pink patches	IPL	500–1200	I–III	550 nm filter 50–75 J/cm² 40–60 ms delay between pulses	Little to no purpura	4–12 weeks	Gradual fading in color	Consider glaucoma, Sturge-Weber syndrome, Klippel-Trenaunay, Cobb, or other associated syndrome
Venous malformation	Blue to violaceous-hued plaques to nodules	Nd:YAG	532/1064	I–VI	Variable, adjust to targeted depth and size of associated vessels	Reduction in nodularity	4–6 weeks	Often requires alternative or adjunctive excision for complete removal	Consider associated syndromes or tissue hypertrophy

(continued)

TABLE 2-1
Laser Treatment of Vascular Lesions[a] *(Continued)*

Diagnosis	Clinical Appearance	Laser	Wavelength (nm)	Skin Phototypes	Settings	Clinical End Point	Treatment Interval	Treatment Expectations	Medical Considerations
Arteriovenous malformation	Initially appears as erythematous patch; develops into plaque or nodules over time; + warmth or bruit often present	Best referred to vascular radiologist for possible embolization or sclerotherapy, or for surgical evaluation	N/A	N/A	N/A	N/A	N/A	N/A	Consider associated syndromes or tissue hypertrophy
Venous lake	2–10 mm blue to purple macules or papules	KTP	532	I–III	7 J/cm², 4 mm, 14 ms	Superficial whitening or purpura	4–6 weeks	Individual lesions typically resolve in 1–2 treatments	Associated with photodamage
Venous lake	2–10 mm blue to purple macules or papules	Nd:YAG	1064	I–VI	120–140 J/cm², 5–7 mm spot size, 0.45 ms pulse duration; pulse stacking may be required	Disappearance of the lesion or superficial whitening	4–6 weeks	Individual lesions typically resolve in 1–2 treatments	Associated with photodamage
Poikiloderma	Telangiectasia, hyperpigmentation, hypopigmentation, and atrophy; usually in sun-exposed skin of neck or chest	PDL	595	I–III	5–7 J/cm², 7–10 mm spot size, 0.45–2 ms pulse width	Purpura	4–6 weeks	Gradual improvement over multiple sessions	Associated with extensive photodamage, occasionally with cutaneous T-cell lymphoma or dermatomyositis
Pyogenic granuloma	0.5–2.0 cm erythematous sessile or pedunculated papule	PDL	595	I–III	6.5–9.0 J/cm², 7–12 mm spot	Use diascopy to flatten lesion; treat to blanching and purple-gray color	Repeat every 3–4 weeks as needed	Most resolve in 1–3 treatments	Shave excision and cautery preferred method of treatment; may be associated with pregnancy, certain medications, trauma, or port-wine stains
Reticular veins	Large blue to violaceous linear to tortuous macular to slightly raised vessels	Nd:YAG	1064	I–VI	125–150 J/cm², 5–7 mm spot, 75–100 ms	Disappearance of vessel or superficial whitening	4–6 weeks	Individual lesions typically improve in 1–2 treatments	On legs evaluate for venous stasis and consider sclerotherapy; consider ocular safety and risk of scarring when treated periorbital veins

[a]Information in this table is provided as a suggested initial consideration only. All treatments should be based on the individual treating physician's knowledge and judgment and individualized appropriately to the patient, lesion, and device used.

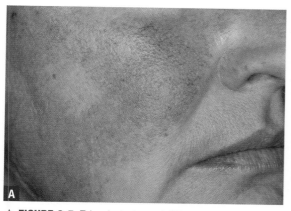
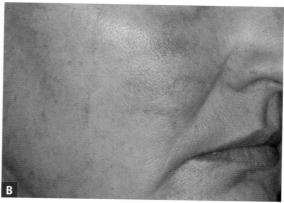

▲ **FIGURE 2-5** Telangiectasias and diffuse erythema. **A.** Rubeosis faciei (red face) in a 45-year-old female patient. **B.** Result after one PDL treatment.

syndrome, esophageal dysmotility, sclerodactyly, and telangiectasia) syndrome, hyperestrogenic states such as pregnancy or liver failure, or other conditions.[32]

Laser treatment is highly effective and remains the standard of care for facial telangiectasias and spider angioma, using the KTP lasers and/or PDLs[33] (Figures 2-5 to 2-8). KTP lasers may provide slightly greater efficacy, though may produce greater erythema and edema than PDL.[34] When using the PDL, conservative pulse stacking may improve efficacy.[35] The nasal

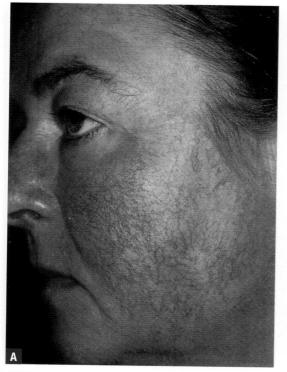
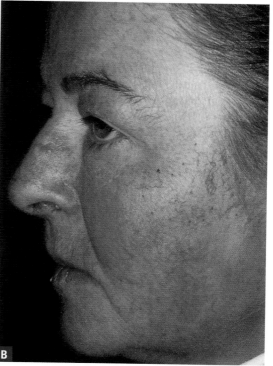

▲ **FIGURE 2-6** **A.** A woman with extensive facial telangiectasia. **B.** Two 585-nm, 450 μsec PDL treatments produced 80% clearing of vessels.

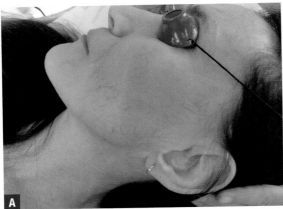
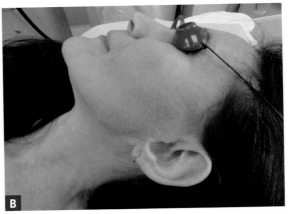

▲ **FIGURE 2-7** Facial telangiectasias immediately before (**A**) treatment show immediate disappearance after (**B**) KTP laser treatment, along with the appearance of erythema and edema that resolves within hours to days.

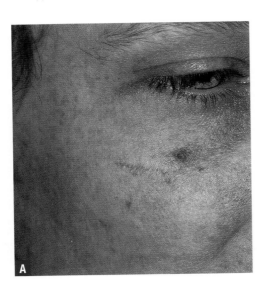
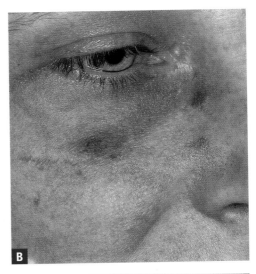

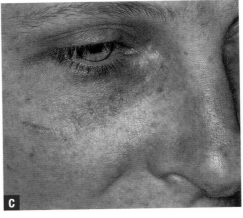

▲ **FIGURE 2-8** Treatment of spider angioma. **A.** Two spider angiomas on the upper right cheek prior to treatment. **B.** Immediately after treatment with a 585-nm PDL using 7.0 J/cm², there is a grayish discoloration of the treated area. **C.** Six weeks later, the angioma under the right eye is completely clear, and the lesion on the right side of the nose has lightened markedly.

ala and alar grooves are at higher risk of atrophic scarring, and caution is advised in these areas with appropriate use of cooling, and potential avoidance of pulse stacking. Lower extremity telangiectasias frequently respond to lasers but are often optimally treated by sclerotherapy, with the exceptions that postsclerotherapy matted telangiectasias, telangiectasias resistant to sclerotherapy, or those present in a needle-phobic patient are best treated by laser therapy.[36] As an alternative option, facial telangiectasias also respond to multiple IPL treatments.[37,38]

Cherry Angioma

Cherry angiomas are small, benign, cherry-red to violaceous dome-shaped superficial vascular papules. They appear with increasing age, usually beginning after age 30. The cause is otherwise poorly understood. For cosmetic removal the KTP lasers or PDLs easily destroy cherry angiomas in 1 or 2 treatments.[39]

Pyogenic Granuloma

Pyogenic granulomas are superficial acquired papular to pedunculated erythematous small (0.5–2.0 cm) vascular lesions. They are typically isolated, frequently occur spontaneously in children, and also appear in association with capillary vascular malformations (CVMs), pregnancy, or trauma, or with use of certain medications including isotretinoin and indinavir.[40,41] Because the lesions frequently bleed, patients seek treatment in the emergency room, often presenting with a bandage over the site (the "band-aid sign").[41] The standard of care is shave excision followed by light electrodessication of the base to prevent recurrence. Laser treatments using argon or carbon dioxide lasers until blanching or photocoagulation occurs, or PDLs with the aid of diascopy and multiple overlapping pulses, are also an option, though with variable effectiveness, frequent need for multiple treatments, and greater recurrence rate.[42–45] Both shave excision with electrodessication and laser treatment generally have good cosmetic results, although mild scarring can occur with either modality.

Venous Lake

Venous lakes are blue to violaceous papules presenting on the head and neck or other sun-exposed areas of middle-aged to elderly adults, most often as solitary lesions. The lesions partially or completely blanch with pressure, suggesting the diagnosis.[46,47] Venous lakes are easily treated with the KTP or Nd:YAG laser alone[48] or in combination with the PDL[46] (Figure 2-9). Diode lasers have also shown effective results in 1 or 2 treatments.[29] PDL alone has shown inconsistent results.[49] Older reports have utilized the argon and carbon dioxide lasers effectively, though with more frequent scarring and pigmentary changes.[46,50,51]

Infantile Hemangioma

IH are the most common vascular tumor in infancy, affecting 8% to 10% of Caucasian patients, more often

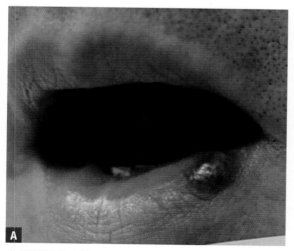
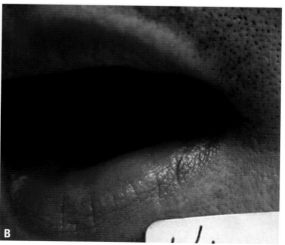

▲ **FIGURE 2-9** Venous lake treated with a potassium-titanyl-phosphate laser. **A.** Before treatment. **B.** After treatment.

females and low-birth-weight infants.[52] The cause remains poorly understood. IH are noticeable at birth in one third of patients, most often appearing as a blanched patch within a few days after birth, with subsequent growth into a red patch or plaque (superficial IH), bluish or skin-colored nodule (deep IH, previously described as cavernous), or both (compound IH). The growth phase typically lasts until 6 to 9 months of age (or corrected age if the child was born premature).[53] The rate of growth and ultimate size are difficult to predict in an individual hemangioma, and cannot be predicted by the initial size.[54] An involution phase, marked by the appearance of dull purple and then central white-gray coloration, invariably follows the growth phase and results in replacement of the IH parenchyma with soft fibrofatty tissue. Fifty percent of IH involute by age 5, 70% by age 7, and nearly all by age 10 to 12. Loose fibrofatty tissue and/or superficial vessels remain permanently after involution in 30% to 80% of cases.[52,55]

IH have a benign (nonmalignant) growth pattern. However, when large, deep, or present in certain anatomic locations, they may result in permanent disfigurement, developmental delay, infection, ulceration, or other adverse effects. Medical evaluation is paramount for large lesions (>5 cm), multiple lesions that may be associated with internal organ involvement, periorbital lesions,[56,57] lesions obstructing the auditory canal, those interfering with the airway,[58] large facial segmental or beard-like distribution IH, sacral hemangiomas,[59,60] and those with associated anomalies (PHACES syndrome).[61] In large hemangiomas, evaluation for iodothyronine deiodinase activity, congestive heart failure, or Kasabach-Merritt syndrome (associated with platelet trapping, anemia, and coagulopathy) may also be warranted.

Early treatment is recommended for IH having significant potential for negative long-term effects. Treatment may be started safely within days after birth. IH should be classified as superficial and/or deep. Laser can effectively treat the superficial component, the portion that appears as pink to red erythematous patches or plaques up to 3 to 4 mm in depth. PDL is the treatment of choice, showing strong efficacy and a good safety profile[62,63] (Figure 2-10). Periorbital skin may be safely and effectively treated with the PDL using an intraocular eye shield to protect the eye[64]

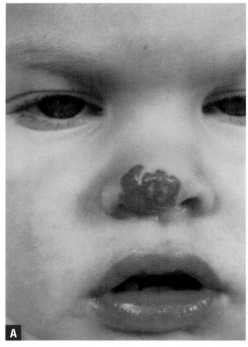 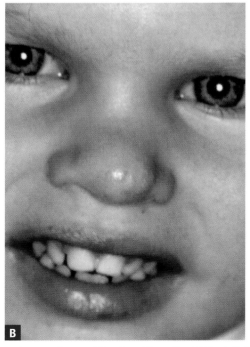

▲ **FIGURE 2-10** Infantile hemangioma. **A.** A partially involuting hemangioma on the nasal tip of an 18-month-old infant. **B.** Following 4 treatments with a 585-nm, 450 μsec PDL using a 5-mm spot at 8 J/cm².

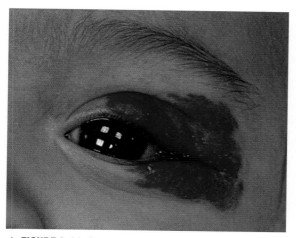 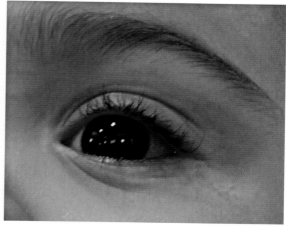

▲ **FIGURE 2-11** Superficial periorbital infantile hemangioma in a 22-week-old infant (left) showing nearly complete clearance (right) after 11 pulsed dye laser treatments performed over 35 weeks. An intraocular eye shield was utilized during treatments to protect the eye. (Reproduced from Hunzeker CM, Geronemus RG. Treatment of superficial infantile hemangiomas of the eyelid using the 595-nm pulsed dye laser. *Dermatol Surg.* 2010;36:590–597.)

(Figure 2-11). Ulcerated hemangiomas are also safely treated with PDL and in fact may show improvement in healing.[65] Common PDL settings range from 5.0 to 9.0 J/cm², 7 to 10 mm spot size, 0.45 to 1.5 milliseconds pulse width, with treatment given at 2- to 4-week intervals depending on the growth rate and stopping once involution is noted. Thick hemangiomas may be alternatively or additionally treated with alexandrite or Nd:YAG lasers to increase depth of penetration and potentially improve treatment response.[66] Laser treatment will typically reduce the growth rate; however, the hemangioma may still grow during the treatment course as long as the growth phase is active and this is not always a sign of treatment failure. The number of sessions required is not predictable, but typically ranges from 2 to 12 depending on the IH thickness, size, and the length of the growth phase. Alternative or adjunctive options for treatment of the superficial component include topical imiquimod[67] or timolol.[68]

The deep portion, a skin-colored, violaceous, or bluish plaque or nodule frequently seen underlying a superficial component, will not respond to surface laser and may require medical or other procedural therapies for control. Options for treatment of deep components of IH include propranolol,[69] systemic or intralesional corticosteroids,[70] or surgical excision.[71] For fibrofatty residuum persistent after IH involution, fractional laser treatment and/or surgery are effective in reducing the excess tissue and improving the appearance.[72–74]

Capillary Vascular Malformations (Also Called Port-Wine Stains)

CVMs are congenital regions of dilated vessels present in 0.3% to 0.5% of the population.[75,76] The underlying cause of vessel dilation is poorly understood, but hypothesized to be the result of a failure of autonomic innervation to the vessels. CVMs are present at birth and appear as dusky pink patches that often darken and/or thicken with age. Dusky pink patches limited to the glabella, eyelid, or posterior neck are likely different from PWS and are best classified as vascular "stains" or nevus flammeus, are common in the population, are less associated with social stigma, and often resolve spontaneously within the first few years of life, so that most often treatment is not recommended. Small vascular papules and pyogenic granulomas frequently develop within PWS over time and spontaneous regression of PWS does not occur.

The head and neck, particularly in the V1 and V2 dermatomes, are affected with greater frequency than the trunk or extremities.[75,76] CVMs are most often an isolated cutaneous abnormality; however, medical evaluation is indicated in particular circumstances. When the V1 dermatome is involved, ophthalmologic examination for glaucoma should be conducted every 3 to 4 months beginning soon after birth, as glaucoma may be present in 10% of patients.[77] Also when the V1 dermatome is involved, there is risk of Sturge-Weber syndrome (SWS), a syndrome of facial CVM, concomitant vascular involvement of the leptomeninges of the brain, and sometimes glaucoma in the ipsilateral eye.[78–80] Neurologic involvement may produce detectable tram-like calcifications in the brain, and risk of seizures or in some cases mental retardation.[80] These changes may not be present at birth or early infancy and for patients at risk of SWS, continued monitoring and/or imaging is warranted over time to detect the syndrome. Other associated syndromes that may present with a CVM are tissue or bony hypertrophy due to increased vascular flow (Klippel-Trenaunay syndrome), sometimes with an underlying arteriovenous malformation contributing to the hypertrophy (Klippel-Trenaunay-Weber syndrome). In addition, midline lumbar CVMs may be associated with an underlying arteriovenous malformation (Cobb syndrome).[81] Patients at risk of or diagnosed with these syndromes typically benefit from multispecialty involvement, patient and family education, and referral to national and international support groups (information available at www.sturge-weber.org and www.birthmark.org).

CVMs can produce physical disfigurement and deformity, especially when untreated as many become darker and thicker over time.[82] Furthermore, hypertrophy, nodular areas, and pyogenic granulomas frequently arise in adulthood in inadequately treated lesions.[83] Risks of psychosocial stigma and effects are well documented.[84–86] Therefore, when the patient or parent desires treatment, there is medical necessity.[83,85] Although some insurance programs may not approve coverage initially,[87] efforts to document medical necessity in letters to the insurer using patient information and evidence-based review of the literature are most often successful in the authors' experience to obtain coverage.

Given the safety and efficacy, the treatment of choice of CVMs is laser.[88] Early treatment, even within days after birth, is recommended for optimal rate and level of clearance, with the additional effect of reduced requirement for sedation to provide safe treatment.[89–92] Intraocular shields should be placed in infants, children, and adults before treating periorbital skin. For treatments away from the periorbital area, the eyes are protected with external shields. With properly trained staff, eye safety can be provided using intraocular shields or external eye protection in an office setting without general anesthesia for infants and small children. When the child is of enough strength to warrant mobility and safety concerns during treatment, general anesthesia should be considered. At any age, ocular safety should be paramount and assured.

Laser treatment is directed at heterogeneous sizes and depth of vessels within any individual CVM. CVM vessel diameter ranges from 10 to 300 μm. The average depth of the dilated PWS vessels is 0.46 to 0.6 mm,[82] with the vessel depth ranging from the superficial papillary dermis downward to nearly 5 mm.[93–95] The ideal pulse duration for CVM treatment (for 20–150 μm vessels) has been estimated as 1 to 10 milliseconds.[96] Because of the heterogeneous vessel sizes and depths, use of multiple or varied laser wavelengths and pulse durations may be required for optimal treatment over time.

PDL is the treatment of choice for early childhood or patch-like pink to red lesions[90,97–99] (Figure 2-12).

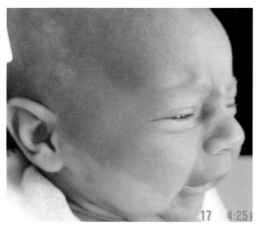
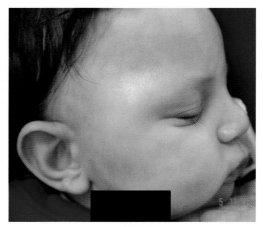

▲ **FIGURE 2-12** Facial capillary vascular malformation in a 4-week-old infant before treatment (left) and at 13 months of age, after 12 pulsed dye laser treatments with an average fluence of 8.9 J/cm² (right). (Reproduced from Chapas AM, Eickhorst KE, Geronemus RG. Efficacy of early treatment of facial port wine stains in newborns: a review of 49 cases. *Lasers Surg Med*. 2007;39:563–568.)

PDL penetrates up to 2 mm into the skin. Very small vessels less than 50 μm in diameter are unlikely to respond to PDL treatment.[100] Lesional areas are most often treated using 0% to 10% overlap. In children, the first treatment generally results in fading of color by half. Each subsequent treatment may show fading of an additional 10%. Most superficial CVMs will fade by 80% after 8 to 10 treatments, although individual results may vary.[101] In adults, 10% clearance is generally seen with each treatment, although as the number of treatments increases a plateau in clinical response is often reached.[102] Many patients may not exhibit more than 90% clearance. Certain locations, such as the peripheral face and neck, respond more rapidly and optimally, while distal and centrofacial lesions are often resistant to treatment[103,104] (Figure 2-13). V2 dermatomes also show less response than the V1, V3, C2, or C3 dermatomes[105] (Figure 2-14). Reasons for these

different rates of clearance based on anatomic location are poorly understood. Size also appears to influence treatment response, with smaller lesions responding better and larger 60 to 100 cm² lesions generally showing incomplete clearance.[106] The safety profile of PDL is generally excellent in skin types I to III, with rates of hyperpigmentation estimated at 1% to 1.7%, hypopigmentation at 0.26% to 2.6%, and atrophic scarring and hypertrophic scarring at 0.1%.[28] KTP lasers have similar effects as PDL and have also been shown to lighten CVM, although safety is slightly reduced and use is limited to Fitzpatrick skin types I to III.[107,108] Plaque-like, thick, dark, or resistant PWS are hypothesized to contain deeper vessels and often respond to PDL, though may also benefit from treatment with longer-wavelength near-infrared lasers including the alexandrite and Nd:YAG lasers[95,109] (Figure 2-15). Alexandrite and Nd:YAG lasers exhibit 50% to 75% deeper

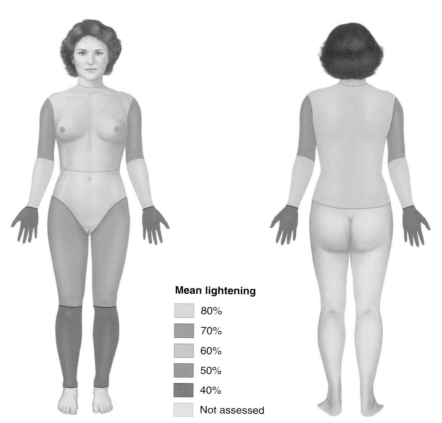

Mean lightening

- 80%
- 70%
- 60%
- 50%
- 40%
- Not assessed

▲ **FIGURE 2-13** Capillary vascular malformation clearance varies by anatomic location, with the trunk and proximal extremities clearing more easily than the distal extremities. (Reproduced from Renfro LR, Geronemus RG, Kauvar AB. Anatomical differences of port-wine stains located on the trunk and extremities in response to treatment with the pulsed dye laser. *Lasers Surg Med*. 1994;14(suppl 6):47.)

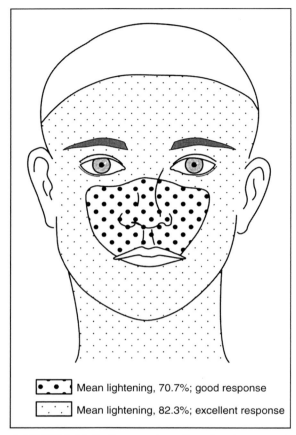
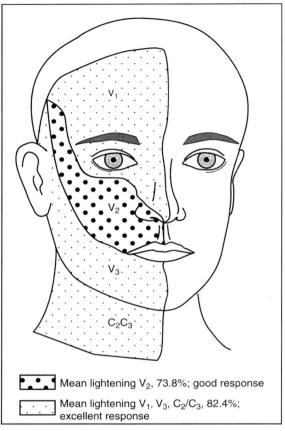

▲ **FIGURE 2-14** Capillary vascular malformation clearance varies by facial region as well as dermatomal distribution. (Reproduced from Renfro LR, Geronemus RG. Anatomical differences of port-wine stains in response to treatment with the pulsed dye laser. *Arch Dermatol.* 1993;129:182–188.)

penetration, but also are less absorbed by hemoglobin, so that higher fluences are required for vessel damage.[109] Pigmentary changes and scarring occur with greater frequency in alexandrite and Nd:YAG treatments than with PDL treatment (0%–4.3% reported risk of scarring).[28,52,110,111] Nd:YAG laser in particular has the lowest therapeutic window compared with PDL or alexandrite lasers, which results from Nd:YAG laser requiring higher fluences for vascular destruction and/or strongly targeting methemoglobin that appears during laser heating of hemoglobin.[112] Pulses spaced 1 to 2 spot diameters apart with filling in of skipped areas after 1 minute of skin cooling have been recommended to reduce bulk heat risks.[5]

The desired clinical end point of laser treatment of CVMs using KTP, pulsed dye, alexandrite, or Nd:YAG lasers is transient gray-blue discoloration of the skin that evolves to lasting purpura. If lasting purpura does not develop, undertreatment is likely, and if persistent gray discoloration appears, overtreatment with risk of scarring is a concern.[5] Traditionally, only 1 vascular-specific laser is used in each treatment session. Occasional reports of concomitant treatment using more than 1 vascular laser per session have been made. This may increase treatment efficacy, though could pose greater risk, and combination laser treatments would benefit from further study.[95]

IPL provides an alternative option for CVMs, particularly when vascular-specific lasers are not available or when seeking to avoid posttreatment purpura.[113,114] Other alternative or adjunctive treatment options that may be discussed with the patient include laser-mediated photodynamic therapy,[115] sclerotherapy, embolization, surgical excision, or cosmetic camouflage.

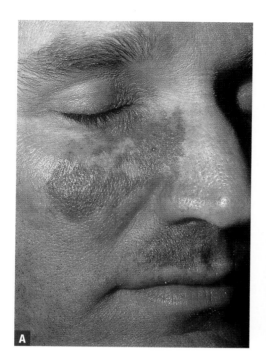

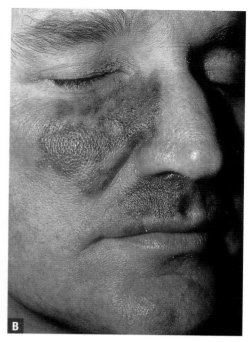

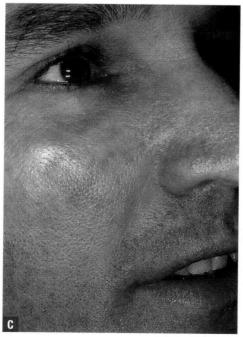

▲ **FIGURE 2-15** Capillary vascular malformations in adults. **A.** A young man with a PWS on the face. **B.** Purplish discoloration immediately after a 585-nm, 450-μsec PDL, using a 5-mm spot and 6 J/cm². **C.** After 4 PDL treatments, there is almost complete clearing with no textural change.

Nevus Simplex (Nevus Flammeus, Salmon Patch, "Angel's Kiss," "Stork Bite")

These are congenital midline CVMs on the glabella, medial upper eyelid, posterior neck, or lumbar skin with a varying prognosis than PWS CVMs.[116] They are sometimes persistent, though often resolve spontaneously within the first 2 years of life, and if treated often respond within 1 or 2 treatments. Because of their benign nature, limited area of involvement, and frequent spontaneous regression, treatment is generally not recommended unless the lesions persist beyond 2 years of age or the family desires earlier treatment.

Reticular Veins

Reticular veins are blue to green-hued, larger, and deeper-situated veins. Facial reticular veins are best treated with the 1064 nm Nd:YAG laser at relatively high fluences. The high fluences required make epidermal cooling important and pigmentary change a frequent side effect. Periorbital reticular veins are amenable to treatment; however, in rare cases eye injuries have occurred with periorbital treatment despite intraocular eye protection.[117] Lower extremity reticular veins and telangiectasias are more often associated with underlying venous stasis, and endovenous ablation and/or sclerotherapy is the treatment of choice.[36] Vascular lasers, including the alexandrite and Nd:YAG lasers, may be used for lower extremity veins as an alternative or adjunctive treatment (Figure 2-16).

Venous Stasis or Varicose Veins

Venous stasis is a condition of dilated veins in the lower extremities or other dependent area caused by incompetent valves that allow prolonged valvular reflux. The condition requires careful history, examination, and frequently imaging prior to diagnosis and selection of therapy. Incompetent lower extremity veins are treated sequentially beginning at the largest, more proximal branches and progressing toward the smaller vessels.[118] Large, deep incompetent veins such as the greater saphenous vein are best treated with endovenous ablation as a first-line choice.[119] An endovenous diode laser is inserted into the vein using a sterile catheter procedure.[120] Reticular, perforating, and telangiectatic veins are best treated with sclerotherapy, typically after an endovenous ablation procedure if one is indicated. However, in the case of matted telangiectasias, veins distal to the ankle, veins resistant to sclerotherapy, or patients with phobia of needles, laser treatment provides the best treatment choice.[118] Small leg telangiectasias or veins may be otherwise treated with PDL or Nd:YAG lasers as a second-line treatment option, since treatment failures, recurrences, and pigmentary changes can be of greater frequency with laser treatment compared with those with sclerotherapy.[36]

Venous Malformations

Venous malformations (VMs) are low-flow regions of dilated veins present at birth and showing progressive dilation with age. They are more frequent on the head and neck but may occur at any site. Treatment consists of laser, sclerotherapy, and/or excision. Given the deep, dilated vessels and venous nature, Nd:YAG laser represents the most effective laser option for cutaneous and/or mucosal VM.[121] Because high fluences are required, contact cooling and large spot sizes are helpful in reducing scarring. Because VMs are deep, Nd:YAG laser does

▲ **FIGURE 2-16** Lower extremity telangiectasias. **A.** Leg telangiectasias before treatment. **B.** After treatment with a 585-nm PDL using a 2 × 7 mm spot and 9 J/cm².

not typically penetrate throughout the lesion and recurrences and need for multiple treatments are common. Despite this, Nd:YAG laser can be a significant first-line option for cutaneous VM, and partial or adjunctive treatment option for deeper VM given surgical excision can be complicated and disfiguring, and also can lead to recurrences and scarring.[121,122]

Kaposi Sarcoma

Kaposi sarcoma is a malignant vascular neoplasm affecting patients with genetic predisposition in the classic form or those with human immunodeficiency virus (HIV–AIDS). Topical and systemic agents are first-line treatments depending on the thickness, depth, and stage. In occasional cases laser treatment using argon,[123] pulsed dye,[123] Nd:YAG,[124] or carbon dioxide lasers[125] has been effective for short-term control, though with frequent recurrence.

Lymphangioma

Lymphangiomas are most often congenital lesions appearing at birth or infancy in 1 in 6000 to 16,000 individuals.[126] They may also be acquired after inflammation, infection, or trauma.[127] The most common location is the axilla or neck, although they may appear anywhere on the skin. The lesion should be classified as superficial (termed lymphangioma circumscriptum, appears as bullae or vesicles with clear or red-orange fluid contents), deep (cystic hygroma), or compound. When congenital, medical evaluation is indicated to search for possible associated chromosomal abnormalities such as Turner syndrome. Asymptomatic lesions most often do not require treatment. Spontaneous regression may occur in up to 15% of deep congenital lymphangioma (cystic hygroma). When treatment is elected, excision or sclerotherapy is most common.[126] In cases having mixed lymphatic fluid and arterial or venous blood (red to orange or violaceous color visualized), selective photothermolysis may be employed.[128] When the fluid is clear and a chromophore is generally not present, selective photothermolysis is not an effective option. Ablative lasers may be used to aid in debulking or excision.[127,129] Scarring and incomplete treatment are frequent occurrences with all of the above modalities.[128,129]

■ CONCLUSION

Laser treatment of cutaneous vascular lesions represents one of the greatest successes in the application of selective photothermolysis. Laser treatment can be performed with excellent efficacy and safety for the majority of cutaneous vascular lesions with the appropriate choice of wavelength, settings, and cooling method for the targeted vessels and skin type of the patient. Vessels beyond the penetration depth of cutaneous lasers, or those with deep feeding vessels or other systemic vascular connection, are unlikely to respond to laser alone. Efficacy and safety continue to improve as technology and medicine advance, and as appropriate adjunctive methods are further developed. Laser treatment by a qualified physician represents a generally highly successful and widely available first-line treatment option for the majority of cutaneous vascular lesions.

REFERENCES

1. Anderson RR, Parrish JA. Selective photothermolysis: precise microsurgery by selective absorption of pulsed radiation. *Science*. 1983;220(4596):524–527.
2. Solomon H, Goldman L, Henderson B, Richfield D, Franzen M. Histopathology of the laser treatment of port-wine lesions. Biopsy studies of treated areas observed up to three years after laser impacts. *J Invest Dermatol*. 1968;50(2):141–146.
3. Black JF, Barton JK. Chemical and structural changes in blood undergoing laser photocoagulation. *Photochem Photobiol*. 2004;80:89–97.
4. Jia W, Sun V, Tran N, et al. Long-term blood vessel removal with combined laser and topical rapamycin antiangiogenic therapy: implications for effective port wine stain treatment. *Lasers Surg Med*. 2010;42(2):105–112.
5. Izikson L, Anderson RR. Treatment endpoints for resistant port wine stains with a 755 nm laser. *J Cosmet Laser Ther*. 2009;11(1):52–55.
6. Garden JM, Tan OT, Kerschmann R, et al. Effect of dye laser pulse duration on selective cutaneous vascular injury. *J Invest Dermatol*. 1986;87(5):653–657.
7. Alves OC, Wajnberg E. Heat denaturation of metHb and HbNO: e.p.r. evidence for the existence of a new hemichrome. *Int J Biol Macromol*. 1993;15(5):273–279.
8. Aguilar G, Choi B, Broekgaarden M, et al. An overview of three promising mechanical, optical, and biochemical engineering approaches to improve selective photothermolysis of refractory port wine stains. *Ann Biomed Eng*. 2012;40(2):486–506.
9. Dreno B, Patrice T, Litoux P, Barriere H. The benefit of chilling in argon-laser treatment of port-wine stains. *Plast Reconstr Surg*. 1985;75(1):42–45.
10. Gilchrest BA, Rosen S, Noe JM. Chilling port wine stains improves the response to argon laser therapy. *Plast Reconstr Surg*. 1982;69(2):278–283.
11. Nelson JS, Milner TE, Anvari B, et al. Dynamic epidermal cooling during pulsed laser treatment of port-wine stain. A new methodology with preliminary clinical evaluation. *Arch Dermatol*. 1995;131(6):695–700.
12. Nelson JS, Milner TE, Anvari B, Tanenbaum BS, Svaasand LO, Kimel S. Dynamic epidermal cooling in

conjunction with laser-induced photothermolysis of port wine stain blood vessels. *Lasers Surg Med*. 1996; 19(2):224–229.

13. Dai T, Diagaradjane P, Yaseen MA, Pikkula BM, Thomsen S, Anvari B. Laser-induced thermal injury to dermal blood vessels: analysis of wavelength (585 nm vs. 595 nm), cryogen spray cooling, and wound healing effects. *Lasers Surg Med*. 2005;37(3):210–218.

14. Anvari B, Milner TE, Tanenbaum BS, Nelson JS. A comparative study of human skin thermal response to sapphire contact and cryogen spray cooling. *IEEE Trans Biomed Eng*. 1998;45(7):934–941.

15. Pfefer TJ, Barton JK, Smithies DJ, et al. Modeling laser treatment of port wine stains with a computer-reconstructed biopsy. *Lasers Surg Med*. 1999;24(2):151–166.

16. Paul BS, Anderson RR, Jarve J, Parrish JA. The effect of temperature and other factors on selective microvascular damage caused by pulsed dye laser. *J Invest Dermatol*. 1983;81(4):333–336.

17. Svaasand LO, Aguilar G, Viator JA, Randeberg LL, Kimel S, Nelson JS. Increase of dermal blood volume fraction reduces the threshold for laser-induced purpura: implications for port wine stain laser treatment. *Lasers Surg Med*. 2004;34(2):182–188.

18. Motley RJ, Lanigan SW, Katugampola GA. Video-microscopy predicts outcome in treatment of port-wine stains. *Arch Dermatol*. 1997;133(7):921–922.

19. Phung TL, Oble DA, Jia W, Benjamin LE, Mihm MC Jr, Nelson JS. Can the wound healing response of human skin be modulated after laser treatment and the effects of exposure extended? Implications on the combined use of the pulsed dye laser and a topical angiogenesis inhibitor for treatment of port wine stain birthmarks. *Lasers Surg Med*. 2008;40(1):1–5.

20. Karen JK, Hale EK, Geronemus RG. A simple solution to the common problem of ecchymosis. *Arch Dermatol*. 2010;146(1):94–95.

21. Reszko A, Sukal SA, Geronemus RG. Reversal of laser-induced hypopigmentation with a narrow-band UV-B light source in a patient with skin type VI. *Dermatol Surg*. 2008;34(10):1423–1426.

22. Achauer BM, Vander Kam VM, Padilla JF 3rd. Clinical experience with the tunable pulsed-dye laser (585 nm) in the treatment of capillary vascular malformations. *Plast Reconstr Surg*. 1993;92(7):1233–1241 [discussion 42–43].

23. Glassberg E, Lask GP, Tan EM, Uitto J. The flashlamp-pumped 577-nm pulsed tunable dye laser: clinical efficacy and in vitro studies. *J Dermatol Surg Oncol*. 1988;14(11):1200–1208.

24. Swinehart JM. Hypertrophic scarring resulting from flashlamp-pumped pulsed dye laser surgery. *J Am Acad Dermatol*. 1991;25(5 pt 1):845–846.

25. Hammes S, Augustin A, Raulin C, Ockenfels HM, Fischer E. Pupil damage after periorbital laser treatment of a port-wine stain. *Arch Dermatol*. 2007;143(3):392–394.

26. Waldorf HA, Kauvar NB, Geronemus RG, Leffel DJ. Remote fire with the pulsed dye laser: risk and prevention. *J Am Acad Dermatol*. 1996;34(3):503–506.

27. Nouri K, Alster T. *Laser Treatment of Acquired and Congenital Vascular Lesions*. Available at http://emedicinemed scapecom/article/1120509-overview. Accessed 1/4/2012.

28. Seukeran DC, Collins P, Sheehan-Dare RA. Adverse reactions following pulsed tunable dye laser treatment of port wine stains in 701 patients. *Br J Dermatol*. 1997;136(5):725–729.

29. Wall TL, Grassi AM, Avram MM. Clearance of multiple venous lakes with an 800-nm diode laser: a novel approach. *Dermatol Surg*. 2007;33(1):100–103.

30. Van Den Bos RR, Neumann M, De Roos KP, Nijsten T. Endovenous laser ablation-induced complications: review of the literature and new cases. *Dermatol Surg*. 2009;35(8):1206–1214.

31. Angiero F, Benedicenti S, Benedicenti A, Arcieri K, Berne E. Head and neck hemangiomas in pediatric patients treated with endolesional 980-nm diode laser. *Photomed Laser Surg*. 2009;27(4):553–559.

32. Goldman MP, Bennett RG. Treatment of telangiectasia: a review. *J Am Acad Dermatol*. 1987;17(2 pt 1):167–182.

33. Geronemus RG. Pulsed dye laser treatment of vascular lesions in children. *J Dermatol Surg Oncol*. 1993;19(4): 303–310.

34. Uebelhoer NS, Bogle MA, Stewart B, Arndt KA, Dover JS. A split-face comparison study of pulsed 532-nm KTP laser and 595-nm pulsed dye laser in the treatment of facial telangiectasias and diffuse telangiectatic facial erythema. *Dermatol Surg*. 2007;33(4):441–448.

35. Rohrer TE, Chatrath V, Iyengar V. Does pulse stacking improve the results of treatment with variable-pulse pulsed-dye lasers? *Dermatol Surg*. 2004;30(2 pt 1): 163–167 [discussion 7].

36. Munia MA, Wolosker N, Munia CG, Chao WS, Puech-Leao P. Comparison of laser versus sclerotherapy in the treatment of lower extremity telangiectases: a prospective study. *Dermatol Surg*. 2011 [Epub ahead of print].

37. Raulin C, Weiss RA, Schonermark MP. Treatment of essential telangiectasias with an intense pulsed light source (PhotoDerm VL). *Dermatol Surg*. 1997;23(10): 941–945 [discussion 5–6].

38. Clementoni MT, Gilardino P, Muti GF, et al. Facial telangiectasias: our experience in treatment with IPL. *Lasers Surg Med*. 2005;37(1):9–13.

39. Dawn G, Gupta G. Comparison of potassium titanyl phosphate vascular laser and hyfrecator in the treatment of vascular spiders and cherry angiomas. *Clin Exp Dermatol*. 2003;28(6):581–583.

40. Calista D, Boschini A. Cutaneous side effects induced by indinavir. *Eur J Dermatol*. 2000;10(4):292–296.

41. Patrice SJ, Wiss K, Mulliken JB. Pyogenic granuloma (lobular capillary hemangioma): a clinicopathologic study of 178 cases. *Pediatr Dermatol*. 1991;8(4):267–276.

42. Arndt KA. Argon laser therapy of small cutaneous vascular lesions. *Arch Dermatol*. 1982;118(4):220–224.

43. Gonzalez E, Gange RW, Momtaz KT. Treatment of telangiectases and other benign vascular lesions with the 577 nm pulsed dye laser. *J Am Acad Dermatol*. 1992;27(2 pt 1):220–226.

44. Goldberg DJ, Sciales CW. Pyogenic granuloma in children. Treatment with the flashlamp-pumped pulsed dye laser. *J Dermatol Surg Oncol*. 1991;17(12): 960–962.

45. Blickenstaff RD, Roenigk RK, Peters MS, Goellner JR. Recurrent pyogenic granuloma with satellitosis. *J Am Acad Dermatol*. 1989;21(6):1241–1244.

46. Roncero M, Canueto J, Blanco S, Unamuno P, Boixeda P. Multiwavelength laser treatment of venous lakes. *Dermatol Surg*. 2009;35(12):1942–1946.

47. Bean WB, Walsh JR. Venous lakes. *AMA Arch Derm.* 1956;74(5):459–463.
48. Bekhor PS. Long-pulsed Nd:YAG laser treatment of venous lakes: report of a series of 34 cases. *Dermatol Surg.* 2006;32(9):1151–1154.
49. Cheung ST, Lanigan SW. Evaluation of the treatment of venous lakes with the 595-nm pulsed-dye laser: a case series. *Clin Exp Dermatol.* 2007;32(2):148–150.
50. del Pozo J, Pena C, Garcia Silva J, Goday JJ, Fonseca E. Venous lakes: a report of 32 cases treated by carbon dioxide laser vaporization. *Dermatol Surg.* 2003;29(3):308–310.
51. Neumann RA, Knobler RM. Venous lakes (Bean-Walsh) of the lips—treatment experience with the argon laser and 18 months follow-up. *Clin Exp Dermatol.* 1990;15(2):115–118.
52. Stier MF, Glick SA, Hirsch RJ. Laser treatment of pediatric vascular lesions: port wine stains and hemangiomas. *J Am Acad Dermatol.* 2008;58(2):261–285.
53. Bivings L. Spontaneous regression of angiomas in children; twenty-two years' observation covering 236 cases. *J Pediatr.* 1954;45(6):643–647.
54. Jackson R. The natural history of strawberry naevi. *J Cutan Med Surg.* 1998;2(3):187–189.
55. Finn MC, Glowacki J, Mulliken JB. Congenital vascular lesions: clinical application of a new classification. *J Pediatr Surg.* 1983;18(6):894–900.
56. Thomson HG, Ward CM, Crawford JS, Stigmar G. Hemangiomas of the eyelid: visual complications and prophylactic concepts. *Plast Reconstr Surg.* 1979;63(5):641–647.
57. Robb RM. Refractive errors associated with hemangiomas of the eyelids and orbit in infancy. *Am J Ophthalmol.* 1977;83(1):52–58.
58. Rahbar R, Nicollas R, Roger G, et al. The biology and management of subglottic hemangioma: past, present, future. *Laryngoscope.* 2004;114(11):1880–1891.
59. Goldberg NS, Hebert AA, Esterly NB. Sacral hemangiomas and multiple congenital abnormalities. *Arch Dermatol.* 1986;122(6):684–687.
60. Albright AL, Gartner JC, Wiener ES. Lumbar cutaneous hemangiomas as indicators of tethered spinal cords. *Pediatrics.* 1989;83(6):977–980.
61. Frieden IJ, Reese V, Cohen D. PHACE syndrome. The association of posterior fossa brain malformations, hemangiomas, arterial anomalies, coarctation of the aorta and cardiac defects, and eye abnormalities. *Arch Dermatol.* 1996;132(3):307–311.
62. Leonardi-Bee J, Batta K, O'Brien C, Bath-Hextall FJ. Interventions for infantile haemangiomas (strawberry birthmarks) of the skin. *Cochrane Database Syst Rev.* 2011;(5):CD006545.
63. Rizzo C, Brightman L, Chapas AM, et al. Outcomes of childhood hemangiomas treated with the pulsed-dye laser with dynamic cooling: a retrospective chart analysis. *Dermatol Surg.* 2009;35(12):1947–1954.
64. Hunzeker CM, Geronemus RG. Treatment of superficial infantile hemangiomas of the eyelid using the 595-nm pulsed dye laser. *Dermatol Surg.* 2010;36(5):590–597.
65. Kim HJ, Colombo M, Frieden IJ. Ulcerated hemangiomas: clinical characteristics and response to therapy. *J Am Acad Dermatol.* 2001;44(6):962–972.
66. Saafan AM, Salah MM. Using pulsed dual-wavelength 595 and 1064 nm is more effective in the management of hemangiomas. *J Drugs Dermatol.* 2010;9(4):310–314.
67. Jiang C, Hu X, Ma G, et al. A prospective self-controlled phase II study of imiquimod 5% cream in the treatment of infantile hemangioma. *Pediatr Dermatol.* 2011;28(3):259–266.
68. Oranje AP, Janmohamed SR, Madern GC, de Laat PC. Treatment of small superficial haemangioma with timolol 0.5% ophthalmic solution: a series of 20 cases. *Dermatology.* 2011;223(4):330–334.
69. Schupp CJ, Kleber JB, Gunther P, Holland-Cunz S. Propranolol therapy in 55 infants with infantile hemangioma: dosage, duration, adverse effects, and outcome. *Pediatr Dermatol.* 2011;28(6):640–644.
70. Chim H, Gosain AK. Discussion: oral prednisolone for infantile hemangioma: efficacy and safety using a standardized treatment protocol. *Plast Reconstr Surg.* 2011;128(3):753–754.
71. Kulbersh J, Hochman M. Serial excision of facial hemangiomas. *Arch Facial Plast Surg.* 2011;13(3):199–202.
72. Brightman L, Brauer J, Terushkin V, et al. Ablative fractional resurfacing for involuted hemangioma residuum. *Arch Dermatol.* 2012 Aug:2021–2025 [Epub ahead of print].
73. Laubach HJ, Anderson RR, Luger T, Manstein D. Fractional photothermolysis for involuted infantile hemangioma. *Arch Dermatol.* 2009;145(7):748–750.
74. Blankenship CM, Alster TS. Fractional photothermolysis of residual hemangioma. *Dermatol Surg.* 2008;34(8):1112–1114.
75. Jacobs AH, Walton RG. The incidence of birthmarks in the neonate. *Pediatrics.* 1976;58(2):218–222.
76. Pratt AG. Birthmarks in infants. *AMA Arch Derm Syphilol.* 1953;67(3):302–305.
77. Iwach AG, Hoskins HD Jr, Hetherington J Jr, Shaffer RN. Analysis of surgical and medical management of glaucoma in Sturge-Weber syndrome. *Ophthalmology.* 1990;97(7):904–909.
78. Enjolras O, Riche MC, Merland JJ. Facial port-wine stains and Sturge-Weber syndrome. *Pediatrics.* 1985;76(1):48–51.
79. Paller AS. The Sturge-Weber syndrome. *Pediatr Dermatol.* 1987;4(4):300–304.
80. Piram M, Lorette G, Sirinelli D, Herbreteau D, Giraudeau B, Maruani A. Sturge-Weber syndrome in patients with facial port-wine stain. *Pediatr Dermatol.* 2012;29(1):32–37.
81. Jessen RT, Thompson S, Smith EB. Cobb syndrome. *Arch Dermatol.* 1977;113(11):1587–1590.
82. Barsky SH, Rosen S, Geer DE, Noe JM. The nature and evolution of port wine stains: a computer-assisted study. *J Invest Dermatol.* 1980;74(3):154–157.
83. Geronemus RG, Ashinoff R. The medical necessity of evaluation and treatment of port-wine stains. *J Dermatol Surg Oncol.* 1991;17(1):76–79.
84. Malm M, Carlberg M. Port-wine stain—a surgical and psychological problem. *Ann Plast Surg.* 1988;20(6):512–516.
85. Wagner KD, Wagner RF Jr. The necessity for treatment of childhood port-wine stains. *Cutis.* 1990;45(5):317–318.
86. Lanigan SW, Cotterill JA. Psychological disabilities amongst patients with port wine stains. *Br J Dermatol.* 1989;121(2):209–215.

87. McClean K, Hanke CW. The medical necessity for treatment of port-wine stains. *Dermatol Surg.* 1997; 23(8):663–667.

88. Alster TS, Railan D. Laser treatment of vascular birthmarks. *J Craniofac Surg.* 2006;17(4):720–723.

89. Ashinoff R, Geronemus RG. Flashlamp-pumped pulsed dye laser for port-wine stains in infancy: earlier versus later treatment. *J Am Acad Dermatol.* 1991;24(3): 467–472.

90. Chapas AM, Eickhorst K, Geronemus RG. Efficacy of early treatment of facial port wine stains in newborns: a review of 49 cases. *Lasers Surg Med.* 2007;39(7): 563–568.

91. Goldman MP, Fitzpatrick RE, Ruiz-Esparza J. Treatment of port-wine stains (capillary malformation) with the flashlamp-pumped pulsed dye laser. *J Pediatr.* 1993; 122(1):71–77.

92. Alster TS, Wilson F. Treatment of port-wine stains with the flashlamp-pumped pulsed dye laser: extended clinical experience in children and adults. *Ann Plast Surg.* 1994;32(5):478–484.

93. Tan OT, Morrison P, Kurban AK. 585 nm for the treatment of port-wine stains. *Plast Reconstr Surg.* 1990;86(6):1112–1117.

94. Troilius A, Svendsen G, Ljunggren B. Ultrasound investigation of port wine stains. *Acta Derm Venereol.* 2000;80(3):196–199.

95. Izikson L, Nelson JS, Anderson RR. Treatment of hypertrophic and resistant port wine stains with a 755 nm laser: a case series of 20 patients. *Lasers Surg Med.* 2009;41(6):427–432.

96. Dierickx CC, Casparian JM, Venugopalan V, Farinelli WA, Anderson RR. Thermal relaxation of port-wine stain vessels probed in vivo: the need for 1-10-millisecond laser pulse treatment. *J Invest Dermatol.* 1995;105(5):709–714.

97. Tan OT, Sherwood K, Gilchrest BA. Treatment of children with port-wine stains using the flashlamp-pulsed tunable dye laser. *N Engl J Med.* 1989;320(7):416–421.

98. Reyes BA, Geronemus R. Treatment of port-wine stains during childhood with the flashlamp-pumped pulsed dye laser. *J Am Acad Dermatol.* 1990;23(6 pt 1):1142–1148.

99. Faurschou A, Olesen AB, Leonardi-Bee J, Haedersdal M. Lasers or light sources for treating port-wine stains. *Cochrane Database Syst Rev.* 2011;(11):CD007152.

100. Shafirstein G, Buckmiller LM, Waner M, Baumler W. Mathematical modeling of selective photothermolysis to aid the treatment of vascular malformations and hemangioma with pulsed dye laser. *Lasers Med Sci.* 2007;22(2):111–118.

101. Kauvar AN, Geronemus RG. Repetitive pulsed dye laser treatments improve persistent port-wine stains. *Dermatol Surg.* 1995;21(6):515–521.

102. Koster PH, van der Horst CM, Bossuyt PM, van Gemert MJ. Prediction of portwine stain clearance and required number of flashlamp pumped pulsed dye laser treatments. *Lasers Surg Med.* 2001;29(2):151–155.

103. Lanigan SW. Port wine stains on the lower limb: response to pulsed dye laser therapy. *Clin Exp Dermatol.* 1996;21(2):88–92.

104. Renfro L, Geronemus RG. Anatomical differences of port-wine stains in response to treatment with the pulsed dye laser. *Arch Dermatol.* 1993;129(2):182–188.

105. Eubanks LE, McBurney EI. Videomicroscopy of port-wine stains: correlation of location and depth of lesion. *J Am Acad Dermatol.* 2001;44(6):948–951.

106. Yohn JJ, Huff JC, Aeling JL, Walsh P, Morelli JG. Lesion size is a factor for determining the rate of port-wine stain clearing following pulsed dye laser treatment in adults. *Cutis.* 1997;59(5):267–270.

107. Pence B, Aybey B, Ergenekon G. Outcomes of 532 nm frequency-doubled Nd:YAG laser use in the treatment of port-wine stains. *Dermatol Surg.* 2005;31(5): 509–517.

108. Chan HH, Chan E, Kono T, Ying SY, Wai-Sun H. The use of variable pulse width frequency doubled Nd:YAG 532 nm laser in the treatment of port-wine stain in Chinese patients. *Dermatol Surg.* 2000;26(7):657–661.

109. Yang MU, Yaroslavsky AN, Farinelli WA, et al. Long-pulsed neodymium:yttrium–aluminum–garnet laser treatment for port-wine stains. *J Am Acad Dermatol.* 2005;52(3 pt 1):480–490.

110. Kelly KM, Nanda VS, Nelson JS. Treatment of port-wine stain birthmarks using the 1.5-msec pulsed dye laser at high fluences in conjunction with cryogen spray cooling. *Dermatol Surg.* 2002;28(4):309–313.

111. McGill DJ, MacLaren W, Mackay IR. A direct comparison of pulsed dye, alexandrite, KTP and Nd:YAG lasers and IPL in patients with previously treated capillary malformations. *Lasers Surg Med.* 2008;40(6): 390–398.

112. Black JF, Wade N, Barton JK. Mechanistic comparison of blood undergoing laser photocoagulation at 532 and 1,064 nm. *Lasers Surg Med.* 2005;36(2):155–165.

113. Faurschou A, Togsverd-Bo K, Zachariae C, Haedersdal M. Pulsed dye laser vs. intense pulsed light for port-wine stains: a randomized side-by-side trial with blinded response evaluation. *Br J Dermatol.* 2009;160(2): 359–364.

114. Babilas P, Schreml S, Eames T, Hohenleutner U, Szeimies RM, Landthaler M. Split-face comparison of intense pulsed light with short- and long-pulsed dye lasers for the treatment of port-wine stains. *Lasers Surg Med.* 2010;42(8):720–727.

115. Yuan KH, Li Q, Yu WL, Huang Z. Photodynamic therapy in treatment of port wine stain birthmarks—recent progress. *Photodiagn Photodyn Ther.* 2009;6(3–4): 189–194.

116. Juern AM, Glick ZR, Drolet BA, Frieden IJ. Nevus simplex: a reconsideration of nomenclature, sites of involvement, and disease associations. *J Am Acad Dermatol.* 2010;63(5):805–814.

117. Biesman BJ. Presentation at Controversies and Conversations in Laser and Cosmetic Surgery; August 2005; Colorado Springs, CO.

118. McCoppin HH, Hovenic WW, Wheeland RG. Laser treatment of superficial leg veins: a review. *Dermatol Surg.* 2011 [Epub ahead of print].

119. Gloviczki P, Comerota AJ, Dalsing MC, et al. The care of patients with varicose veins and associated chronic venous diseases: clinical practice guidelines of the Society for Vascular Surgery and the American Venous Forum. *J Vasc Surg.* 2011;53(5 suppl):2S–48S.

120. Johnson CM, McLafferty RB. Endovenous laser ablation of varicose veins: review of current technologies and clinical outcome. *Vascular.* 2007;15(5):250–254.

121. Glade RS, Richter GT, James CA, Suen JY, Buckmiller LM. Diagnosis and management of pediatric cervicofacial venous malformations: retrospective review from a vascular anomalies center. *Laryngoscope*. 2010;120(2):229–235.

122. Scherer K, Waner M. Nd:YAG lasers (1,064 nm) in the treatment of venous malformations of the face and neck: challenges and benefits. *Lasers Med Sci*. 2007;22(2):119–126.

123. Wheeland RG, Bailin PL, Norris MJ. Argon laser photocoagulative therapy of Kaposi's sarcoma: a clinical and histologic evaluation. *J Dermatol Surg Oncol*. 1985;11(12):1180–1185.

124. Rosenfeld H, Wellisz T, Reinisch JF, Sherman R. The treatment of cutaneous vascular lesions with the Nd:YAG laser. *Ann Plast Surg*. 1988;21(3):223–230.

125. Tur E, Brenner S. Treatment of Kaposi's sarcoma. *Arch Dermatol*. 1996;132(3):327–331.

126. Acevedo JL, Shah RK, Brietzke SE. Nonsurgical therapies for lymphangiomas: a systematic review. *Otolaryngol Head Neck Surg*. 2008;138(4):418–424.

127. Lanjouw E, de Roos KP, den Hollander JC, Prens EP. Acquired scrotal lymphangioma successfully treated using carbon dioxide laser ablation. *Dermatol Surg*. 2011;37(4):539–542.

128. Lai CH, Hanson SG, Mallory SB. Lymphangioma circumscriptum treated with pulsed dye laser. *Pediatr Dermatol*. 2001;18(6):509–510.

129. Eliezri YD, Sklar JA. Lymphangioma circumscriptum: review and evaluation of carbon dioxide laser vaporization. *J Dermatol Surg Oncol*. 1988;14(4):357–364.

CHAPTER 3

Treatment of Pigmented Lesions and Tattoos

Jeremy A. Brauer, Melanie A. Warycha, and Elizabeth K. Hale

▮ TREATMENT OF PIGMENTED LESIONS

Introduction

Laser treatment of pigmented lesions has evolved into a highly selective and relatively safe procedure being increasingly performed in dermatology practices. Although earlier attempts at treating pigmented lesions with ablative continuous wave CO_2 and argon lasers were complicated by scarring and pigmentary alteration, the introduction of short-pulsed lasers, namely, quality-switched (QS) mode lasers, has enabled a more direct targeting of pigment with a low risk of damage to surrounding tissue. While these lasers remain the standard treatment for pigmented lesions, more recently, ablative and nonablative fractionated devices and lasers of picosecond pulse durations have been added to the armamentarium for the treatment of pigmented lesions.

Destruction of pigmented lesions through laser technology is based on the principle of selective photothermolysis. According to this theory, a target chromophore can be preferentially heated and destroyed without harm to adjacent tissues by selection of a wavelength of maximum absorption and a pulse duration that is shorter than the thermal relaxation time of the target.[1]

Although several lasers are currently available for the treatment of pigmented lesions and pigmentary disorders, it is of utmost importance that the clinical diagnosis of the lesion be certain.[2] If not, biopsy is recommended to rule out a dysplastic nevus or melanoma, as the effect of laser irradiation on malignant degeneration is not fully understood, and therefore laser treatment of these lesions is not recommended by the authors. In fact, controversy still remains over laser treatment of nevocellular and congenital melanocytic nevi given their premalignant potential.

Choosing the Appropriate Light Source

Pigmented lesions can be epidermal, dermal, or combined, and can differ in both the overall quantity and the density of pigment distribution. The location of pigment guides the selection of the appropriate wavelength for treatment, as lesions with deeper pigment, in general, will be more amenable to treatment with longer wavelengths. The chromophore targeted in the treatment of pigmented lesions is the melanosome, with a thermal relaxation time ranging from 50 to 500 nanoseconds.[1] Melanosomes are typically destroyed at pulse durations between 40 and 750 nanoseconds, with an absorption spectrum ranging from 351 to 1064 nm.[3,4] QS mode lasers have pulse durations in the nanosecond range and are thus recommended for the treatment of pigmented lesions. Nonpulsed, quasi-continuous wave green light lasers such as copper vapor (511 nm), krypton (520–530 nm), and variable pulse with KTP (532 nm) lasers do not work consistently because thermal relaxation time of the melanosome is exceeded. While not always possible, all attempts should be made to avoid lasers with absorption peaks of other commonly targeted chromophores found in the skin, namely, hemoglobin and oxyhemoglobin.

While fractional ablative and nonablative devices tend to target water as their main chromophore, the resultant microscopic treatment zones (MTZs) create distinct columns of epidermal and dermal injury[5] with resultant transepidermal elimination of microscopic epidermal necrotic debris (MENDs) including pigment.[6]

In addition to finding the appropriate device for treatment, equally important is the need for education regarding sun avoidance and protection prior to as well as after treatment to minimize postprocedural pigmentary alteration.

Laser Treatment of Epidermal Pigmented Lesions

Epidermal pigmented lesions, with pigment mainly located at or above the dermoepidermal junction, in general, respond well to laser treatment with minimal risk of scarring, hyperpigmentation, or hypopigmentation, and usually clear in a single treatment session.

EPHELIDES AND SOLAR LENTIGINES Ephelides, or freckles, are characterized by increased epidermal melanin and present clinically as uniform, small, tan to pale brown macules in sun-exposed areas. They often begin in early childhood and may become more apparent during the months of summer. While lentigines can have a similar appearance to ephelides, they are typically larger in size, can exhibit subtle variations in color, and tend to increase in number with age and sun damage. On histopathologic examination, lentigines contain increased melanin in the basal layer of the epidermis with a background of solar elastosis.

Nearly 25 years ago, initial laser treatment of epidermal lesions involved the use of ablative CO_2 and argon devices in the treatment of solar lentigines, with encouraging results. In 1 report of 5 patients, higher energy treatments with an ablative CO_2 device resulted in substantial lightening or total clearance in 81% of treated lentigines.[7] Years later, a study of 83 lentigines treated with either a continuous wave or superpulsed CO_2 laser reported complete clearance of all treated lesions, while another comparing argon and CO_2 lasers yielded good to excellent results in 87% and 84% of 300 treated lentigines, respectively.[8,9]

As mentioned above, with the theory of selective photothermolysis and development of reliable nanosecond pulse duration QS lasers, Q-switched Nd:YAG lasers (QSNYL), Q-switched alexandrite lasers (QSAL), and Q-switched ruby lasers (QSRL) have been very well studied and regularly used in the treatment of epidermal pigmented lesions. In a study of skin type V individuals with ephelides and lentigines, treatment with a frequency-doubled 532 nm QSNYL resulted in greater than 50% improvement in 10 of 14 (71%) patients with ephelides and 6 of 6 (100%) patients with lentigines. Four of the patients with ephelides experienced partial recurrence within 2 years, and no lentigines recurred. Transient hypopigmentation in 25% of patients and hyperpigmentation in 10% of patients were reported, with complete resolution within 2 to 6 months.[10] A second study evaluating varying fluences of the frequency-doubled QSNYL in the treatment of lentigines demonstrated a dose response, where 15 of 37 cases (40%) treated at 2 J/cm^2 had 76% to 100% improvement compared with 22 of 37 (59%) cases at 5 J/cm^2.[11]

In a randomized controlled trial, treatment of lentigines of the hands with several different lasers was shown to be more efficacious than treatment with cryotherapy. At 6 weeks posttreatment, the frequency-doubled 532 nm QSNYL demonstrated the greatest improvement in color, followed by the 521 nm krypton laser, 532 nm diode-pumped vanadate laser, and cryotherapy.[12] Another randomized controlled trial investigating the use of QSAL or intense pulse light (IPL) in the treatment of ephelides and lentigines in patients with skin type III and IV found that QSAL was more effective in the treatment of ephelides. Of note, 1 session of QSAL was shown to be more effective than 2 of IPL. In those with lentigines, efficacy was similar between the 2 interventions; however, 47% of patients developed postinflammatory hyperpigmentation following QSAL.[13] An evaluation of differing fluences and pulse durations in a single treatment session with QSAL found that lighter lentigines required higher fluences for comparable clearance rates compared with darker lesions, but varying the pulse duration had no effect on overall efficacy.[14]

The QSRL has also been proven effective in the treatment of ephelides and lentigines. Specifically, 1 study demonstrated 76% to 100% clearance of lentigines after 1 treatment in 24 of 36 (63.2%) patients with skin type II, 24 of 41 (58.5%) patients with skin type III, and 6 of 12 (50%) patients with skin type IV. A second treatment resulted in complete clearance of all lesions, with transient postinflammatory hyperpigmentation in 16.6% of patients with skin type IV that resolved within 6 months.[15] In a study comparing the QSRL and QSNYL, 6 patients with lentigines were treated, with an average of 67% of lesions cleared after treatment with the QSRL compared with 58% with the QSNYL.[16] The QSRL has also been studied in the treatment of labial melanotic macules, with 1 study showing 5 of 8 patients cleared after 1 treatment, the remaining 3 clearing after a second treatment session. No recurrences were noted at a follow-up time of 2 years[17] (Figures 3-1A and B and 3-2A and B).

CAFÉ AU LAIT MACULES Café au lait macules (CALMs) are uniformly pigmented, well-demarcated epidermal lesions that can vary in shades of brown. These can present as benign isolated lesions or as a manifestation of neurocutaneous disease. While clearance of CALMs following laser treatment has been previously reported, clearance is typically more difficult to achieve compared with the treatment of lentigines, with variable treatment response. Recurrences, as well as pigment darkening, are common with the treatment of CALMs.[18] In 1 study with greater than a year of follow-up posttreatment with a QSRL, 6 of 12 (50%) patients experienced repigmentation.[19] In a multicentered trial using a frequency-doubled QSNYL in the treatment of various pigmented lesions, Kilmer et al found that only 2 of 7 CALMs had an excellent

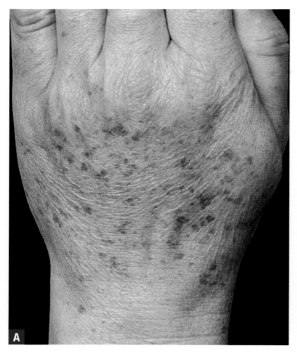 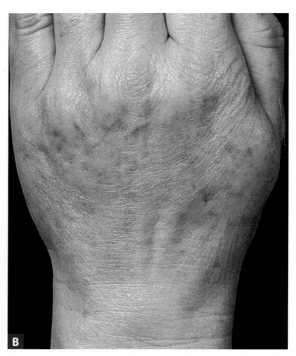

▲ **FIGURE 3-1** **A.** Lentigines, or sunspots, of hand prior to treatment. **B.** Lentigines, or sunspots, of hand after 1 treatment with quality-switched ruby laser.

response (>75% lightening) at a higher fluence (5 J/cm²) compared with 1 of 7 CALMs at a low fluence (2 J/cm²). The remaining 4 CALMs treated at a low fluence showed minimal response (0%–25% lightening).[11] One case report documented successful treatment of segmental CALMs in a patient with the 1064 nm QSNYL; however, 10 treatments were required.[20] In a study examining the predictive value of the presence or absence of melanocyte hyperplasia on histologic examination on treatment response, Grossman et al reported resolution of CALMs in 1 of 8 patients at a 6-month follow-up time after treatment with either 532 nm frequency-doubled QSNYL or QSRL. Histologic findings were found not to be predictive of treatment outcome.[21] In a comparison of normal-mode ruby laser and QSRL in the treatment of CALMs in 33 patients, a 42.4% recurrence rate was observed with the normal-mode ruby laser compared with 81.8% recurrence rate in those treated with the QSRL at 3-month follow-up.[22]

SEBORRHEIC KERATOSES Seborrheic keratoses (SK) are common benign epidermal proliferations that present as brown "stuck-on" papules or plaques. In individuals of darker Fitzpatrick skin types, clinically similar lesions known as dermatosis papulosa nigra (DPN) may be seen on the face and around the eyes. Many patients find these lesions to be cosmetically unacceptable and often request removal. In addition to cryosurgery, electrodesiccation and curettage, and dermabrasion, ablative lasers, such as CO_2 and erbium:YAG lasers, have shown efficacy in the treatment of SK.[23,24] There has also been a report of successful treatment of SK using an alexandrite laser.[25] In a study employing 532 nm diode lasers, a clearance rate of 93% was achieved after color enhancement with a red marker.[26] Regarding the treatment of DPN, 70% to 90% resolution was reported in 2 patients with DPN after 1 treatment with a long-pulsed Nd:YAG, and in a second report of 1 patient, greater than 75% improvement was seen after a series of 3 treatments with the 1550 nm fractionated erbium-doped fiber laser.[27,28] In a study of 14 patients with skin types IV, V, or VI treated with a KTP laser, 75% noted between 76% and 100% improvement, 21% had 51% to 75% improvement, and 4% had 26% to 50% improvement.[29]

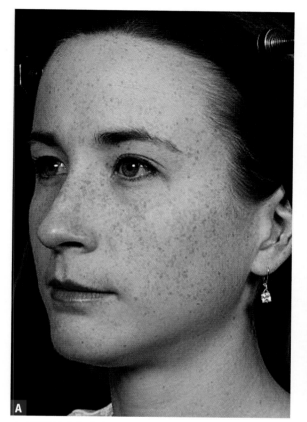 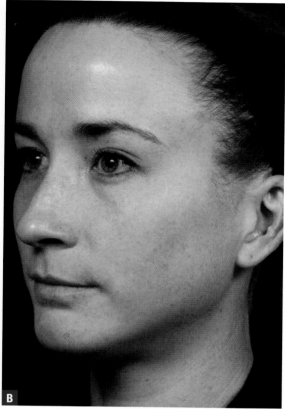

▲ **FIGURE 3-2 A.** Facial ephelides, or freckling, prior to treatment. **B.** Facial ephelides, or freckling, after 1 treatment with quality-switched ruby laser. (Courtesy of Solta Medical)

NEVUS SPILUS Nevus spilus most often presents on the trunk or extremities as a cluster of darkly pigmented macules scattered on the background of a larger lighter tan patch. Given that greater than 20 cases of melanoma have been documented to have arisen from these lesions, laser treatment is not routine.[30] Nevertheless, complete and partial clearances have been reported with many laser modalities. Several cases have been reported describing 50% clearance of a large congenital facial nevus spilus after 16 treatments with a QSAL, as well as a report showing marked clearance without recurrence at 6 months following treatment with IPL.[31,32] Results with the QSRL have been mixed, in 1 study achieving complete or near complete response in 6 nevus spilus lesions, while in a case report only successfully removing the junctional or compound nevi component.[33,34]

Laser Treatment of Dermal–Epidermal Pigmented Lesions

BECKER NEVI Becker nevi present in adolescence or early adulthood on the shoulders, chest, or back as brown, usually hypertrichotic, well-demarcated plaques, often several centimeters in diameter. While successful lightening with ablative and QS lasers has been reported, adverse effects and recurrences are common.[24] A small series of individuals with Becker nevus of skin types III, IV, or V were treated an average of 4 times with an alexandrite laser and showed excellent (75%–100% pigment lightening) response in 2 of 11, good (50%–75% pigment lightening) response in 5 of 11, and fair (25%–50% pigment lightening) response in 4 of 11. Hypopigmentation and textural changes were noted in a few of these patients.[35]

In another series of patients with Becker nevus, 11 were treated with 2940 nm Er:YAG and another 11 with the QSNYL. Fifty-four percent, 6 of 11, of patients treated with the Er:YAG laser showed complete clearance 2 years posttreatment, with all patients experiencing at least 50% clearance. Only 1 patient treated with the QSNYL had 51% to 99% clearance, while 45.5% had 26% to 50% clearance and 27.3% had 1% to 25% clearance. Numerous sessions with the QSNYL were required to achieve these results compared with only 1 Er:YAG treatment, although transient erythema was more common with Er:YAG.[36] Treatment of 2 patients with Becker nevus with a nonablative 1550 nm laser resulted in greater than 75% lightening in color up to 6 months after treatment, but without improvement in hypertrichosis.[37]

ACQUIRED MELANOCYTIC NEVI Acquired melanocytic nevi are most prevalent in early adulthood as brown, often symmetric macules, usually 2 to 6 mm in diameter. Junctional nevi tend to be darker with shades of medium to dark brown, although still uniform and small in size. Compound nevi are elevated papules and usually lighter in color. As mentioned previously, given premalignant potential of some nevi, laser treatment of these lesions remains controversial. If treated with laser, these lesions typically require 1 to 3 sessions to achieve complete clearance, although more elevated lesions with nests of dermal melanocytes tend to be more resistant. While recurrences are uncommon, long-term follow-up studies are lacking. In 14 patients with 28 nevi and skin types II or III, a single session with the short-pulse Er:YAG laser resulted in clinical and histopathologic resolution of all but 1 lesion without scarring.[38] One to 3 treatments with a QS, followed by a normal-mode ruby laser, resulted in the complete clearance of almost all acquired melanocytic nevi in a study of 12 patients, without evidence of scarring or postinflammatory hyperpigmentation. Minimally elevated nevi or histologically proven compound nevi, as well as red-brown nevi, did not respond as well.[39] In another study of the QSRL, 12 of 18 acquired nevi (67%) showed complete response and 6 (33%) showed partial response. On histologic examination, residual nevomelanocytic nests were noted in the superficial reticular dermis of the partially responding nevi.[40]

CONGENITAL NEVI It has been estimated that between 1% and 6% of infants are born with a congenital nevus.[41]. Clinically they present as well-circumscribed brown plaques with the presence of deep dermal nevomelanocytes that on histology extend to hair follicles, exocrine ducts, and neurovascular structures. Congenital nevi have been classified by their predicted adult size into small (<1.5 cm in diameter), medium (1.5–19.9 cm in diameter), and giant (≥20 cm in diameter), with a 6% to 12% risk of developing melanoma in large congenital nevi compared with a 1% to 2% risk in small congenital nevi.[42,43] In addition to this potential for malignant transformation, congenital nevi can be cosmetically and psychologically disfiguring, thus prompting patients to seek removal at an early age. At present, the best treatment modality for removal remains controversial as resultant scarring and the underlying potential for melanoma development in deep dermal and subcutaneous tissues needs to be considered. In addition to surgical excision, dermabrasion, chemical peels, and curettage, laser treatment of congenital melanocytic nevi has been well documented in the literature, with case reports and small case series reporting improvement with both ablative and QS lasers. Of importance regarding laser therapy, age at initiation of treatment has not been shown to impact the final clearance of lesions.[44] Repigmentation remains problematic after laser therapy given presence of deeper melanocytes. The reported maximum depth of destruction as measured from the papillary dermis is only 0.2 mm for the QSNYL and 0.4 mm for the QSRL.[45] Scarring is also more common with ablative CO_2 and Er:YAG lasers compared with treatment with short-pulse QS lasers. Therefore, the QSRL is often the device of choice in the removal of congenital melanocytic nevi. Regardless of the treatment utilized, however, long-term follow-up of all lesions is recommended to monitor for malignant transformation.

In a trial of 10 giant congenital melanocytic nevi treated with a 2940 nm Er:YAG laser, good to excellent results in pigment lightening were achieved; however, 6 patients experienced areas of mild repigmentation at the periphery and 2 developed hypertrophic scarring.[46] A median of 3 treatments with a combination of the normal mode followed by QSRL were performed on medium-sized facial congenital melanocytic nevi in 14 patients, with only a partial improvement in lightening, with eventual repigmentation in all lesions after several months.[47] In a separate case series of 18 patients, 1 month to 14 years old, with congenital nevi less than or equal to 5 cm in size, an average of 8 treatments with the QSRL resulted in an average improvement in pigmentation in greater than 75% of lesions. Within an average of 5 months, partial repigmentation occurred in all but 1 case.[48] These results are in contrast to a smaller case series of 9 patients with medium to giant congenital melanocytic nevi also treated with a QSRL. Pigmentation was reduced to 0% to 20% of baseline, with most patients having only mild repigmentation within 1 year, and 1 patient experiencing repigmentation to 70% of the baseline color within 2 weeks.[49] The superior results of this study compared with others may be a matter of the number of treatment sessions performed. The QSAL in combination with an ablative CO_2 laser has also been studied in the treatment of congenital nevi, with a report of 61% to 100% improvement in pigmentation in 30 of 53 (56.6%) patients, but with repigmentation in 83% of patients.[50] In a study comparing the results of treatment with the QSRL and QSNYL, 5 congenital nevi were treated with the QSRL-treated areas resulting in greater pigmentation lightening.[45]

Laser Treatment of Dermal Pigmented Lesions

NEVUS OF OTA AND RELATED CONDITIONS Most commonly seen in the Asian population, nevus of Ota is a unilateral dermal melanocytic lesion presenting clinically as a speckled blue to gray-brown lesion of the periorbital area innervated by the first and second branches of the trigeminal nerve.[51] Approximately 50% are congenital, with the remainder acquired presenting by the second decade of life. Acquired bilateral nevus of Ota (Hori nevus), while clinically similar, presents later in life, with melanocytes restricted to the papillary and mid dermis, not throughout as seen in nevus of Ota. Nevus of Ito also has a similar clinical appearance, but is located on the shoulder.

In a case series of 15 patients with nevus of Ota, treatment with the QSRL resulted in complete clearance in 4 of 15 (26.7%) patients, and at least 50% clearance in the remainder, all without evidence of scarring.[52] Of importance, a study using the QSRL in the treatment of 46 Japanese children and 107 adults with nevus of Ota showed that fewer sessions are required for clearance if treatment is initiated at a younger age. The children, with a mean age of 2.8 years, required an average of 3.5 sessions to achieve 75% or more improvement, while adults with a mean age of 30.2 years required an average of 5.9 sessions.[53] Regarding potential complications of treatment with the QSRL, a retrospective analysis of 101 nevus of Ota patients treated with the QSRL found hypopigmentation to be the most common, occurring in 16.8% of patients with a mean follow-up time of 33 months, followed by hyperpigmentation in 5.9% of patients.[54]

While most reports detail use of the QSRL, the QSAL was also examined in a large study of 602 Chinese patients with nevus of Ota. While clearance rates were not reported, a positive correlation was noted between response and the number of treatment sessions obtained. Presence of the lesion on the eyelid also made it harder to treat.[55]

Despite differing histology, the QSRL has also been proven effective in the treatment of acquired bilateral nevus of Ota. Treatment of 131 patients with the QSRL resulted in complete clearance in all patients after an average of 2.3 sessions, with no recurrence seen at mean follow-up time of 2.5 years. Ten of the 131 (7.6%) patients developed hyperpigmentation that responded to hydroquinone, while 8 patients (6.1%) had either prolonged or persistent hypopigmentation.[56] In a split-face study of 13 women with skin type III, IV, or V and acquired bilateral nevus of Ota, results of treatment with QSRL were compared with results in those treated with a scanner CO_2 laser followed by QSRL. At an average of 16-month follow-up, improved pigmentation was more apparent on the combination treatment side, with no cases of persistent erythema or difference in healing time.[57] In a small series evaluating the QSNYL, 15 patients with acquired bilateral nevus of Ota were treated a median of 11 times at 1- to 2-week intervals. On conclusion of the study, 76% to 100% improvement was noted in 7 of 15 (46.7%) patients, 51% to 75% improvement in 5 of 15 (33.3%) patients, and 26% to 50% improvement in 3 of 15 (20%) patients.[58] A report of 1 patient achieved complete clearance after 2 treatments with a fractionated 1440 nm Nd:YAG laser.

DERMAL MELANOCYTOSIS Dermal melanocytosis, or Mongolian spot, most commonly presents at birth or within a few weeks of life usually in children of Asian or African descent as confluent blue-gray patches in the lumbosacral area. In a retrospective analysis of babies born at 2 hospitals in Tehran between 2004 and 2006, dermal melanocytosis was diagnosed in 11.4% and 37.3%.[59] These lesions have been reported in up to 100% of Asian children.[60] While these lesions often resolve spontaneously over the first few years of life, lesions outside of the sacral area, extrasacral dermal melanocytosis, are more likely to persist. Fifty-three of these patients with 57 extrasacral dermal melanocytosis were treated with a QSRL comparing treatment response of distal extremity lesions (exposed) with that of proximal extremity and trunk lesions (nonexposed). Improvement in pigmentation was found to be statistically significantly better for exposed lesions compared with that for nonexposed lesions (P = .0005).[61] The QSAL has also been examined, with a good therapeutic outcome for infants and children compared with a fair response in adults. Postinflammatory hyperpigmentation was noted in 3 of 26 patients.[62]

BLUE NEVI Blue nevi are benign, blue to black macules or papules. Three main variants of blue nevi have been described, including the common blue, cellular blue, and combined blue nevi. These lesions tend to be most common in Asian patients. Limited data are available regarding outcomes of laser treatment of blue nevi; however, 1 report described complete clearance of histologically confirmed blue nevi in 2 patients with the QSRL after 3 treatment sessions, a response which was maintained 2 years later.[63]

MELASMA Often refractory to treatment with a high risk of recurrence, melasma is a common condition characterized by symmetric hyperpigmented patches mainly on the face that may involve the epidermis, dermis, or both. On histology, melanocytes tend to be larger, more metabolically active, and dendritic, but without absolute increase in number.[64] Melasma is more commonly seen in young women of darker Fitzpatrick skin types, and also tends to persist longer in these individuals. Worsening of the condition, especially with risk of postinflammatory pigmentation, is common and if treating with lasers, the authors recommend a regimen that includes use of topical hydroquinone before and after treatment. Lasers that have been studied with variable success and often limited long-term efficacy include the QSRL, QSAL, and QSNYL, ablative Er:YAG and CO_2 lasers, as well as the nonablative fractional devices including the 1550 and 1927 nm wavelength lasers, often in combination with topical or oral therapies. Anecdotally, the authors have also had preliminary success with a 1440 nm nonablative fractional laser.

In an observational study, 27 women of skin types II to V with refractory melasma were treated with a low-fluence QSNYL immediately following microdermabrasion every 4 weeks, average of 2.6 treatments, with monthly follow-ups from 3 to 12 months. At 3 months, 23 patients (85%) had at least 75% clearance and 12 (44%) had greater than 95% clearance. Of 9 subjects seen at 12-month follow-up, 8 (89%) maintained clearance. No dyspigmentation was recorded.[65]

Comparing 15% trichloroacetic acid chemical peel with a single treatment with 1550 nm fractional erbium-doped laser, 18 Korean women were randomized in a split-face comparative study. No differences were noted between the 2 interventions, with both equally safe and effective, without lasting benefit. At 4 weeks, improvement in pigmentation was noted, but recurrence of melasma occurred by 12-week follow-up. Postinflammatory hyperpigmentation occurred in 28% of patients at 4 weeks, resolving in all but 1 by 12-week follow-up.[66] Twenty-five women of Fitzpatrick skin types III to IV in a pilot study of the 1927 nm fractional thulium fiber laser, 14 patients had 3 to 4 treatments, 4 weeks apart, and evaluated at 1, 3, and 6 months. Results showed statistically significant improvement at 1 month, with 51% reduction in the melasma area and severity index (MASI). While not statistically significant, reductions of 33% and 34% were reported at 3 and 6 months, respectively.[67]

■ TATTOO REMOVAL

Tattoos consist of small exogenous pigment particles roughly 40 to 300 nm in size, situated in membrane-bound organelles within fibroblasts, macrophages, and mast cells.[68] According to a 2004 survey of US college students, 24% admit to having at least 1 tattoo, of which approximately 6% will seek removal in the future.[69,70] Tattoo removal has a storied past, with early techniques including dermabrasion, chemical peels, cryotherapy, and surgical excision, all of which have fallen out of favor given the associated risks of scarring, textural changes, and pigmentary abnormalities. With the theory of selective photothermolysis and development of highly selective, short-pulsed lasers, the mainstay of treatment has shifted to laser tattoo removal.

Since the first report of laser tattoo removal in 1967, much has been learned regarding the procedure; however, the exact mechanism of laser tattoo clearance is still under investigation.[71] It is believed that laser energy ruptures pigment-containing cells through photoacoustic and photomechanical injury, with resultant fragmented particles subsequently removed through macrophages and fibroblasts via the vascular or lymphatic system.[72–75] Alternatively, particles can be eliminated through the epidermis, with resultant pigment lightening. Tattoo pigment is typically composed of a mixture of inorganic and/or organic compounds, such as chromium, mercury, cobalt, iron, titanium, and copper. Given the variety of available tattoo compounds, not FDA approved, 1 wavelength may not effectively account for all pigment particles present within a multicolored tattoo, thus complicating laser tattoo removal.

Several types of tattoos exist as well, including professional, amateur, cosmetic, medicinal, and traumatic.

Professional tattoos are composed of manufactured ink pigments that are situated deep in the dermis and are often more stable compared with amateur pigments. These tattoos generally necessitate more treatment sessions, often as many as 10 to 20 treatments, to achieve clearance. Amateur tattoos tend to require fewer treatments as the pigment, often carbon-based, is located more superficially in the dermis. Cosmetic tattoos are frequently used to create permanent eye or lip liner, or to cover scars or pigmentary conditions such as melasma or vitiligo. These tattoos tend to be off-white, tan, red-brown, or flesh-colored, and are often made with iron pigments that are subject to paradoxical darkening on treatment. For this reason, as well as to identify ideal parameters, a test spot is recommended prior to complete laser treatment. Traumatic tattoos are often black or blue in color and can result from carbon, graphite, dust, dirt, sand, gunpowder, or other debris that penetrates the skin.[68] The presence of multiple elements within the tattoo as described above and their stability, as well as how and where the ink is deposited within the skin, account for why tattoos of the same color may have different rates of clearance when treated with the same laser and settings.

Choosing the Appropriate Light Source

Due to the size of tattoo pigment particles, the pulse duration of the selected laser should ideally be in the range of nanoseconds. Currently available nanosecond QS lasers have become the preferred treatment for laser tattoo removal, as the pulse duration is similar to the thermal relaxation time of tattoo pigment, or approximately 10 nanoseconds.[76] At the time of publication, new lasers with even shorter pulse durations, in the picosecond and femtosecond range, are currently in development as well as in limited use, and may optimize tattoo removal in the future.[77,78] In addition to pulse duration, one must also consider the wavelength needed to selectively target the particular color of tattoo pigment. According to an in vitro analysis of tattoo pigment, red had a maximum absorption spectrum of 500 to 570 nm, orange 420 to 540 nm, yellow 470 to 485 nm, green 615 to 654 nm, blue pigment 590 to 770 nm, and black pigment 600 to 800 nm. An important limitation, however, was the lack of measurements up to 1064 nm, the wavelength of the QSNYL.[79] Based on these data, one could use the QSRL at 694 nm for treatment of black, blue, green, and dark brown pigments; the QSNYL is effective at 532 nm for removal of red, orange, yellow, and purple pigments, while at the 1064 nm mode, it is effective at removal of black, blue, and dark brown pigments. The QSAL at 755 nm could be used for black, blue, green, and dark brown pigments. In an ongoing prospective clinical trial at our center using a picosecond alexandrite 755 nm laser, preliminary findings have shown near complete clearance of blue and green tattoo pigments after 1 to 2 treatment sessions in multicolored tattoos, or those with persistent pigment after at least 10 previous treatments[78] (Figure 3-3A and B).

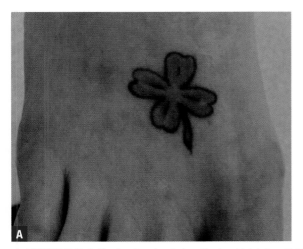
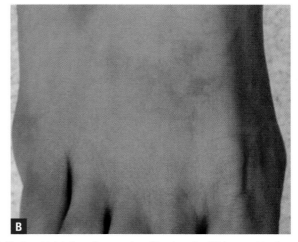

▲ **FIGURE 3-3 A.** Previously untreated multicolored ink tattoo. **B.** Multicolored ink tattoo after a series of treatments utilizing combination of quality-switched ruby and picosecond lasers.

The QSRL is extremely effective in the removal of black, blue, and green pigments. Studies have shown the QSRL to be as good, if not better, at the removal of these colors when compared with the QSNYL.[80,81] In a case series of blue and black tattoos treated with the QSAL, QSNYL, or QSRL, the QSRL was shown to have the highest clearance rate. Of importance, it also had the highest incidence of hypopigmentation when compared with the adverse effects of treatment with the QSAL or QSNYL.[82] In a separate study, hypopigmentation was found to be the most common adverse event after treatment with the QSRL, though usually transient.[83] Scarring and textural changes are not commonly encountered.

The QSNYL can be used to treat blue, black, and dark brown pigments at the 1064 nm wavelength setting. Red, orange, yellow, and purple pigments can be targeted when using the 532 nm wavelength. The QSNYL at 1064 nm has a better safety profile for dark-skinned individuals compared with other QS lasers because of its long wavelength and decreased targeting of and absorption by epidermal melanin.[84] In the treatment of cosmetic eyebrow tattoos, initial treatment with the QSNYL at 1064 nm at lower fluences has been recommended in order to minimize darkening of ink particles as well as absorption by hair, followed by treatment at higher fluences.[85] Successful removal of an orange eyebrow cosmetic tattoo has also been reported using a QSNYL at 532 nm.[86] Unlike the QSRL, the QSNYL does carry a small risk of textural change in addition to hyperpigmentation.

The QSAL works best on blue, black, green, and dark brown tattoo pigments, and several reports have described the efficacy of this laser in professional, amateur, and traumatic tattoos. A series of 31 patients with 42 tattoos (24 professional and 18 amateur) were treated every 6 to 8 weeks with the 755 nm QSAL or in the event of red pigment, at the 510 nm wavelength setting, with clearance achieved on average within 4.6 treatment sessions in amateur tattoos and within 8.5 treatment sessions for professional tattoos. In general, amateur tattoos were able to be treated at lower fluences compared with professional tattoos. Transient hypopigmentation was observed in 2 patients, resolving by 3 months.[87] The QSAL has also proven successful in the treatment of traumatic tattoos in 9 patients, with 78% pigment lightening after an average of 6 treatment sessions, without scarring or dyspigmentation.[88] An examination of amateur tattoos treated an average of 4 times with the QSAL resulted in greater than 75% lightening in 15 of 20 patients with skin types III or IV, without side effects.[89] Although many of these studies

reported low rates of complications, transient hypopigmentation was noted in as many as 50% of patients in 1 case series of 17 professional and amateur tattoos treated with the QSAL.[90]

Although ablative carbon dioxide lasers are no longer considered the preferred treatment for the majority of tattoos, they continue to be particularly effective in the removal of cosmetic tattoos, many of which are subject to paradoxical darkening after treatment with QS lasers. Fractional ablative and nonablative lasers have recently been used in conjunction with QS lasers in the treatment of tattoos demonstrating enhancement of tattoo removal outcomes. In a case series of 3 patients, tattoos were completely treated with a QSRL, and then one half received additional immediate resurfacing with either an ablative fractionated carbon dioxide laser (AFR) or a nonablative fractionated 1550 nm laser (NAFR). In the first case, the patient had 6 such treatments with AFR, and at 12-week follow-up, had greater pigment clearance on the combination side. The second subject had 1 treatment with QSRL and AFR, and at 3-day follow-up, diffuse blistering and bullae were present on the QSRL—only half of the tattoo and not on the combination side. Nonablative fractionated resurfacing was used in combination with QSRL for 9 treatments of the third patient's tattoo. Seven weeks afterward the last treatment, hypopigmentation was present throughout, but considerably less prominent on the combination side[91] (Figure 3-4A and B).

Paradoxical Pigment Darkening

Paradoxical pigment darkening occurs when ferric oxide is irreversibly reduced to ferrous oxide and is often noted following QS laser treatment of cosmetic tattoos, which are shades of red, pink, tan, or white and contain iron oxide or titanium. In an analysis of tattoo pigments, darkening was more common after treatment with a wavelength of 532 nm than with a 752 nm wavelength.[79] The resultant pigment darkening can be relatively resistant to treatment, although successful treatment with the CO_2 and QS lasers can be accomplished. The pulsed CO_2 laser has been shown to effectively treat cosmetic tattoos without resultant scarring or pigmentary changes.[92] This is likely the safest laser to use for cosmetic tattoos given that it does not lead to paradoxical darkening. While treatment with QS lasers can lead to paradoxical darkening, once present, these lasers have also been demonstrated to improve it. Blue-green pigment darkening that occurred secondary to QSRL treatment of a flesh-colored cosmetic tattoo was effectively treated with the QSAL

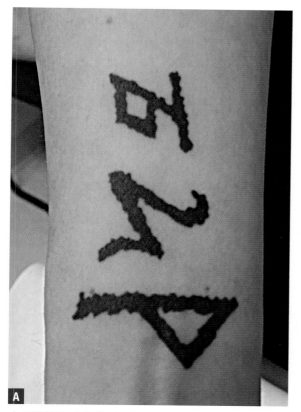
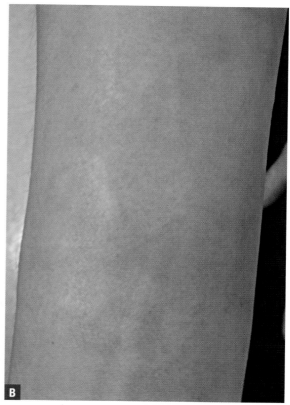

▲ **FIGURE 3-4** **A.** Previously untreated black ink tattoo. **B.** Black ink tattoo after a series of treatments utilizing combination of quality-switched ruby and ablative and nonablative fractional lasers.

with greater than 90% improvement after 12 treatment sessions. Interestingly, pigment lightening was not appreciated until the 10th treatment session. Continued treatment with the 1064 nm QSNYL ultimately achieved greater than 99% clearance after a total of 26 treatment sessions.[93] Successful treatment of paradoxical black pigment within a cosmetic tattoo of the lips was also achieved with 2 treatments of a QSNYL. Paradoxical yellow, orange, and green pigments have also been reported to clear after treatment with a combination of the QSRL and QSNYL.[94]

Drug-induced Hyperpigmentation

Drug-induced hyperpigmentation has been reported with use of antimalarials, tricyclic antidepressants, minocycline, amiodarone, as well as other psychotropic medications. Treatment with the QSAL resulted in complete resolution of minocycline-induced hyperpigmentation of the face and legs in 6 patients after an

average of 4 treatment sessions, without scarring or dyspigmentation.[95] Treatment with the QSAL resulted in the progressive lightening of facial hyperpigmentation in 2 patients taking combinations of perphenazine, desipramine, and amitriptyline. In 1 case report, imipramine-induced hyperpigmentation of the dorsal hands initially worsened with treatment using a QSNYL but then successfully treated with the QSRL.[96] The use of a 1550 nm fractionated erbium-doped fiber laser has also led to pigment lightening in a patient with minocycline-induced facial hyperpigmentation after a series of 4 sessions.[97]

Treatment Considerations

Prior to initiating laser tattoo treatment, it is important to obtain a medical history including propensity for keloidal scarring, as well as medication history including use of Accutane, as this may impact the rate of complications. Potential risks, including but not limited to dyspigmentation, scarring, infection, and textural changes, should be discussed. Topical anesthesia or lidocaine injections should be offered for pain control. Postoperatively, sunblock should be applied, with strict sun avoidance of the treatment area. Two-dimensional photography before and after should be obtained and stored for clinical monitoring and comparison.

Patients should also be aware that several treatment sessions will most likely be required for pigment lightening, with an understanding that complete clearance of all pigment may not be feasible. In a retrospective analysis of 238 patients undergoing tattoo removal treatment over a 10-year period, total clearance was achieved in only 1.26% of patients, which was attributed to poor patient compliance.[73] This emphasizes the importance of maintaining treatment sessions until satisfactory results are achieved. While previously the interval between treatment sessions was thought to ideally be between 1 and 2 months, new techniques including the "R20" and "R0" methods have been proposed.[98,99] In a prospective study of 18 tattoos on 12 Greek individuals, tattoos were split and randomized to receive either a single treatment pass with a QSAL or 4 treatment passes with an interval of 20 minutes between them with the same laser. This 20-minute interval is based on the duration of time required for the decreased penetration from immediate whitening to resolve. Interestingly, the authors found less immediate whitening after each subsequent pass. The tattoos were evaluated and biopsied at 3-month follow-up. Based on blinded comparison, the "R20" method resulted in an average of 88% lightening compared with 18% lightening with the single pass, representing the standard treatment. This was shown to be a statistically significantly difference in the lightening of pigment. No scarring was noted.[98]

Despite the impressive results of the above study, to date they have not been reliably reproducible and the time involved is considered to be quite prohibitive, particularly in a high-volume practice setting. Due in part to the limited practicality of this technique, a small study was conducted at our center, in which a total of 31 tattoos were exposed to perfluorodecalin (PFD), an inert, nontoxic liquid fluorocarbon with gas-carrying capacity. This liquid was evaluated in an effort to expedite clearance of the immediate whitening, potentially eliminating the need for 20-minute intervals. Twenty-two of the tattoos were treated with 4 passes of either a QSRL or QSNYL, in which PFD was applied immediately after each pass—the "R0" method, resulting in dissolution of the whitening

within seconds. This permitted for the execution of 3 successive passes to be performed within a matter of minutes. A second group of 6 tattoos were divided in half and were treated with a single pass with and without application of PFD afterwards. The remaining 3 tattoos were also split, where one half was treated with the aforementioned "R20" method and the other half with the "R0" method. All tattoos demonstrated fading, with pigment resolution noted to be equivalent between the 2 methods. No scarring or other adverse events were reported.[99] The question remains as to whether there is benefit to multiple treatment passes in a single session, and we anticipate further evaluation of the benefit of multiple passes in efficacy and efficiency of laser tattoo removal.

REFERENCES

1. Anderson RR, Parrish JA. Selective photothermolysis: precise microsurgery by selective absorption of pulsed radiation. *Science*. 1983;220(4596):524–527.
2. Stankiewicz K, Chuang G, Avram M. Lentigines, laser, and melanoma: a case series and discussion. *Lasers Surg Med*. 2012;44:112–116.
3. Goldberg DJ. Laser removal of pigmented and vascular lesions. *J Cosmet Dermatol*. 2006;5:204–209.
4. Goldberg DJ. Laser treatment of pigmented lesions. *Dermatol Clin*. 1997;15:397–407.
5. Manstein D, Herron GS, Sink RK. Fractional photothermolysis: a new concept of cutaneous remodeling using microscopic patterns of thermal injury. *Lasers Surg Med*. 2004;34:426–438.
6. Hantash BM, Bedi VP, Sudireddy V, et al. Laser-induced transepidermal elimination of dermal content by fractional photothermolysis. *J Biomed Opt*. 2006;11(4):041115.
7. Dover JS, Smoller BR, Stern RS, et al. Low-fluence carbon dioxide laser irradiation of lentigines. *Arch Dermatol*. 1988;124;1219–1224.
8. Fitpatrick RE, Goldman MP, Ruiz-Esparza J. Clinical advantage of the CO_2 laser superpulsed mode. Treatment of verruca vulgaris, seborrheic keratoses, lengitigines, and actinic cheilitis. *J Dermatol Surg Oncol*. 1994;20:449–456.
9. Stern RS, Dover JS, Levin JA, et al. Laser therapy versus cryotherapy of lentigines: a comparative trial. *J Am Acad Dermatol*. 1994;30:985–987.
10. Rashid T, Hussain I, Haider M, et al. Laser therapy of freckles and lentigines with quasi-continuous, frequency-doubled, Nd:YAG (532 nm) laser in Fitzpatrick skin type IV: a 24-month follow-up. *J Cosmet Laser Ther*. 2002;4:81–85.
11. Kilmer SL, Wheeland RG, Goldberg DJ, et al. Treatment of epidermal pigmented lesions with the frequency-doubled Q-switched Nd:YAG laser. A controlled, single-impact, dose-response, multicenter trial. *Arch Dermatol*. 1994;130(12):1515–1519.
12. Todd MM, Rallis TM, Gerweis JW, et al. A comparison of 3 lasers and liquid nitrogen in the treatment of solar lentigines: a randomized, controlled, comparative trial. *Arch Dermatol*. 2000;136:841–846.

13. Wang CC, Sue YM, Yang CH, et al. A comparison of Q-switched alexandrite laser and intense pulsed light for the treatment of freckles and lentigines in Asian persons: a randomized, physician-blinded, split-face comparative trial. *J Am Acad Dermatol.* 2006;54:804–810.

14. Trafeli JP, Kwan JM, Meehan KJ, et al. Use of a long-pulse alexandrite laser in the treatment of superficial pigmented lesions. *Dermatol Surg.* 2007;33:1477–1482.

15. Sadighha A, Saatee S, Muhaghegh-Zahed G. Efficacy and adverse effects of Q-switched ruby laser on solar lentigines: a prospective study of 91 patients with Fitzpatrick skin type II, III, and IV. *Dermatol Surg.* 2008;34:11:1465.

16. Tse Y, Levine VJ, McClain SA, et al. The removal of cutaneous pigmented lesions with the Q-switched ruby laser and the Q-switched neodymium:yttrium aluminum garnet laser. A comparative study. *J Dermatol Surg Oncol.* 1994;20:795–800.

17. Gupta G, MacKay IR, MacKie RM. Q-switched ruby laser in the treatment of labial melanotic macules. *Lasers Surg Med.* 1999;25:219–222.

18. Kagami S, Asahina A, Watanabe R, et al. Treatment of 153 Japanese patients with Q-switched alexandrite laser. *Lasers Med Sci.* 2007;22:159–163.

19. Shimbashi T, Kamide R, Hashimoto T. Long-term follow-up in treatment of solar lentigo and café-au-lait macules with Q-switched ruby laser. *Aesthetic Plast Surg.* 1997;21:445–448.

20. Kim JS, Kim MJ, Cho SB. Treatment of segmental café-au-lait macules using 1064-nm Q-switched Nd:YAG laser with low pulse energy. *Clin Exp Dermatol.* 2009; 34(7):e223–e224.

21. Grossman MC, Anderson RR, Farinelli W, et al. Treatment of café au lait macules with lasers. A clinicopathologic correlation. *Arch Dermatol.* 1995;131:1416–1420.

22. Chan HH, Kono T. The use of lasers and intense pulsed light sources for the treatment of pigmentary lesions. *Skin Therapy Lett.* 2004;9(8):5–7.

23. Khatri KA. Ablation of cutaneous lesions using an erbium:YAG laser. *J Cosmet Laser Ther.* 2003;5:150–153.

24. Polder KD, Landau JM, Vergilis-Kalner IJ, et al. Laser eradication of pigmented lesions: a review. *Dermatol Surg.* 2011;37:572–595.

25. Mehrabi D, Brodell RT. Use of alexandrite laser for treatment of seborrheic keratoses. *Dermatol Surg.* 2002; 28(5):437.

26. Culbertson GR. 532-nm diode laser treatment of seborrheic keratoses with color enhancement. *Dermatol Surg.* 2008;34(4):525–528.

27. Schweiger ES, Kwasniak L, Aires DJ. Treatment of dermatosis papulosa nigra with a 1064 nm Nd:YAG laser: report of two cases. *J Cosmet Laser Ther.* 2008;10: 120–122.

28. Katz TK, Goldberg LH, Friedman PM. Dermatosis papulosa nigra treatment with fractional photothermolysis. *Dermatol Surg.* 2009;35:1840–1843.

29. Kundu RV, Joshi SS, Suh KY, et al. Comparison of electrodessication and potassium titanyl phosphate laser for treatment of dermatosis papulosa nigra. *Dermatol Surg.* 2009;35:1079–1083.

30. Haenssle HA, Kaune KM, Buhl T, et al. Melanoma arising in segmental nevus spilus: detection by sequential digital dermatoscopy. *J Am Acad Dermatol.* 2009;61:337.

31. Moreno-Arias GA, Bulla F, Vilata-Corell JJ, et al. Treatment of widespread segmental nevus spilus by Q-switched alexandrite laser (755 nm, 100 nsec). *Dermatol Surg.* 2001;27(9):841.

32. Gold MH, Foster TD, Bell MW. Nevus spilus successfully treated with an intense pulsed light source. *Dermatol Surg.* 1999;25:254–255.

33. Grevelink JM, González S, Bonoan R, et al. Treatment of nevus spilus with the Q-switched ruby laser. *Dermatol Surg.* 1997;23(5):365–369.

34. Taylor CR, Anderson RR. Treatment of benign pigmented epidermal lesions by Q-switched ruby laser. *Int J Dermatol.* 1993;32:908–912.

35. Choi JE, Kim JW, Seo SH, et al. Treatment of Becker's nevi with a long-pulse alexandrite laser. *Dermatol Surg.* 2009;35(7):1105–1108.

36. Trelles MA, Allones I, Moreno-Arias GA, et al. Becker's naevus: a comparative study between erbium: YAG and Q-switched neodymium:YAG; clinical and histopathological findings. *Br J Dermatol.* 2005;152(2): 308–313.

37. Glaich AS, Goldberg LH, Dai T, et al. Fractional resurfacing: a new therapeutic modality for Becker's nevus. *Arch Dermatol.* 2007;143(12):1488.

38. Baba M, Bal N. Efficacy and safety of the short-pulse erbium:YAG laser in the treatment of acquired melanocytic nevi. *Dermatol Surg.* 2006;32:256–260.

39. Westerhof W, Gamei M. Treatment of acquired junctional melanocytic naevi by Q-switched and normal mode ruby laser. *Br J Dermatol.* 2003;148:80–85.

40. Vibhagool C, Byers HR, Grevelink JM. Treatment of small nevomelanocytic nevi with a Q-switched ruby laser. *J Am Acad Dermatol.* 1997;36:738–741.

41. Marghoob AA. Congenital melanocytic nevi. Evaluation and management. *Dermatol Clin.* 2002;20:1–10.

42. Kopf AW, Bart RS, Hennessey P. Congenital nevocytic nevi and malignant melanomas. *J Am Acad.* 1979;1: 123–130.

43. Rhodes AR, Melski JW. Small congenital nevocellular nevi and the risk of cutaneous melanoma. *J Pediatr.* 1982;100:219–224.

44. Zitelli JA, Grant MG, Abell E, et al. Histologic patterns of congenital nevocytic nevi and implications for treatment. *J Am Acad Dermatol.* 1984;11:402–409.

45. Grevelink JM, van Leeuwen RL, Anderson RR, et al. Clinical and histological responses of congenital melanocytic nevi after single treatment with Q-switched lasers. *Arch Dermatol.* 1997;133:349–353.

46. Ostertag JU, Quaedvlieg PJ, Kerchkhoffs FE, et al. Congenital naevi treated with erbium:YAG laser (Derma K) resurfacing in neonates: clinical results and review of the literature. *Br J Dermatol.* 2006;154: 889–895.

47. Helsing P, Mork G, Sveen B. Ruby laser treatment of congenital melanocytic naevi—a pessimistic view. *Acta Derm Venereol.* 2006;86:235–237.

48. Waldorf HA, Kauvar AN, Geronemus RG. Treatment of small and medium congenital nevi with the Q-switched ruby laser. *Arch Dermatol.* 1996;132:301–304.

49. Kishi K, Okabe K, Ninomiya R, et al. Early serial Q-switched ruby laser therapy for medium-sized to giant congenital melanocytic naevi. *Br J Dermatol.* 2009; 161:345–352.

50. Kim S, Kang WH. Treatment of congenital nevi with the Q-switched alexandrite laser. *Eur J Dermatol.* 2005;15: 92–96.
51. Hidano A, Kajima H, Ikeda S, et al. Natural history of nevus of Ota. *Arch Dermatol.* 1967;95(2):187–195.
52. Geronemus RG. Q-switched ruby laser therapy of nevus of Ota. *Arch Dermatol.* 1992;128:1618–1622.
53. Kono T, Chan HH, Ercocen AR, et al. Use of Q-switched ruby laser in the treatment of nevus of Ota in different age groups. *Lasers Surg Med.* 2003;32:391–395.
54. Kono T, Nozaki M, Chan HH, et al. A retrospective study looking at the long-term complications of Q-switched ruby laser in the treatment of nevus of Ota. *Lasers Surg Med.* 2001;29:156–159.
55. Wang HW, Liu YH, Zhang GK, et al. Analysis of 602 Chinese cases of nevus of Ota and the treatment results treated by Q-switched alexandrite laser. *Dermatol Surg.* 2007;33:455–460.
56. Kunachak S, Leelaudomlipi P, Sirikulchayanonta V. Q-switched ruby laser therapy of acquired bilateral nevus of Ota-like macules. *Dermatol Surg.* 1999;25:938–941.
57. Manuskiatti W, Sivayathorn A, Leelaudomlipi P, et al. Treatment of acquired bilateral nevus of Ota-like macules (Hori's nevus) using a combination of scanned carbon dioxide laser followed by Q-switched ruby laser. *J Am Acad Dermatol.* 2003;48:584–591.
58. Cho SB, Park SJ, Kim MJ, et al. Treatment of acquired bilateral nevus of Ota-like macules (Hori's nevus) using 1064-nm Q-switched Nd:YAG laser with low fluence. *Int J Dermatol.* 2009;48:1308–1312.
59. Reza AM, Farahnaz GZ, Hamideh S, et al. Incidence of Mongolian spots and its common sites at two university hospitals in Tehran, Iran. *Pediatr Dermatol.* 2010;27(4): 397–398.
60. Cordova A. The Mongolian spot: a study of ethnic differences and a literature review. *Clin Pediatr.* 1981;20(11): 714–719.
61. Shirakawa M, Ozawa T, Ohasi N, et al. Comparison of regional efficacy and complications in the treatment of aberrant Mongolian spots with the Q-switched ruby laser. *J Cosmet Laser Ther.* 2010;12:138–142.
62. Kagami S, Asahina A, Watanabe R, et al. Laser treatment of 26 Japanese patients with Mongolian spots. *Dermatol Surg.* 2008;34:1689–1694.
63. Milgraum SS, Cohen ME, Auletta MJ. Treatment of blue nevi with the Q-switched ruby laser. *J Am Acad Dermatol.* 1995;32(2):307–310.
64. Grimes PE, Yamada N, Bhawan J. Light microscopic immunohistochemical and ultrastructural alterations in patients with melasma. *Am J Dermatopathol.* 2005;27: 96–101.
65. Kauvar ANB. Successful treatment of melasma using a combination of microdermabrasion and q-switched Nd:YAG lasers. *Lasers Surg Med.* 2012;44:117–124.
66. Hong SP, Han SS, Choi SJ, et al. Split-face comparative study of 1550 nm fractional photothermolysis and trichloroacetic acid 15% chemical peeling for facial melasma in Asian skin. *J Cosmet Laser Ther.* 2012;14(2): 81–86.
67. Polder KD, Bruce S. Treatment of melasma using a novel 1927nm fractional thulium fiber laser: a pilot study. *Dermatol Surg.* 2012;38(2):199–206.
68. Baumler W, Eibler ET, Hohenleutner U, et al. Q-switched laser and tattoo pigments: first results of the chemical

69. and photophysical analysis of 41 compounds. *Lasers Surg Med.* 2000;26(1):13–21.
69. Armstrong ML, Roberts AE, Owen DC, et al. Contemporary college students and body piercing. *J Adolesc Health.* 2004;35(1):58–61.
70. Mayers LB, Judelson DA, Moriarty BW, et al. Prevalence of body art (body piercing and tattooing) in university undergraduates and incidence of medical complications. *Mayo Clin Proc.* 2002;77(1):29–34.
71. Goldman L, Rockwell RJ, Meyer R, et al. Laser treatment of tattoos. A preliminary survey of three year's clinical experience. *JAMA.* 1967;201:841–844.
72. Ferguson JE, Andrew SM, Jones CJ, et al. The Q-switched neodymium:YAG laser and tattoos: a microscopic analysis of laser–tattoo interactions. *Br J Dermatol.* 1997;137(3): 405–410.
73. Jow T, Brown A, Goldberg DJ. Patient compliance as a major determinant of laser tattoo removal success rates: a 10-year retrospective study. *J Cosmet Laser Ther.* 2010; 12:166–169.
74. Ara G, Anderson R, Mandel K, et al. Irradiation of pigmented melanoma cells with the high intensity pulsed radiation generates acoustic waves and kills cells. *Lasers Surg Med.* 1990;10(1):52–59.
75. Kent KM, Graber EM. Laser tattoo removal: a review. *Dermatol Surg.* 2012;38(1):1–13.
76. Graber E, Iyengar V, Rohrer T, et al. Laser treatment of tattoos and pigmented lesions. In: Robinson JK, Hanke CW, Siegel DM, Fratila A, eds. *Surgery of the Skin: Procedural Dermatology.* 2nd ed. China: Mosby; 2010: 537–548.
77. Ross V, Naseef G, Lin G, et al. Comparison of responses of tattoos to picosecond and nanosecond Q-switched neodymium: YAG lasers. *Arch Dermatol.* 1998;134:167–171.
78. Brauer JA, Reddy KK, Weiss ET, et al. Successful and rapid treatment of blue and green tattoo pigment with a novel picoseconds laser. *Arch Dermatol.* 2012;148(7): 820–823.
79. Beute TC, Miller CH, Timko AL, et al. In vitro spectral analysis of tattoo pigments. *Dermatol Surg.* 2008;34: 508–516.
80. Levine VJ, Geronemus RG. Tattoo removal with the Q-switched ruby laser and the Q-switched Nd:YAG laser: a comparative study. *Cutis.* 1995;55(5):291–296.
81. Lin T, Jia G, Rong H, et al. Comparison of a single treatment with Q-switched ruby laser and Q-switched Nd:YAG laser in removing black-blue Chinese tattoos. *J Cosmet Laser Ther.* 2009;11(4):236–239.
82. Leuenberger ML, Mulas MW, Hata TR, et al. Comparison of the Q-switched alexandrite, Nd:YAG, and ruby lasers in treating blue-black tattoos. *Dermatol Surg.* 1999;25:10–14.
83. Taylor CR, Gange RW, Dover JS, et al. Treatment of tattoos by Q-switched ruby laser. A dose-response study. *Arch Dermatol.* 1990;126:893–899.
84. Grevelink JM, Duke D, van Leeuwen RL, et al. Laser treatment of tattoos in darkly pigmented patients: efficacy and side effects. *J Am Acad Dermatol.* 1996;34:653–656.
85. Lee CN, Bae EY, Park JG, et al. Permanent makeup removal using Q-switched Nd:YAG laser. *Clin Exp Dermatol.* 2009;34:e594–e596.
86. Guedes R, Leite L. Removal of orange eyebrow tattoo in a single session with the Q-switched Nd:YAG 532-nm laser. *Lasers Med Sci.* 2010;25:465–466.

87. Alster TS. Q-switched alexandrite laser treatment (755 nm) of professional and amateur tattoos. *J Am Acad Dermatol.* 1995;33:69–73.

88. Moreno-Arias GA, Casals-Andreu M, Camps-Fresneda A. Use of Q-switched alexandrite laser (755 nm, 100 nsec) for removal of traumatic tattoo of different origins. *Lasers Surg Med.* 1999;25:445–450.

89. Bukhari IA. Removal of amateur blue-black tattoos in Arabic women of skin type (III–IV) with Q-switched alexandrite laser. *J Cosmet Dermatol.* 2005;4:107–110.

90. Fitzpatrick RE, Goldman MP. Tattoo removal using the alexandrite laser. *Arch Dermatol.* 1994;130(12):1508–1514.

91. Weiss ET, Geronemus RG. Combining fractional resurfacing and q-switched ruby laser for tattoo removal. *Dermatol Surg.* 2010;37:97–99.

92. Mafong EA, Kauvar AN, Geronemus RG. Surgical pearl: removal of cosmetic lip-liner tattoo with the pulsed carbon dioxide laser. *J Am Acad Dermatol.* 2003;48(2):271–272.

93. Fitzpatrick RE, Lupton JR. Successful treatment of treatment-resistant laser-induced pigment darkening of a cosmetic tattoo. *Lasers Surg Med.* 2000;27:358–361.

94. Jimenez G, Weiss E, Spencer JM. Multiple color changes following laser therapy of cosmetic tattoos. *Dermatol Surg.* 2002;28(2):177–179.

95. Alster TS, Gupta SN. Minocycline-induced hyperpigmentation treated with a 755-nm Q-switched alexandrite laser. *Dermatol Surg.* 2004;30:1201–1204.

96. Izikson L, Anderson RR. Delayed darkening of imipramine-induced hyperpigmentation after treatment with a Q-switched Nd:YAG laser followed by a Q-switched ruby laser. *Dermatol Surg.* 2009;35:527–529.

97. Izikson L, Anderson RR. Resolution of blue minocycline pigmentation of the face after fractional photothermolysis. *Lasers Surg Med.* 2008;40:399–401.

98. Kossida T, Rigopoulos D, Katsambas A, et al. Optimal tattoo removal in a single laser session based on the method of repeated exposures. *J Am Acad Dermatol.* 2012;66:271–277.

99. Reddy KK, Brauer JA, Anolik R, et al. Topical perfluorodecalin resolves immediate whitening reactions and allows rapid effective multiple pass treatment of tattoos. *Lasers Surg Med.* 2012 [Epub ahead of print].

CHAPTER 4

Lasers and Light Devices for Hair Removal

Kira Minkis and Leonard J. Bernstein

INTRODUCTION

The achievement of permanent or semipermanent hair removal has been a goal for over a century. As early as the 19th century, physicians have attempted to achieve permanent hair removal with employment of electrolysis, initially for the treatment of trichiasis.[1] With the development of laser technology, the field of hair epilation has vastly expanded in recent years. Laser hair removal (LHR) has revolutionized the field of hair removal in large part due to the ability to selectively target and destroy hair follicles, leading to more long-lasting hair removal, requiring less operator dependency, and decreasing the potential side effects compared with other methods of hair removal. However, despite these advantages, it is of paramount importance for safe, effective LHR that the laser/light device operator has a basic understanding of laser–skin interactions including proper patient/laser selection as well as an understanding of hair anatomy, growth, and physiology.

THE HISTORY OF LASER HAIR REMOVAL

The earliest anecdotal evidence of hair destruction by laser light was by Goldman et al who first described ruby laser injury to pigmented hair follicles in 1964.[2] Later observations of hair loss were made as an indirect side effect during treatment of tattoos and nevi with quality-switched (QS) 694-nm ruby lasers. Lasers were initially used with the target goal of hair removal in the field of ophthalmology and urology for the treatment of trichiasis and urethral grafts.[3–5] The lasers utilized for these early treatments did not specifically target the hair follicles.

The theory of selective photothermolysis, introduced by Anderson and Parrish in 1983, revolutionized the field of lasers with the concept of selectively targeting a particular chromophore based on its absorption spectra and size.[6] In selective photothermolysis, energy is delivered at a wavelength well absorbed by the target, within a time period less than or equal to the thermal relaxation time of the target. Based on this theory, Grossman et al began the search for a means to specifically eliminate hair utilizing light energy. They selectively targeted melanin in hair follicles using normal-mode, long-pulsed ruby lasers to achieve long-term hair removal.[7] The preliminary studies with the ruby laser on hair follicles revealed the ability to induce a growth delay and permanent hair removal in some individuals. These early results opened a flood gate of research into the study of various wavelengths and a more in-depth look at laser–tissue interactions in the pursuit of long-term hair removal utilizing lasers and light devices.[7–10]

Since the introduction of the first Food and Drug Administration (FDA)–approved hair removal laser system in 1996, the field of laser-assisted hair removal has grown tremendously. Currently, multiple lasers and light sources are available and marketed for the treatment of unwanted or excessive hair in both a clinical environment and, more recently, the home setting. The goals of ideal laser epilation are for the treatment to be practical and efficient, have long-lasting results or permanence, produce only minimal discomfort, avoid epidermal injury, and be available for all skin phototypes and hair colors.

HAIR ANATOMY

The pilosebaceous unit is a very important adnexal structure of the skin consisting of the hair follicle and sebaceous glands. It serves many roles in the proper homeostasis of the skin as well as a source of epithelial cells during wound healing. The hair follicle can exist in 2 phenotypes, terminal hairs and vellus hairs. Terminal hairs include the androgen-independent hair (eyebrows, lashes) as well as hormone-dependent regions including the scalp, beard, chest, axilla, and pubic region. These hairs are long (>2 cm), thick (>60 μm in diameter), and pigmented. Terminal hair usually extends more than 3 mm deep into the subcutis.

The hair bulb of terminal anagen hairs is located in the subcutis. In contrast, vellus hairs, which cover a large portion of the remainder of the body, are short (<2 cm), thin (<30 μm in diameter), often not pigmented, and extend just 1 mm into the dermis.

The hair follicle consists of 3 anatomic units: the infundibulum, the isthmus, and the inferior segments. The infundibulum is the region of the hair follicle from the orifice of the follicle to the entrance of the sebaceous duct. The epithelium of the infundibulum is contiguous with the epidermis. The isthmus is the region between the entrance of the sebaceous duct and immediately above the insertion of the arrector pili muscle at the "bulge." The inferior portion of the isthmus contains the bulge area of the hair follicle at the insertion of the arrector pili muscle and extends downward to form the hair bulb at its base during the anagen phase of the hair cycle.

The hair bulb is at the deepest portion of the hair follicle that surrounds the dermal papilla. It is composed of matrix cells and melanocytes. The dermal papilla contains the neurovascular structure that supplies the hair matrix. The differentiation of the matrical cells forms the various layers of the hair follicle that include, from the outer layers, the outer root sheath, the inner root sheath (composed of the Henle layer, the Huxley layer, and the cuticle), and the 3 layers of the hair shaft, namely, the cuticle, cortex, and medulla (Figures 4-1 and 4-2).

The bulge area is a contiguous part of outer root sheath that provides the insertion point for arrector pili muscle and marks the bottom of the permanent portion of hair follicles. The cells within the bulge area and the surrounding follicular cells possess stem cell properties, such as high proliferative capacity and multipotency, which is the ability to regenerate not

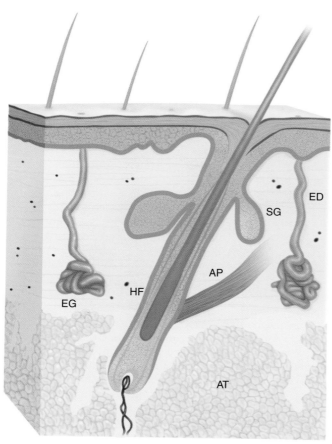

EG - Eccrine gland

SG - Sebaceous gland

ED - Eccrine duct

AT - Adipose tissue

AP - Arrector pili muscle

HF - Hair follicle

▲ **FIGURE 4-1** The skin in vertical section: the pilosebaceous unit, the eccrine glands, and the adipose tissue.

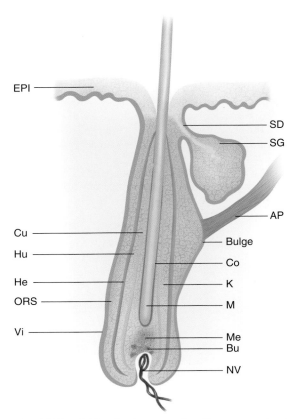

EPI

SD

SG

AP

Cu

Bulge

Hu

Co

He

K

ORS

M

Vi

Me

Bu

NV

▲ **FIGURE 4-2** The pilosebaceous unit and its component parts: epidermis (EPI), sebaceous duct (SD), sebaceous gland (SG), arrector pili muscle (AP), bulge, cortex (Co), keratinocytes (K), medulla (M), melanocytes (Me), bulb (Bu), neurovascular bundle (NV), vitreous membrane (Vi), outer root sheath (ORS), Henle layer of inner root sheath (He), Huxley layer of inner root sheath (Hu), and cuticle of inner root sheath (Cu).

hair growth in each body site. Bulbar matrix cells differentiate to make up the hair shaft and inner root sheath, which leads to hair lengthening by outward migration. Catagen phase follows anagen and is a transition period lasting 2 to 4 weeks. During this time the bulbar portion of the hair follicle undergoes degradation through apoptosis. The follicle regresses with a shortening in length, with a more superficial placement of the hair bulb. The telogen phase, the last in the hair cycle, follows catagen and is marked by a period of inactivity lasting 2 to 4 months. Subsequently, the hair cycle continues with new hair growth resuming in a new anagen phase.

The hair follicle is regenerated through differentiation of stem cells. Despite the previously held belief that hair follicle stem cells reside in the bulbar area of hair follicles, accumulated evidence indicates that keratinocyte stem cells reside in and around the bulge area of the hair follicle, which migrate downward with anagen hair growth.[11] Recent studies by Festa et al have described the role of immature adipocytes during the activation of hair growth.[12] Adipocyte precursors are able to induce progression of the follicle from telogen to anagen and thus affect follicular cycling and communicate with follicular stem cells.

The duration of anagen determines the final length of the hair, and this varies depending on body site. Body sites with long hair such as the scalp have a lengthy anagen phase, whereas body sites with short hair have a short anagen phase and a lengthy telogen phase. In adults, the hairs of the scalp and body are not synchronous and are at various stages of growth. Hence, there is a continual shedding of telogen hairs and renewal of anagen hairs on a daily basis leading to a steady state of hair density.

Hair color is determined by melanin pigmentation within keratinocytes of the hair fiber. The hair melanin is produced by melanocytes that are located in the hair bulb epithelium. The density of bulbar melanocytes is greater than in the epidermis with approximately 1 melanocyte to 4 basal keratinocytes in the upper hair bulb compared with 1:10 in the basal layer of the epidermis. Two types of melanin are present in hair: eumelanin is the brown-black pigment and pheomelanin is the yellow-red pigment. Fire-red hair color contains the highest levels of pheomelanin with other hair colors containing melanocytes with eumelanosomes. Melanogenic activity in the hair follicle is closely linked to the hair cycle with melanogenesis occurring within the early part of the anagen phase of the hair cycle and ceasing with the onset of catagen.

only hair follicles but also sebaceous glands and epidermis.[11]

Hair follicles are self-renewing structures that reconstitute themselves through the hair cycle. They can be subdivided into the permanent and nonpermanent portions. The upper and middle portions of the follicle are permanent, but the lower region regenerates with each hair cycle. The follicular bulge forms the lowermost aspect of the permanent follicular structure. Hair undergoes a cyclic growth pattern that consists of 3 phases, namely, anagen, catagen, and telogen. Anagen is the period of active growth during the hair cycle. The duration of anagen will vary greatly for different body regions and accounts for the varying length of

■ HAIR REMOVAL METHODS

The cosmetic and functional desire to remove or minimize the appearance of hair has prompted the development of a wide array of modalities to achieve this goal prior to the introduction of lasers. With the exception of electrical epilation, or electrolysis, these techniques have produced transient solutions. Cosmetic procedures, such as bleaching, are used to diminish the appearance of unwanted hair by reducing the pigmentation in the exposed hair shaft. Mechanical hair removal methods, such as trimming, shaving, plucking, threading, and waxing, as well as chemical depilatories, provide temporary methods of hair removal (Table 4-1).

Probably the most popular method of mechanical hair removal is shaving. Despite the misconception that hair will grow faster if it has been shaven, the act of shaving or trimming does not lead to an increased hair length, width, or density. A drawback to this simple mechanical method is the need for frequent and regular use to maintain a desired clinical appearance. Moreover, associated complications can include cuts, irritation of the skin, and pseudofolliculitis barbae.

Unlike shaving, which only removes hair above the surface of the skin, epilation removes the entire hair shaft. Methods of epilation include plucking, waxing, threading, abrasives, sugaring, and use of mechanical devices. Sugaring is an ancient method of temporary hair removal similar to waxing in which a warm mixture composed of sugar and lemon juice is applied and pressed into large hair-bearing areas with the subsequent removal of the attached hair shafts, in addition to a superficial skin exfoliation.[13] Epilation has the advantage over shaving of repetitive trauma to the hair follicle, which can lead to matrix damage and finer hair growth over time. However, the disadvantages of mechanical epilation may include pseudofolliculitis barbae, the requirement that the hair be allowed to grow to a sufficient length for effective removal, and in the case of hot waxing techniques, there exists the possibility of thermal injury. All means of mechanical epilation should be used with caution in patients on systemic or topical retinoids, where epidermal injury from excessive, unexpected exfoliation is possible.

Chemical depilation removes the hair shaft including its external projection from the surface and a small portion within the upper infundibulum. Common chemical depilatory agents consist of sodium thioglycolate or calcium thioglycolate. These agents work by disruption of disulfide bonds of hair keratin, causing hair breakage.[14] Adverse reactions to these agents include skin irritation, allergic contact dermatitis, and pseudofolliculitis barbae.

In 1886, the first attempt at permanent hair removal by electrosurgical epilation, or electrolysis, was performed.[15] Electrolysis works by the insertion of a fine needle into the hair follicle and the application of an electrical current in an effort to damage and eventually destroy the hair follicle.[16] There are 2 types of electrolysis, galvanic (direct current electrolysis) and thermolysis (alternating current electrolysis). Although electrolysis does offer the potential for permanent hair removal, it is highly operator dependent and has the potential for associated side effects/risks. These include scarring, postinflammatory pigmentary alteration, pain, and the possibility for infection due to the transmission of bacterial or viral elements. Furthermore, limited efficacy, described as 30% to 40%, for destroying individual hair follicles and the time-consuming nature of electrolysis provide for an impractical means of hair removal when treating large surface areas or in individuals with extensive hair.

In addition to the physical removal of unwanted hair, one can address hair growth itself through medical management with an attempt to slow or repress it. The goal is to suppress ovarian or adrenal androgen secretion or block the effects of androgens on the hair follicle. Thus, these medical treatment options are appropriate for patients with androgen-dependent hirsutism, rather than simple hypertrichosis. Systemic medications used for such purposes include cyproterone acetate, flutamide, spironolactone, and finasteride. Although antiandrogen therapy is most efficient, if the serum testosterone concentration is elevated, the addition of an oral contraceptive improves the likelihood

TABLE 4-1
Methods of Hair Removal

METHODS OF HAIR REMOVAL	DURATION
Mechanical	
Waxing	Short term
Plucking	Short term
Threading	Short term
Shaving	Short term
Trimming	Short term
Chemical	
Depilatory	Short term
Electrical	
Electrolysis	Long term
Photothermal	
Lasers/light devices	Long term

of response.[17] A more recent newcomer to the field of medical management for hair removal is topical eflornithine, an irreversible inhibitor of the enzyme ornithine decarboxylase. Eflornithine is thought to slow hair growth by inhibiting this enzyme in hair follicles. Use of this cream should be combined with other hair removal practices as it slows the growth of hair rather than removing hair. The combination of mechanical removal and medical therapy offers a better likelihood of improvement of hirsutism.[18]

The advent of lasers for epilation has revolutionized the field of hair removal. Compared with the mechanical or chemical epilation techniques, lasers are more effective and faster, and produce a longer-lasting result. Prior to the development of lasers for epilation, electrolysis had been the mainstay of long-term hair removal. In a comparative study by Görgü et al, electrolysis was compared with laser epilation using an alexandrite laser on axillary hair. The results revealed clearance rates of 74% for the areas treated with the alexandrite laser and 35% for the areas treated with electrolysis at 6 months after the initial treatment. Moreover, the treatment duration for the laser was 60 times shorter than that for electrolysis and the laser treatment was felt to be less painful.[19]

MECHANISMS OF LASER HAIR REMOVAL

The theory of selective photothermolysis underlies the mechanism of LHR. This theory enables selective targeting of pigmented hair follicles by utilizing the melanin of the hair shaft as a chromophore. Melanin functions as a chromophore for wavelengths spanning the visible and near-infrared portion of the electromagnetic spectrum.[20] The hair follicle components that contain melanin include the hair shaft and matrix. Although the ideal targets for LHR should be the follicular stem cells, these cells do not contain an appreciable amount of melanin or other chromophore that may serve as a target for light energy interactions. As a result, an extended theory of selective photothermolysis was proposed, which requires diffusion of heat from the chromophore to the desired target for destruction.[21] Applying the extended theory of selective photothermolysis, follicular stem cells could be damaged by heat diffusion from the hair shaft or the matrix cells.

Based on the clinical findings of LHR/light-based hair removal, one would expect complete or partial destruction of the hair follicle following the application of sufficient thermal energy to eliminate hair growth. Histological evaluations of hair follicles, having been treated with typical laser parameters to induce clinical hair loss, have revealed puzzling results with regard to the direct visible effect on the follicle. After laser treatment, there is evidence of thermal injury to the hair shaft with a distortion of its normal appearance. The internal root sheath remains mostly unchanged with only focal areas of damage. There is barely any visible damage in the outer root sheath, hair bulb, or dermal papilla. In fact, recent immunohistochemical evaluations of the hair follicle postlaser treatment revealed little change in the suspected stem cells in and around the bulge area of the follicle. In particular, cytokeratin 15 and 19, which are believed to be biomarkers for the follicular stem cells, showed persistent staining after laser treatment, suggesting the viability of these cells. It is possible that there is a thermal effect that essentially turns off the proper functioning of these cells without their complete destruction.[22]

On the other hand, the desire to destroy the hair follicle in order to prevent further hair growth may lead to a concern that proper wound healing following laser/light therapy would be affected. As the repaired epithelium is partly derived from the follicular epithelium, one would anticipate that there could be a significant delay in wound healing following laser destruction of the follicle. In fact, in the clinical setting of successful hair removal with lasers, we do find normal wound healing after minor surgical procedures.[23]

As the underlying principle of LHR/light hair removal treatment is dependent on the presence of hair shafts within the follicle, one would conclude that only anagen hair follicles are affected. This would imply that multiple treatments at frequent intervals are necessary to effectively treat every follicle due to the absence of a target in a percentage of follicles not in anagen phase at any given time. This was further investigated by Lin et al, who studied the effects of a ruby laser on hair follicles throughout the varying phases of the hair cycle. Using both histological assessment and gross observations of the injury and regrowth of hair, the authors concluded that actively growing and pigmented anagen stage hair follicles were sensitive to hair removal by normal-mode ruby laser exposure, whereas catagen and telogen stage hair follicles were resistant to laser irradiation.[24] In fact, in clinical practice the interval between laser/light device treatment sessions is based on the presence of some regrowth from the previous session and will vary for both individuals and body sites. Treatment intervals of

4 to 8 weeks may be average for facial sites of hair removal while 8 to 12 weeks may be needed for the body and extremities, which have a slower follicular regeneration time. Treating regions prior to the presence of hair within the follicle will have no effect on these follicles.

Attempts to utilize exogenous chromophores have been explored, such as the topical application of phosphatidylcholine-based liposomes, Meladine (Creative Technologies, Inc, Chesapeake, Virginia). This is a topical melanin-encapsulated liposomal spray that was approved by the FDA to enhance the effects of lasers in nonpigmented hair. By binding these liposomal products onto blonde or gray hairs, it will create a pigmented target for lasers.[25] However, the efficacy of this molecule in this setting has not been well demonstrated. A similar liposomal melanin product, Lipoxome (Dalton Medicare, The Netherlands), has been studied on the head and bodies of 16 patients. Results showed a 14% reduction in hair counts after diode laser treatment compared with a 10% reduction in hair counts in control patients.[26]

 ## PREOPERATIVE ASSESSMENT AND PREPARATION

Prior to initiation of treatment, patients requesting LHR should have a physical examination and a review of pertinent medical history. A pretreatment consultation is essential to establish patient and physician expectations prior to initiation of treatment. Potential risks of the procedure should be entirely reviewed and an informed consent should be obtained (Table 4-2).

Medical History

A medical history is important, particularly to determine if the patient may have a familial pattern of excess hair growth or a contributing medical condition. If the latter is suspected, a workup should be obtained in order to eliminate the underlying cause of hair growth and improve the outcome of laser treatment. Additional historical inquiries should include a past history of herpes simplex virus, previous systemic gold therapy, or the recent use of oral retinoids. If there is a past history of herpes simplex virus at or near the treatment site, the use of prophylactic antiviral therapy may be considered. A patient with a past history of gold therapy should not be treated with lasers for hair removal due to the risk of induction of cutaneous chrysiasis, which has been reported to occur with various laser

TABLE 4-2
Preoperative Assessment

Preoperative assessments/review
Medical history
    Familial hair growth patterns
    Menstrual cycle (in women)
    Herpes simplex infections
    Isotretinoin
    Oral gold therapy
    Previous laser/light therapy
Physical examination
    Skin phototype
    Hair density
    Hair color
    Hair coarseness
    Presence of vellus hairs
Patient expectations
    Pain management
    Posttreatment effects on skin
        Erythema
        Edema—perifollicular
        Hair shaft discharge/char
    Multiple treatments
    Risks of procedure

wavelengths.[27,28] This troubling discoloration of the skin is noted abruptly after laser interaction with the skin that contains gold salts. Although extremely troubling for patients, this dyspigmentation has been treated successfully in the past with QS pigment lasers and pulsed dye lasers over several sessions. The use of oral retinoids in the recent past may lead one to postpone treatment due to concerns regarding a higher risk of hypertrophic/keloid scarring following laser treatment. Although the risks are clearly evident with ablative laser treatments, recent observations in small sample groups of patients using oral retinoids while undergoing LHR revealed no adverse effects.[29–31] An inquiry into past LHR treatment is likewise important to determine the previous course, parameters, and response to treatment, as these details may influence the treatment plan.

Physical Examination

The patient's hair color and skin tone should be noted, as these characteristics will significantly influence both the success of treatment and potential side effects. The ideal candidate for LHR would have a lighter skin phototype (Fitzpatrick I and II) with dark terminal hair. The least ideal patient would have darker skin phototypes (Fitzpatrick III and VI) and a lighter hair phenotype. Patients with blonde, gray, red, or white hair are poor candidates due to reduced melanin content in the hair shafts. Darker skin phototypes (Fitzpatrick V and VI) may have an increased risk for complications due to the significant increase in the competing epidermal melanin if care is not taken with laser selection. In these individuals, epidermal melanin will absorb a portion of the laser energy intended for the dermal follicular structures and can increase the potential for side effects including vesiculation, prolonged erythema, and postoperative pigmentary alteration.

During the preoperative examination, the presence of a tan should be noted. A tan in all skin phototypes increases the risk of epidermal injury. A decision to postpone treatment until the tan fades or to utilize a longer-wavelength device, such as the 1064-nm neodymium:yttrium-aluminum garnet (Nd:YAG) laser, should be considered to avoid potential side effects such as dyspigmentation. Patients should be counseled to avoid tanning or significant sun exposure prior to or during the treatment course.

The presence of vellus hairs in the treatment field may preclude the use of laser/light devices for the treatment of unwanted hairs. The risk for the development of paradoxical hypertrichosis rises significantly when blonde, fine-textured vellus hairs are irradiated with laser/light energy. The poor absorption of the light energy, due to the lack of melanin, leads to only a minor thermal effect on these hairs, which could actually induce differentiation of these hairs to terminal hairs. This effect is often seen along the jawline and neck of women, but has been reported in men as well.

Patient Expectations

TREATMENT DISCOMFORT Patients should be counseled on the expectation that the procedure may induce a variable degree of discomfort. The use of topical anesthetics prior to laser therapy can help to minimize this effect. Patients should be discouraged from applying these topical anesthetic creams without the explicit direction from their physician. Although these agents are available over the counter at most pharmacies, the application of large quantities over a large surface area can lead to significant toxicity and even death.[32] The use of cold air blowers during the LHR treatment can add a significant degree of comfort and distraction to the patient. This technique should not be used in combination with

▲ **FIGURE 4-3** Perifollicular edema following laser hair removal on a patient's back.

laser devices that utilize a dynamic cooling device, as the blowing air will disrupt the coolant flow to the skin and may prevent adequate epidermal protection.

TREATMENT EFFECTS Patients should be made aware of the expected posttreatment presence of perifollicular edema, erythema, acneiform eruptions, and charred hair stubble (Figure 4-3). The perifollicular edema will have a variable duration lasting minutes to 1 or 2 days. The use of cool compresses or ice will hasten its regression. When treating body sites with very dense and coarse hairs or follicles with pili multigemini, one can expect a greater degree of edema, in some cases lasting for up to 1 week following treatment. The use of oral corticosteroids can help to minimize the perifollicular edema and aid in patient comfort. Acneiform eruptions are often transient, if these should arise, and can be treated with standard acne preparations.

TREATMENT OUTCOMES Establishing realistic goals of treatment is important prior to initiation of treatment. Patients should understand the wide range of outcomes with LHR. Lasers offer a method to significantly delay hair growth and will result in finer hair growth. Through the induction of catagen and telogen, temporary hair loss is achievable for most patients. However, the degree to which hair removal is long term is dependent on a patient's physical characteristics as well as treatment parameters. In the ideal candidate with light skin and dark hair, a 20% to 30% hair loss has been observed with each treatment when effective fluences are used (Figure 4-4). This percentage decreases significantly when less than optimal fluences are utilized.

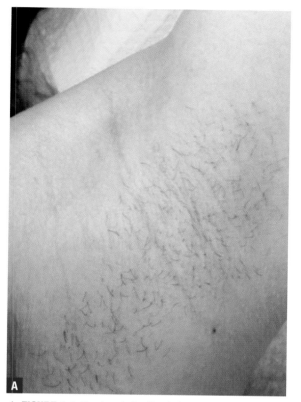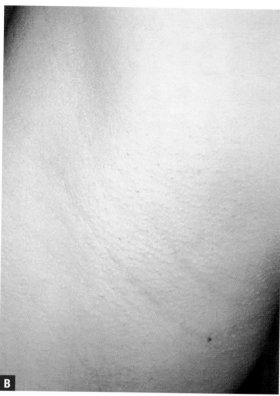

▲ **FIGURE 4-4** Treatment of axillary hair in a patient with Fitzpatrick skin phototype II. Before treatment (**A**) and 3 months after 5 bimonthly treatments with an alexandrite laser (**B**).

The potential for permanent, complete hair removal in this later situation is very low.

HAIR MAINTENANCE Prior to treatment, patients should be instructed to avoid excessive sun exposure for 6 weeks prior to treatment and to protect the area throughout the entire treatment course with the use of daily broad-spectrum sunscreen. Hair removal methods, which remove the hair shaft, such as plucking, waxing, threading, sugaring, and electrolysis, should be avoided before any treatment session, as these methods remove the target chromophore for LHR. However, it is safe for the patient to continue to shave, bleach, or use depilatory creams between treatment sessions.

Patients who are pregnant are not precluded from being treated with lasers for hair removal. However, the use of topical anesthetic agents should be avoided during pregnancy or while lactating in the postpartum period to avoid toxicity to the fetus or infant.

LASER TECHNOLOGY

Q-switched Nd:YAG Laser

The first laser-assisted hair removal device was made commercially available in 1996 when the US FDA approved a patented laser process (SoftLight, Thermolase Corp, La Jolla, California) for hair removal that included the use of a QS Nd:YAG laser after pretreatment wax epilation and the application of a carbon-based solution. Since then, the FDA has approved multiple laser systems, which are currently on the market (Table 4-3).

Goldberg et al initially reported that use of the QS Nd:YAG laser treatment and application of a suspension of carbon mineral oil provided a reduction in hair growth for up to 6 months.[33] The process consisted of epilating the hair from the follicle and filling the empty follicle with a carbon-containing substance that acts as an energy-absorbing chromophore. This method was

TABLE 4-3
Lasers for Hair Removal

LASER	MANUFACTURER	LASER	MANUFACTURER
Ruby laser—694 nm			
EpiLaser	Palomar		
Alexandrite laser—755 nm			
Harmony	Alma Lasers	Light A/A Star	Quanta
GentleLase/Max	Candela/Syneron	Arion	Quantel
Apogee	Cynosure	ClearScan ALX	Sciton
Elite/Elite MPX	Cynosure		
Diode laser—800–810 nm			
Soprano	Alma Lasers	LEDA EPI	Quantel Derma
MeDioStar	Eclipse Aesthetics	eMax/eLaser	Candela/Syneron
LightSheer Duet	Lumenis		
Nd:YAG (long pulsed)—1064 nm			
LightPod Neo	Aerolase	Elite	Cynosure
Harmony	Alma Laser	Gemini	Iridex/Cutera
GentleYag/Max	Candela/Syneron	Light B/A Star	Quanta
CoolGlide	Cutera	ClearScan YAG	Sciton
Intense pulsed light—variable from 500–1200 nm			
Prowave	Cutera	Icon MaxR	Palomar
Elite MPX	Cynosure	Prolite III	Quantel
Eclipse SmoothCool	Eclipse	BBL	Sciton
Lumenis One	Lumenis	eMax	Candela/Syneron

subsequently described and used successfully in a patient with congenital hypertrichosis lanuginosa.[34] Later studies comparing this method of hair removal with treatment in the absence of the carbon solution indicated that, although the combination of pretreatment wax epilation and topical carbon solution application was effective, laser irradiation alone also provided a significant delay in hair growth (although no permanent hair removal was achieved with either modality).[35]

Ruby Laser

The ruby laser emits light at a wavelength of 694 nm. This wavelength penetrates relatively deeply into the dermis, and is better absorbed by melanin than by surrounding skin structures. A normal-mode ruby laser was designed to maximize delivery of light to the reticular dermis while minimizing epidermal injury. The EpiLaser from Palomar Medical Technologies was the first long-pulsed 694-nm ruby laser system approved for hair removal by the FDA. Grossman et al first reported a delay in hair growth using ruby laser pulses delivered through a cold sapphire lens to minimize epidermal injury.[7] In individuals with fair skin and dark hair, high-fluence ruby laser pulses (6-mm spot size, fluences of 20–60 J/cm², and pulses of 0.27-millisecond duration) induced growth delay lasting 1 to 3 months in all patients. Multiple studies have since evaluated the efficacy of this laser, which has been shown to be safe and effective, with laser exposures producing a hair growth delay consistent with induction of telogen. Prolonged as well as permanent hair loss was subsequently reported in some subjects.[8,10,36] Histological assessment of immediate posttreatment ruby laser sites demonstrated selective thermal damage to pigmented hair follicles, with vaporization of hair shafts and apoptosis of follicular epithelial cells. Subjects who exhibited permanent hair loss demonstrated a reduction in large terminal hairs with a reciprocal increase in small vellus-like hairs as well as a decreased average hair shaft diameter without the presence of fibrosis.[8,37] The long-pulsed ruby laser can be safely used in Fitzpatrick skin phototypes I to III. Despite efficacy associated with the ruby laser, there are significant dose-related side effects (vesiculation, crusting, and dyspigmentation), mainly as a result of epidermal injury. Therefore, the ruby laser is best used on patients with lighter skin phototypes (Fitzpatrick types I–III).

Alexandrite Lasers

The alexandrite laser is also a red light laser system with a wavelength of 755 nm. The safety and efficacy of the long-pulsed alexandrite laser has been well established for hair removal in Fitzpatrick skin phototypes I to VI.[38–42] The longer wavelength of the alexandrite laser, compared with that of the ruby laser, allows for a slightly greater depth of penetration while its slightly lower melanin absorption decreases the risk of epidermal damage. Great care must be used when utilizing this laser in the darker skin phototypes including the use of longer pulse durations and lower fluences.

Treatment efficacy for the alexandrite laser varies with the anatomic location, pulse duration, and number of treatments. McDaniel et al found maximum hair reductions of 15% to 56% at 6 months, depending on body site (with greatest hair reduction using 10 milliseconds pulse duration at 20 J/cm^2).[43] Other groups, using average fluences of 30 to 40 J/cm^2, have found efficacy rates with a 3-millisecond alexandrite laser to be between 60% and 75% after a mean of 5.6 treatments.[40] Histologically, alexandrite laser–treated skin demonstrates moderate follicular damage immediately, and cystic formation of hair follicles and foreign body giant cells along with follicular apoptosis 1 month following laser treatment.[44] A recent randomized, investigator-blinded clinical trial of subjects with Fitzpatrick skin phototypes III to IV comparing treatment with a long-pulsed alexandrite laser (12 and 18 mm spot size, 1.5 milliseconds pulse duration, and fluences of 20 or 40 J/cm^2) either alone or in combination with long-pulsed Nd:YAG for 4 sessions showed mean hair reduction of 76% to 84% for the alexandrite laser, 74% for the Nd:YAG laser, and 78% for the combination therapy 18 months after the last treatment.[45] Combination treatment of alexandrite and Nd:YAG lasers did not provide any additional benefit and increased adverse effects.

Diode Laser

The diode lasers (800–810 nm) reside at the far end of the visible light spectrum and at the near end of the infrared spectrum. They have demonstrated good long-term results for hair removal in skin phototypes I to V.[46–48] In the earliest evaluation of the diode laser, Lou noted a 25% hair count reduction extending through a 20-month follow-up period. The longer pulse durations and longer wavelength of this laser allow for the treatment of all Fitzpatrick skin types due to a lower absorption by epidermal melanin. A limiting factor with the traditional diode laser is the small spot size, the need for higher fluences and the associated discomfort. A recent study by Ibrahimi and Kilmer using an 800-nm long-pulsed diode laser with a large spot size (22 × 35 mm), lower average fluences of 10 to 12 J/cm^2, and vacuum-assisted suction (LightSheer Duet HS, Lumenis, Santa Clara, California) demonstrated hair clearance of 54% at 6 months and 42% at 15 months following 3 treatment sessions.[49,50] Another attempt to address patient comfort was evaluated in a recent study by Braun, who compared the effectiveness of a high-fluence single-pass diode laser with a low-fluence, multiple-pass in-motion technique. The efficacy was similar; however, the perception of treatment discomfort was considerably less with the lower-fluence system.[51] The histological evaluation of this low-fluence, multiple-pass method in patients with darker skin phototypes has been described by Trelles et al. A significant perifollicular edema, hair shaft detachment from the sheath, and follicular inflammation were noted. This demonstrates that the effect on hair follicles was sufficient to cause focal damage with a laser utilizing a lower-than-average fluence, but with multiple passes.[52]

Nd:YAG Lasers

The long-pulsed 1064-nm Nd:YAG laser has a deeply penetrating wavelength in the infrared spectrum resulting in a reduction of melanin absorption. These lasers require higher fluences for adequate follicular injury. They offer the best combination of safety and efficacy for darker skin phototypes (Fitzpatrick V and VI). Alster et al reported a 70% to 90% reduction of facial, axillary, and leg hair growth 1 year after 3 monthly treatments with a 1064-nm Nd:YAG laser (pulse duration of 50 milliseconds, fluences of 40–50 J/cm^2) with a histological assessment showing evidence of selective follicular injury without epidermal disruption.[53] Further histological evaluation of laser-treated skin found that laser exposure caused damage to follicular epithelium seen as increased cytoplasmic eosinophilia and nuclear elongation with no damage to the perifollicular epidermis.[54] In general, the Nd:YAG laser is an effective device for hair removal in patients with darker skin phototypes; however, it is thought to be less efficacious than the alexandrite and diode lasers for hair removal in patients with light skin phototypes and light hair phenotypes.[45,55]

Intense Pulsed Light Devices

Flashlamp-powered intense pulsed light (IPL) sources emit noncoherent, multiwavelength energy with an output spectrum extending across the 500- to 1200-nm range. Filters are utilized to cut off undesired wavelengths and target specific chromophores (such as melanin), allowing for a more selective treatment. Several studies have demonstrated the efficacy of IPL with 1 study demonstrating a 33% reduction in hair growth after 2 treatments at 6 months (2.8–3.2 milliseconds pulse duration for 3 pulses with thermal relaxation intervals of 20–30 milliseconds; 615-nm filter for Fitzpatrick types I and II or 645-nm filter for Fitzpatrick types III and above).[56] Comparative studies of IPL versus other lasers for hair removal (long-pulsed alexandrite and Nd:YAG) have demonstrated superiority of laser devices.[57,58]

Combination treatment of IPL and a radio-frequency source has also been explored.[59,60] Sadick and Shaoul examined the long-term photoepilatory effect of this electro-optical synergy (ELOS) technology, which combines an IPL source (680–980 nm) with a bipolar radio-frequency device (Aurora Syneron Medical, Yokneam, Israel). The theory behind this technology is to decrease optical energy to a level that is safe for all skin phototypes while compensating for the lower light energy by combining it with radio-frequency heating of the mid dermal layer. Patients were treated over 4 sessions with IPL fluences of 15 to 26 J/cm^2 and RF energy of 10 to 20 J/cm^3, producing an average clearance rate of 75% at 18 months. Histological evaluation revealed thermal damage to hair follicles with vacuolar degeneration.[60] Sochor et al evaluated a similar device comparing it with both a diode laser and an IPL alone. The results showed similar efficacy with the combined IPL and RF device and the diode laser, both of which were significantly better than the IPL alone.[61] This combined technology of IPL and RF was thought to be the answer for the successful treatment of light hair phenotypes as the RF component is pigment-blind. Despite early reports of its success, subsequent evaluations proved no significant long-term hair removal for lighter hair phenotypes.

Microwave

A microwave-based hair removal system (Microwave Delivery System, MW Medical, Scottsdale, Arizona) was FDA approved in 1999 for the removal of unwanted body hair. However, to date, no data have been available regarding the safety or efficacy of this device.

TREATMENT PROTOCOL

Either immediately before or within a short time prior to the treatment session, patients should be instructed to remove the hair extending from the surface of the skin by shaving, trimming, or chemical depilatory. This will help to prevent complications from contact burns due to draping of longer hairs with the laser/light device handpiece over the skin surface while pulsing, as well as to insure that the energy is delivered to the desired, deeper target. Patients should be instructed to avoid the mechanical epilation of hairs in the treatment area by plucking, waxing, threading, or other physical methods for at least 2 to 3 weeks prior to treatment. The hair shaft within the dermal portion of the hair follicle is necessary for the laser/light and hair interaction to be successful. The use of bleaching agents is permitted, as they will not alter the deeper dermal hair shaft pigmentation.

The use of topical anesthetic creams can help to minimize patient discomfort during the procedure. These agents are applied to the treatment areas 0.5 to 1 hour prior to treatment. Popular prescribed and OTC topical anesthetics include a eutectic mixture of lidocaine 2.5% and prilocaine 2.5% cream (EMLA cream) or topical 4% lidocaine cream (LMX cream). One study comparing these 2 found no statistically significant difference in pain control.[62] Stronger topical anesthetics can include compounded prescriptions containing lidocaine, tetracaine, and/or betacaine. Caution should be exercised in using these topical anesthetics on large skin surface areas, as systemic toxicity has previously been reported in this setting.[32] A study evaluating the use of piroxicam gel found a significant decrease in discomfort during a laser procedure compared with that of a control agent.[63] Use of modified tumescent anesthesia has also been described, but adds a significant procedure to a rather uncomplicated process.[64]

Other methods to minimize discomfort during the procedure can include the use of cold air blowing on the adjacent skin surface, cold compresses applied to treated skin surfaces, the application of prechilled rollers in advance of the laser/light pulse, and pneumatic skin flattening (PSF) devices. PSF technology helps to reduce treatment discomfort based on the principles of the gate control theory, which asserts that activation of non-nociceptive nerve fibers can interfere with signal transmission from pain fibers, thereby inhibiting pain. The PSF suction device works by generating contact and compression between a transparent sapphire window and the skin. It activates the tactile and pressure receptors on skin before the laser irradiation and thereby blocks the transmission of pain to the brain when the laser is shot. This technology has been employed with IPL devices as well as various lasers with successful decrease in patient discomfort.[65–68]

Immediately prior to initiating a treatment session, the patient should be situated in a comfortable position and proper protective eyewear should be secured to prevent inadvertent injury to the eyes. The laser/light device should be calibrated to insure proper energy delivery. The use of a vacuum to remove smoke plume from vaporized hair is important to minimize the potentially toxic inhalation of smoke and the malodorous scent of burnt hair. Any topical anesthetic agent should be thoroughly removed from the treatment site.

In general, properly trained personnel should be employed to perform LHR/light device hair removal. They should have a clear understanding of the proper use of laser/light devices and an ability to monitor the skin surface for the occurrence of undesirable side effects and to address any complications should they arise. The treatment should be done in a manner to avoid missed or skipped areas and prevent excessive overlap of pulses.

Following the laser/light treatment, the skin can be gently scrubbed with cool compresses to alleviate any discomfort and remove any burnt hair stubble from the surface of the skin. If a significant degree of perifollicular edema is present, the application of a low-potency topical corticosteroid is helpful. The patient should be instructed to avoid topical agents that can be irritating for a few days following treatment, to use proper sun protection during the immediate postoperative period, and to expect the discharge of follicular hair shafts for several days following the treatment session.

TREATMENT PARAMETERS

There are many parameters to be considered in the use of laser/light devices for the purpose of hair removal. These parameters include wavelength, fluence, pulse duration, spot size, and the use of epidermal cooling systems. Each of these parameters should be selected after a careful evaluation of the patient with regard to hair thickness, skin phototype, presence or absence of a tan, and skin location.

Wavelength

As noted above, there are many devices that are available for LHR/light hair removal. The choice of which

wavelength to use on a patient is dependent on the native skin phototype and the presence of a tan. Patients with lighter skin phototypes will have better outcomes with shorter wavelengths, such as the ruby, alexandrite, or diode lasers, where there is a higher absorption of energy by melanin. These same wavelengths may produce excessive heating in darker skin phototypes. The long-pulsed 1064-nm Nd:YAG lasers or the long-pulsed diode lasers are more favorable choices for darker skin phototypes.

Fluence

Fluence is the amount of energy delivered to a given unit of skin surface. Higher fluences have been shown to improve long-term hair removal; however, increased fluence is more likely to cause side effects.[69] Clinical monitoring of a patient's response to laser pulses is important in determining what the appropriate fluence should be. The highest tolerated fluence, which yields perifollicular erythema and edema, without any adverse effects, is often the best fluence for treatment. The fluences associated with each laser/light system vary widely. Recent exceptions to the rule for the use of higher fluences have been shown in the use of PSF and with low-fluence, multipass techniques.[49–51]

Pulse Duration

Pulse duration is defined as the duration in seconds of laser exposure. Optimal pulse durations for a given target can be determined by calculating the thermal relaxation time of the target based on the theory of selective photothermolysis. Although the desired target for LHR/light hair removal is the follicular stem cell, these cells do not contain an adequate chromophore. Terminal hairs, which rest against the surface of our desired target, contain an abundance of melanin, which can be selectively targeted. These hair shafts are roughly 300 μm in diameter, and thus the calculated TRT of a terminal hair follicle is roughly 100 milliseconds.[70] Given the spatial separation of melanin within the hair shaft and the stem cells in the bulge, which require destruction for permanent hair removal, the expanded theory of selective photothermolysis proposes a longer thermal damage time than the TRT. In real practice, the pulse durations are considerably shorter than these suggested times. One should choose pulse durations based on the particular device being used and the patient's skin type. In general, longer pulse durations in darker skin phototypes offer better epidermal protection from excessive heating.

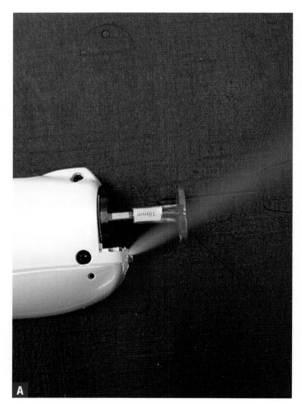
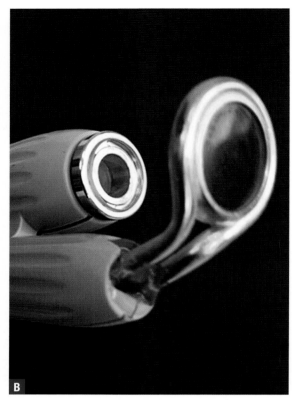

▲ **FIGURE 4-5** Cooling systems in hair removal: dynamic cooling device (DCD) (**A**) and cold water chilled sapphire tip window (**B**).

Spot Diameter

The spot size is the diameter in millimeters of the laser beam. A larger spot size appears to be more effective for laser-assisted hair removal.[71,72] This may in part be due to decreased photon scatter at the outer border of the laser spot and an additive effect in the center of the beam with larger spot sizes based on the Monte Carlo model of laser–tissue interaction.[70] In addition, a larger beam spot size will shorten the overall treatment time and minimize patient discomfort.[63]

Epidermal Cooling

Cooling of the skin surface can be used to minimize epidermal damage, while permitting treatment with higher fluences, by minimizing thermal destruction of epidermal melanin. Various cooling methods exist—use of an aqueous cold gel, copper-plated cooling surfaces, chilled water sapphire window surfaces, forced chilled air, as well as built-in dynamic cooling systems

in commercially available lasers (Figure 4-5). Cooling can be controlled to be utilized prepulse, postpulse, or throughout the laser pulse. Contact cooling, usually with a sapphire tip, provides skin cooling just before and during a laser pulse. Dynamic cooling with cryogen liquid spray precools the skin with a spray of cryogen just milliseconds before the laser pulse. Post-cooling is also possible with delivery of a second spray immediately after the laser pulse; however, it has been associated with a greater risk of postinflammatory hyperpigmentation.

COMPLICATIONS

In general, LHR is safe with rare adverse effects that are often transient with very low incidence of permanent sequelae. The majority of adverse effects seen with LHR are a result of epidermal injury.[73] These side effects include blistering, hypopigmentation, hyperpigmentation, and rarely scarring. Other less common side

TABLE 4-4
Complications of Laser/Light Hair Removal

Dyspigmentation
   Hyperpigmentation
   Hypopigmentation
Epidermal vesiculation/burning
Paradoxical hypertrichosis
Acneiform eruptions
Hyperhidrosis
Urticaria
Reticulate erythema
Ocular injury

leukotrichia, paradoxical hypertrichosis, and folliculitis as the major side effects.[74] Skin containing a greater amount of melanin has a greater risk of side effects; therefore, avoidance of sun tanning prior to treatment and selecting the proper wavelength and/or device to utilize is essential. A comparative study of alexandrite laser, diode laser, and IPL revealed a greater frequency of side effects with the diode laser and lowest frequency of side effects with the alexandrite laser. In all cases, the side effects were reported as temporary.[75]

Dyspigmentation

Dyspigmentation can consist of either hyperpigmentation or hypopigmentation (Figure 4-6). Hyperpigmentation is usually reversible and results from the stimulation of melanin production from epidermal melanocytes due to an inflammatory injury. In addition, there is an increase in melanin within macrophages of the dermis due to epidermal disruption. The use of bleaching

effects of LHR, which have been described, include acneiform eruptions, hyperhidrosis, urticaria, and reticulate erythema (Table 4-4). One study evaluating the side effects of IPL hair removal therapy among 2541 female hirsute patients reported epidermal injury,

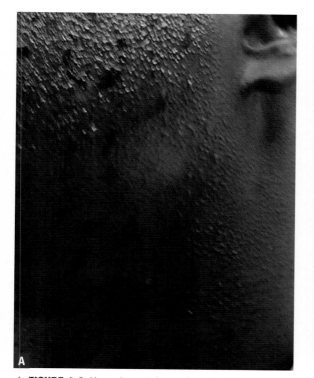
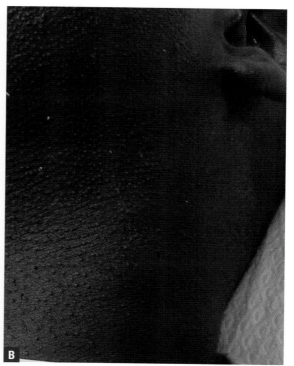

▲ FIGURE 4-6 Hyperpigmentation and crusting following mismatch of laser light and DCD cooling device during treatment in a patient with Fitzpatrick skin phototype VI. Note the typical arc pattern produced by excessive heating of epidermal pigmentation due to inadequate surface cooling (**A**). This pigmentation often resolves spontaneously with proper wound care. The same patient 2 months later (**B**).

agents such as hydroquinone can help minimize the development of hyperpigmentation when an epidermal injury occurs in darker skin phototypes.

Hypopigmentation may be transient or permanent. If there is significant epidermal melanin present, such as from a tan, there is often a transient hypopigmentation resulting from the thermal destruction of the excess epidermal pigments. An area of skin that has a normal variant of hyperpigmentation compared with baseline skin is the genital area. Caution should be used with wavelength and fluence considerations when there are variations in skin color in a given individual. Normal repigmentation often will occur in areas of hypopigmentation over a variable time period, ranging from weeks to months. If there is a very significant thermal injury to the melanocytes, preventing melanin production, the hypopigmentation may be permanent. This is more often seen when there is an inappropriate selection of a shorter-wavelength laser/light device for darker skin phototypes. Appropriate treatment parameters, including proper selection of wavelength, fluence, and proper epidermal cooling, can reduce this risk.

Hypopigmentation can occasionally be observed after laser-assisted hair removal in combination with dynamic cryogen spray cooling systems. The pathophysiology of this dyspigmentation is somewhat controversial—whether it is a cold-induced injury from the cryogen agent or a laser-induced thermal injury. When using any cooling device, epidermal protection is complete only when the cooling device is held perpendicular to the skin surface and in contact when using contact cooling systems. In the case of dynamic cooling devices, if the handpiece is angled 6° or more from perpendicular, there will be incomplete cryogen coverage of the laser spot resulting in a crescent-shaped burn matching the not adequately cooled edge of the laser spot.[76]

This may lead to a transient hypopigmented or hyperpigmented area matching the thermal injury. Although this typical pattern of injury is more likely due to thermal injury from a mismatch of laser beam spot dimension and adequate cryogen, a prolonged cryogen spray duration using these dynamic cooling devices can also lead to hyperpigmentation most notably in darker skin phototypes. This injury is due to a cold-induced inflammatory injury and subsequent postinflammatory hyperpigmentation.

Paradoxical Hypertrichosis

Paradoxical hypertrichosis, or the induction of terminal hair from vellus hair, as a side effect of LHR has been well documented[77,78] (Figure 4-7). The incidence of this very troubling side effect has been reported to range from 5% to as high as 10% in some studies, affecting all skin phototypes. This increased hair growth occurred within the treated areas as well as in the adjacent, nontreated skin. The most common sites for this phenomenon are the jawline, neck, and cheeks of women with darker skin phototypes. These locations contain finer vellus hairs, which are converted to terminal hairs most likely due to thermal induction of follicular maturation. These changes have also been reported on the torso. The hair appears coarser and darker than the hairs initially treated.[79,80] Treatment of the paradoxical hypertrichosis consists of further laser treatment of the involved areas. Reports of cooling the skin adjacent to the treatment area as well as confining the laser energy to the target area have shown a decrease in the incidence of this side effect.

Acneiform Eruptions

Acneiform eruptions, consisting of small pustules in a follicular distribution, have been reported to have an incidence of 6%, occurring most commonly on the face in younger women. Treatment with standard acne therapies often helps resolve this, often, transient problem.

Hyperhidrosis

Hyperhidrosis, or excessive sweating, is an uncommon side effect. When it follows LHR, it is most often noted to occur in the axilla. One study reported hyperhidrosis that developed following treatment with a 1064-nm Nd:YAG laser and persisted for at least 1 year.[81] It appears to be a transient problem, as the symptoms seem to abate with the regrowth of hair in the involved area.

Urticaria

There have been several case reports of severe, symptomatic urticaria in the treated areas lasting for up to several days after laser treatment[82,83] (Figure 4-8). These cases represent patients being treated with a variety of lasers for hair removal. Many of these individuals have had previous laser treatments without consequence. The urticaria responded to both topical and systemic corticosteroids. The etiology of the urticaria is unclear.

Reticulate Erythema

A very rare but troubling side effect of LHR was reported in 10 patients treated with an 800-nm diode laser described as a reticulate erythema most noted on the lower extremities. The patterned erythema,

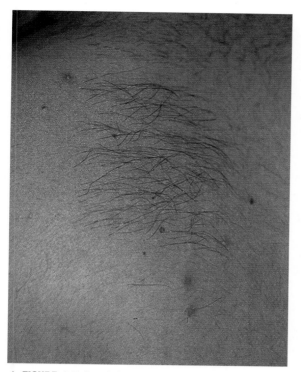
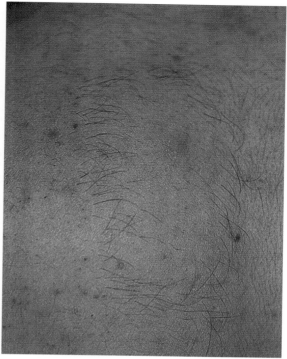

▲ **FIGURE 4-7** Paradoxical hypertrichosis. New terminal hair growth is noted in the area immediately surrounding the treated area of unwanted hair in an area previously noted to consist of fine vellus hairs. (photograph—courtesy of Eric Bernstein, MD) (From Bernstein EF. Hair growth induced by diode laser treatment. *Dermatol Surg.* 2005;31(5):584–586.)

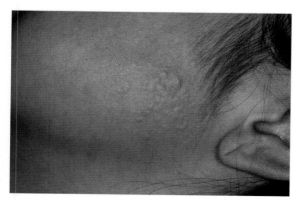

▲ **FIGURE 4-8** Urticaria noted on lateral cheek of young woman immediately following laser treatment utilizing a long-pulsed Nd:YAG 1064 nm laser for unwanted hair of the sideburn area. (photograph—courtesy of Eric Bernstein, MD) (From Bernstein EF. Severe urticaria after laser treatment for hair reduction. *Dermatol Surg.* 2010;36(1):147–151.)

consisting of reddish blue lace-like pattern that was nonblanching with pressure, appeared in these individuals after an average of 2.7 treatments. The etiology is unclear, but a variant of erythema ab igne is strongly considered.

Ocular Injury

The least common, but most important, side effect of LHR is ocular injury. Caution should be exercised in treatment of hair in the periorbital region. Laser injuries to the eye are very serious and often permanent. These injuries can include destruction of the retina, iris, and ocular epithelium.[84] Blindness, either partial or complete, can result from these injuries to an eye. The use of longer-wavelength lasers for hair removal makes ocular injury especially more likely in the orbital area due to their greater depth of penetration. Use of these laser/light devices within the orbital rim should be avoided. There has been a case report of diode laser epilation on the upper eyelid in the absence of protective eyewear that led to iris atrophy and cataract.[84]

LASERS IN THE TREATMENT OF HAIR-SPECIFIC PATHOLOGIES

Although LHR has become a means to eliminate undesired hair for cosmetic reasons or for simple convenience in everyday grooming, a significant role for this laser technology has evolved into treating hair that has a pathologic basis. Conditions, once difficult to manage including hirsutism associated with polycystic ovarian syndrome, pilonidal cysts, pseudofolliculitis barbae, and hair growth on transplanted free flaps or grafts, are now managed in a large part with LHR.

Hirsutism

Hirsutism is defined as growth of terminal hair in women at androgen-dependent sites where normally only men develop coarse hair. It is one of the most common conditions for which patients seek the benefits of permanent hair removal. However, establishing the underlying cause, whether it is due to hormonal imbalance, genetic patterns, or drug-induced, is important to instate a disease-targeted treatment in addition to LHR. Polycystic ovary syndrome (PCOS) is one of the more common causes of hirsutism. Excess terminal hair growth is estimated to occur in approximately 75% of patients with this syndrome.[85] Several trials have evaluated the efficacy of LHR in the treatment of unwanted hair in the setting of hormonal-induced hirsutism. A recent randomized control trial, comparing the efficacy and safety of IPL and long-pulsed diode laser treatment of facial hairiness in a population of hirsute women, reported a 40% hair reduction in patients treated with an IPL and a 34% hair reduction for patients treated with a diode laser at the 6-month follow-up visit.[86] The long-term effects of laser therapy on the severity of facial hirsutism and on the psychological morbidity to women with PCOS have been investigated in a randomized trial. Laser treatments appear to reduce the severity of facial hair and time spent on hair removal in addition to alleviating depression and anxiety in women with PCOS.[87]

Pilonidal Cysts

Based on the presumed role of hair in pilonidal cyst pathogenesis, the use of laser epilation has proven to be an effective adjunct to surgery in the treatment of recurrent recalcitrant disease. Results of studies using various lasers for the epilation of hair near the sacrum in patients with pilonidal sinus disease have shown a significant resolution of disease at long-term follow-up in a majority of these patients.[88-91]

Pseudofolliculitis Barbae and Follicular-based Disease

Another troubling condition in both men and women that has been shown to respond well to LHR is pseudofolliculitis barbae[92] (Figure 4-9). This condition, also known as razor bumps or ingrown hairs, is an inflammatory condition of the hair follicle due to irritation of the follicular channel by a broken/trimmed hair shaft below the follicular orifice. Clinically, it presents as erythematous, follicular, inflammatory papules with or without an obvious hair fragment. In individuals, it is more common in areas where the hair is more naturally curved. As a result of the inflammatory response, these

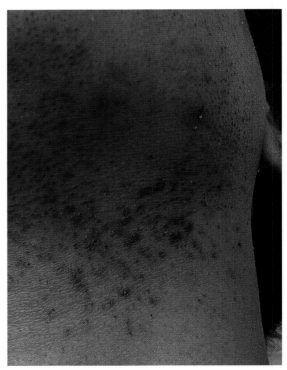

▲ **FIGURE 4-9** Pseudofolliculitis barbae. Hyperpigmented follicular-based papules and macules resulting from the inflammatory response of ingrown hairs on the neck.

patients will often develop postinflammatory hyperpigmentation. Laser treatment of the affected area will help to decrease the dyspigmentation, inflammatory papules, as well as cobblestoning of the skin surface by eliminating the source of the problem.[93] In addition, there have been several reports of LHR successfully used in the treatment of other follicular-based diseases, such as congenital hypertrichosis, Becker nevi, nevoid hypertrichosis, hidradenitis suppurativa, dissecting cellulitis of the scalp, folliculitis decalvans, and trichostasis spinulosa.[34,75,94–98]

Surgical Flaps and Grafts

The advancement in surgical technique has made it possible to repair difficult defects following surgical procedures in the treatment of cancer or due to traumatic injury. The use of skin grafts and free flaps to repair defects utilizing hair-bearing skin in areas traditionally devoid of hair adds an element of morbidity not previously imagined. Although the presence of terminal hair on a skin graft placed on a nose may provide a mere cosmetic problem for an individual, the presence of hair on an intraoral free flap transplanted within the oral cavity following a tumor resection creates an uncomfortable problem when there is persistent hair growth (Figure 4-10). The use of laser

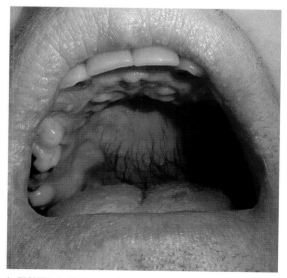

▲ **FIGURE 4-10** Intraoral terminal hair growth, as a result of the transferring of a hair-bearing free flap, in oral reconstruction following the resection of a cancerous growth.

epilation on these transplanted tissues has been well described.[99–102]

LASERS FOR HAIR GROWTH

Paradoxical terminal hair growth following treatment for LHR has been well described.[103] These observations have led to the development of laser devices designed for hair growth induction. One such device, the HairMax LaserComb® 655-nm laser device, was evaluated in a randomized, double-blind, sham device–controlled, multicenter trial in male patients with androgenetic alopecia. The device uses a technique of parting the user's hair by combs that are attached to the device. This improves delivery of distributed laser light to the scalp. The authors found an increase in mean terminal hair density in subjects treated with the HairMax LaserComb® device over the sham device and a subjective improvement in overall hair regrowth at 26 weeks over baseline.[104] This device received clearance for marketing by the FDA in 2007. Other laser technologies are also being explored in this setting, including a recent small study investigating the 1550-nm fractional erbium-glass laser.[105] Lee et al studied the degree of hair regrowth in 28 South Korean women suffering from female pattern hair loss after stimulation with a fractional 1550-nm laser.[106] The patients were treated biweekly for 5 months with low laser fluences (6 mJ) and a small density pattern (800 spots/cm^2). The results showed a roughly 50% increase in hair count/cm^2 as well as an increase in hair thickness.

HOME-USE HAIR REMOVAL DEVICES

A growing trend in laser technology for hair removal has been the introduction of home-use lasers; these include a lower-energy, portable, handheld IPL device (475–1200 nm Silk'n, Home Skinovations, Kfar Saba, Israel) as well as a battery-powered, handheld, portable diode laser (810 nm Tria, SpectraGenics, Inc, Pleasanton, California). Home-use LHR devices utilize lower fluences compared with professional devices. Efficacy of home-use IPL and lasers ranges from 40% to 60% hair reduction, lasting approximately 3 months for most at-home devices. The lower fluences of these devices make the likelihood of long-term or permanent hair removal relatively small, while at the same time decreasing the risk of adverse reactions. The movement from professional oversight to individual consumer use raises certain safety issues, particularly those of ocular safety.[107–109]

REFERENCES

1. Benson A. On the treatment of partial trichiasis by electrolysis. *Br Med J.* 1882;16(2):1203–1204.
2. Goldman L, Blaney DJ, Kindel DJ Jr, Richfield MF, Owens P, Homan EL. Effect of the laser beam on the skin. III. Exposure of cytological preparations. *J Invest Dermatol.* 1964;42:247–251.
3. Gossman MD, Yung R, Berlin AJ, Brightwell JR. Prospective evaluation of the argon laser in the treatment of trichiasis. *Ophthalmic Surg.* 1992;23(3):183–187.
4. Finkelstein LH, Blatstein LM. Epilation of hair-bearing urethral grafts using the neodymium:YAG surgical laser. *J Urol.* 1991;146(3):840–842.
5. Bartley GB, Bullock JD, Olsen TG, Lutz PD. An experimental study to compare methods of eyelash ablation. *Ophthalmology.* 1987;94(10):1286–1289.
6. Anderson RR, Parrish JA. Selective photothermolysis: precise microsurgery by selective absorption of pulsed radiation. *Science.* 1983;220(4596):524–527.
7. Grossman MC, Dierickx C, Farinelli W, Flotte T, Anderson RR. Damage to hair follicles by normal-mode ruby laser pulses. *J Am Acad Dermatol.* 1996;35(6):889–894.
8. Dierickx CC, Grossman MC, Farinell WA, Anderson RR. Permanent hair removal by normal-mode ruby laser. *Arch Dermatol.* 1998;134(7):837–842.
9. Finkel B, Eliezri YD, Waldman A, Slatkine M. Pulsed alexandrite laser technology for noninvasive hair removal. *J Clin Laser Med Surg.* 1997;15(5):225–229.
10. Lask G, Elman M, Slatkine M, Waldman A, Rozenberg Z. Laser-assisted hair removal by selective photothermolysis. Preliminary results. *Dermatol Surg.* 1997;23(9):737–739.
11. Ohyama M. Hair follicle bulge: a fascinating reservoir of epithelial stem cells. *J Dermatol Sci.* 2007;46(2):81–89.
12. Festa E, Fretz J, Berry R, et al. Adipocyte lineage cells contribute to the skin stem cell niche to drive hair cycling. *Cell.* 2011;146(5):761–771.
13. Tannir D, Leshin B. Sugaring: an ancient method of hair removal. *Dermatol Surg.* 2001;27(3):309–311.
14. Natow AJ. Chemical removal of hair. *Cutis.* 1986;38(2):91–92.
15. Smith G. The removal of superfluous hairs by electrolysis. *Br Med J.* 1886;1(1308):151–152.
16. Richards RN, Meharg GE. Electrolysis: observations from 13 years and 140,000 hours of experience. *J Am Acad Dermatol.* 1995;33(4):662–666.
17. Crosby PD, Rittmaster RS. Predictors of clinical response in hirsute women treated with spironolactone. *Fertil Steril.* 1991;55(6):1076–1081.
18. Rittmaster RS. Hirsutism. *Lancet.* 1997;349(9046):191–195.
19. Görgü M, Aslan G, Aköz T, Erdoğan B. Comparison of alexandrite laser and electrolysis for hair removal. *Dermatol Surg.* 2000;26(1):37–41.
20. Anderson RR, Parrish JA. The optics of human skin. *J Invest Dermatol.* 1981;77(1):13–19.
21. Altshuler GB, Anderson RR, Manstein D, Zenzie HH, Smirnov MZ. Extended theory of selective photothermolysis. *Lasers Surg Med.* 2001;29(5):416–432.
22. Orringer JS, Hammerberg C, Lowe L, et al. The effects of laser-mediated hair removal on immunohistochemical staining properties of hair follicles. *J Am Acad Dermatol.* 2006;55(3):402–407.
23. Sellheyer K. Mechanisms of laser hair removal: could persistent photoepilation induce vitiligo or defects in wound repair? *Dermatol Surg.* 2007;33(9):1055–1065.
24. Lin TY, Manuskiatti W, Dierickx CC, et al. Hair growth cycle affects hair follicle destruction by ruby laser pulses. *J Invest Dermatol.* 1998;111(1):107–113.
25. Hoffman RM. Topical liposome targeting of dyes, melanins, genes, and proteins selectively to hair follicles. *J Drug Target.* 1998;5(2):67–74.
26. Sand M, Bechara FG, Sand D, Altmeyer P, Hoffmann K. A randomized, controlled, double-blind study evaluating melanin-encapsulated liposomes as a chromophore for laser hair removal of blond, white, and gray hair. *Ann Plast Surg.* 2007;58(5):551–554.
27. Trotter MJ, Tron VA, Hollingdale J, Rivers JK. Localized chrysiasis induced by laser therapy. *Arch Dermatol.* 1995;131(12):1411–1414.
28. Almoallim H, Klinkhoff AV, Arthur AB, Rivers JK, Chalmers A. Laser induced chrysiasis: disfiguring hyperpigmentation following Q-switched laser therapy in a woman previously treated with gold. *J Rheumatol.* 2006;33(3):620–621.
29. Khatri KA. The safety of long-pulsed Nd:YAG laser hair removal in skin types III–V patients during concomitant isotretinoin therapy. *J Cosmet Laser Ther.* 2009;11(1):56–60.
30. Khatri KA, Garcia V. Light-assisted hair removal in patients undergoing isotretinoin therapy. *Dermatol Surg.* 2006;32(6):875–877.
31. Khatri KA. Diode laser hair removal in patients undergoing isotretinoin therapy. *Dermatol Surg.* 2004;30(9):1205–1207 [discussion 1207].
32. Elsaie ML. Cardiovascular collapse developing after topical anesthesia. *Dermatology.* 2007;214(2):194.
33. Goldberg DJ, Littler CM, Wheeland RG. Topical suspension-assisted Q-switched Nd:YAG laser hair removal. *Dermatol Surg.* 1997;23(9):741–745.
34. Littler CM. Laser hair removal in a patient with hypertrichosis lanuginosa congenita. *Dermatol Surg.* 1997;23(8):705–707.
35. Nanni CA, Alster TS. Optimizing treatment parameters for hair removal using a topical carbon-based solution and 1064-nm Q-switched neodymium: YAG laser energy. *Arch Dermatol.* 1997;133(12):1546–1549.
36. Sommer S, Render C, Sheehan-Dare R. Facial hirsutism treated with the normal-mode ruby laser: results of a 12-month follow-up study. *J Am Acad Dermatol.* 1999;41(6):974–979.
37. McCoy S, Evans A, James C. Long-pulsed ruby laser for permanent hair reduction: histological analysis after 3, 4 1/2, and 6 months. *Lasers Surg Med.* 2002;30(5):401–405.
38. Aldraibi MS, Touma DJ, Khachemoune A. Hair removal with the 3-msec alexandrite laser in patients with skin types IV–VI: efficacy, safety, and the role of topical corticosteroids in preventing side effects. *J Drugs Dermatol.* 2007;6(1):60–66.
39. Boss WK Jr, Usal H, Thompson RC, Fiorillo MA. A comparison of the long-pulse and short-pulse alexandrite laser hair removal systems. *Ann Plast Surg.* 1999;42(4):381–384.
40. Eremia S, Li CY, Umar SH, Newman N. Laser hair removal: long-term results with a 755 nm alexandrite laser. *Dermatol Surg.* 2001;27(11):920–924.

41. Laughlin SA, Dudley D. Long-term hair removal using a 3-millisecond alexandrite laser. *J Cutan Med Surg.* 2000; 4(2):83–88.

42. Goldberg DJ, Ahkami R. Evaluation comparing multiple treatments with a 2-msec and 10-msec alexandrite laser for hair removal. *Lasers Surg Med.* 1999;25(3):223–228.

43. McDaniel DH, Lord J, Ash K, Newman J, Zukowski M. Laser hair removal: a review and report on the use of the long-pulsed alexandrite laser for hair reduction of the upper lip, leg, back, and bikini region. *Dermatol Surg.* 1999;25(6):425–430.

44. Kato T, Omi T, Naito Z, Hirai T, Kawana S. Histological hair removal study by ruby or alexandrite laser with comparative study on the effects of wavelength and fluence. *J Cosmet Laser Ther.* 2004;6(1):32–37.

45. Davoudi SM, Behnia F, Gorouhi F, et al. Comparison of long-pulsed alexandrite and Nd:YAG lasers, individually and in combination, for leg hair reduction: an assessor-blinded, randomized trial with 18 months of follow-up. *Arch Dermatol.* 2008;144(10):1323–1327.

46. Campos VB, Dierickx CC, Farinelli WA, Lin TY, Manuskiatti W, Anderson RR. Hair removal with an 800-nm pulsed diode laser. *J Am Acad Dermatol.* 2000; 43(3):442–447.

47. Kopera D. Hair reduction: 48 months of experience with 800nm diode laser. *J Cosmet Laser Ther.* 2003; 5(3–4):146–149.

48. Lou WW, Quintana AT, Geronemus RG, Grossman MC. Prospective study of hair reduction by diode laser (800 nm) with long-term follow-up. *Dermatol Surg.* 2000;26(5):428–432.

49. Ibrahimi OA, Kilmer SL. Long-term clinical evaluation of a 800-nm long-pulsed diode laser with a large spot size and vacuum-assisted suction for hair removal. *Dermatol Surg.* 2012;38(6):912–917.

50. Halachmi S, Lapidoth M. Low-fluence vs. standard fluence hair removal: a contralateral control non-inferiority study. *J Cosmet Laser Ther.* 2012;14(1):2–6.

51. Braun M. Comparison of high-fluence, single-pass diode laser to low-fluence, multiple-pass diode laser for laser hair reduction with 18 months of follow up. *J Drugs Dermatol.* 2011;10(1):62–65.

52. Trelles MA, Urdiales F, Al-Zarouni M. Hair structures are effectively altered during 810 nm diode laser hair epilation at low fluences. *J Dermatolog Treat.* 2010;21(2):97–100.

53. Alster TS, Bryan H, Williams CM. Long-pulsed Nd:YAG laser-assisted hair removal in pigmented skin: a clinical and histological evaluation. *Arch Dermatol.* 2001; 137(7):885–889.

54. Goldberg DJ, Silapunt S. Histologic evaluation of a millisecond Nd:YAG laser for hair removal. *Lasers Surg Med.* 2001;28(2):159–161.

55. Li R, Zhou Z, Gold MH. An efficacy comparison of hair removal utilizing a diode laser and an Nd:YAG laser system in Chinese women. *J Cosmet Laser Ther.* 2010; 12(5):213–217.

56. Weiss RA, Weiss MA, Marwaha S, Harrington AC. Hair removal with a non-coherent filtered flashlamp intense pulsed light source. *Lasers Surg Med.* 1999;24(2):128–132.

57. Goh CL. Comparative study on a single treatment response to long pulse Nd:YAG lasers and intense pulse light therapy for hair removal on skin type IV to VI—is longer wavelengths lasers preferred over shorter wavelengths lights for assisted hair removal. *J Dermatolog Treat.* 2003;14(4):243–247.

58. McGill DJ, Hutchison C, McKenzie E, McSherry E, Mackay IR. A randomised, split-face comparison of facial hair removal with the alexandrite laser and intense pulsed light system. *Lasers Surg Med.* 2007; 39(10):767–772.

59. Yaghmai D, Garden JM, Bakus AD, Spenceri EA, Hruza DJ, Kilmer SL. Hair removal using a combination radio-frequency and intense pulsed light source. *J Cosmet Laser Ther.* 2004;6(4):201–207.

60. Sadick NS, Shaoul J. Hair removal using a combination of conducted radiofrequency and optical energies—an 18-month follow-up. *J Cosmet Laser Ther.* 2004;6(1):21–26.

61. Sochor M, Curkova AK, Schwarczova Z, Sochorova R, Simaljakova M, Buchvald J. Comparison of hair reduction with three lasers and light sources: prospective, blinded and controlled study. *J Cosmet Laser Ther.* 2011;13(5):210–215.

62. Guardiano RA, Norwood CW. Direct comparison of EMLA versus lidocaine for pain control in Nd:YAG 1,064 nm laser hair removal. *Dermatol Surg.* 2005;31(4): 396–398.

63. Akinturk S, Eroglu A. Effect of piroxicam gel for pain control and inflammation in Nd:YAG 1064-nm laser hair removal. *J Eur Acad Dermatol Venereol.* 2007;21(3): 380–383.

64. Krejci-Manwaring J, Markus JL, Goldberg HA, Friedman PM, Markus RF. Surgical pearl: tumescent anesthesia reduces pain of axillary laser hair removal. *J Am Acad Dermatol.* 2004;51(2):290–291.

65. Fournier N. Hair removal on dark-skinned patients with pneumatic skin flattening (PSF) and a high-energy Nd:YAG laser. *J Cosmet Laser Ther.* 2008;10(4):210–212.

66. Yeung CK, Shek SY, Chan HH. Hair removal with neodymium-doped yttrium aluminum garnet laser and pneumatic skin flattening in Asians. *Dermatol Surg.* 2010;36(11):1664–1670.

67. Lask G, Friedman D, Elman M, Fournier N, Shavit R, Slatkine M. Pneumatic skin flattening (PSF): a novel technology for marked pain reduction in hair removal with high energy density lasers and IPLs. *J Cosmet Laser Ther.* 2006;8(2):76–81.

68. Bernstein EF. Pneumatic skin flattening reduces pain during laser hair reduction. *Lasers Surg Med.* 2008; 40(3):183–187.

69. Campos VB, Dierickx CC, Farinelli WA, Lin TY, Manuskiatti W, Anderson RR. Ruby laser hair removal: evaluation of long-term efficacy and side effects. *Lasers Surg Med.* 2000;26(2):177–185.

70. Ibrahimi OA, Avram MM, Hanke CW, Kilmer SS, Anderson RR. Laser hair removal. *Dermatol Ther.* 2011; 24(1):94–107.

71. Baumler W, Scherer KA, Abels C, Neff S, Landthaler M, Szeimies RM. The effect of different spot sizes on the efficacy of hair removal using a long-pulsed diode laser. *Dermatol Surg.* 2002;28(2):118–121.

72. Nouri K, Chen H, Saghari S, Ricotti CA Jr. Comparing 18- versus 12-mm spot size in hair removal using a gentlease 755-nm alexandrite laser. *Dermatol Surg.* 2004;30(4 pt 1):494–497.

73. Lim SP, Lanigan SW. A review of the adverse effects of laser hair removal. *Lasers Med Sci.* 2006;21(3):121–125.

74. Radmanesh M, Azar-Beig M, Abtahian A, Naderi AH. Burning, paradoxical hypertrichosis, leukotrichia and folliculitis are four major complications of intense pulsed light hair removal therapy. *J Dermatolog Treat.* 2008;19(6):360–363.

75. Toosi S, Ehsani AH, Noormohammadpoor P, Esmaili N, Mirshams-Shahshahani M, Moineddin F. Treatment of trichostasis spinulosa with a 755-nm long-pulsed alexandrite laser. *J Eur Acad Dermatol Venereol.* 2010;24(4):470–473.

76. Kelly KM, Svaasand LO, Nelson JS. Further investigation of pigmentary changes after alexandrite laser hair removal in conjunction with cryogen spray cooling. *Dermatol Surg.* 2004;30(4 pt 1):581–582.

77. Desai S, Mahmoud BH, Bhatia AC, Hamzavi IH. Paradoxical hypertrichosis after laser therapy: a review. *Dermatol Surg.* 2010;36(3):291–298.

78. Alajlan A, Shapiro J, Rivers JK, MacDonald N, Wiggin J, Lui H. Paradoxical hypertrichosis after laser epilation. *J Am Acad Dermatol.* 2005;53(1):85–88.

79. Willey A, Torrentegui J, Azpiazu J, Landa N. Hair stimulation following laser and intense pulsed light photoepilation: review of 543 cases and ways to manage it. *Lasers Surg Med.* 2007;39(4):297–301.

80. Kontoes P, Vlachos S, Konstantinos M, Anastasia L, Myrto S. Hair induction after laser-assisted hair removal and its treatment. *J Am Acad Dermatol.* 2006;54(1):64–67.

81. Aydin F, Pancar GS, Senturk N, et al. Axillary hair removal with 1064-nm Nd:YAG laser increases sweat production. *Clin Exp Dermatol.* 2010;35(6):588–592.

82. Bernstein EF. Severe urticaria after laser treatment for hair reduction. *Dermatol Surg.* 2010;36(1):147–151.

83. Moreno-Arias GA, Tiffon T, Marti T, Camps-Fresneda A. Urticaria vasculitis induced by diode laser photoepilation. *Dermatol Surg.* 2000;26(11):1082–1083.

84. Brilakis HS, Holland EJ. Diode-laser-induced cataract and iris atrophy as a complication of eyelid hair removal. *Am J Ophthalmol.* 2004;137(4):762–763.

85. Lapidoth M, Dierickx C, Lanigan S, et al. Best practice options for hair removal in patients with unwanted facial hair using combination therapy with laser: guidelines drawn up by an expert working group. *Dermatology.* 2010;221(1):34–42.

86. Haak CS, Nymann P, Pedersen AT, et al. Hair removal in hirsute women with normal testosterone levels: a randomized controlled trial of long-pulsed diode laser vs. intense pulsed light. *Br J Dermatol.* 2010;163(5):1007–1013.

87. Clayton WJ, Lipton M, Elford J, Rustin M, Sherr L. A randomized controlled trial of laser treatment among hirsute women with polycystic ovary syndrome. *Br J Dermatol.* 2005;152(5):986–992.

88. Abbas O, Sidani M, Rubeiz N, Ghosn S, Kibbi AG. Letter: 755-nm alexandrite laser epilation as an adjuvant and primary treatment for pilonidal sinus disease. *Dermatol Surg.* 2010;36(3):430–432.

89. Lindholt-Jensen CS, Lindholt JS, Beyer M, Lindholt JS. Nd-YAG laser treatment of primary and recurrent pilonidal sinus. *Lasers Med Sci.* 2012;27(2):505–508.

90. Oram Y, Kahraman F, Karincaoğlu Y, Koyuncu E. Evaluation of 60 patients with pilonidal sinus treated with laser epilation after surgery. *Dermatol Surg.* 2010;36(1):88–91.

91. Lukish JR, Kindelan T, Marmon LM, Pennington M, Norwood C. Laser epilation is a safe and effective therapy for teenagers with pilonidal disease. *J Pediatr Surg.* 2009;44(1):282–285.

92. Ross EV, Cooke LM, Overstreet KA, Buttolph GD, Blair MA. Treatment of pseudofolliculitis barbae in very dark skin with a long pulse Nd:YAG laser. *J Natl Med Assoc.* 2002;94(10):888–893.

93. Schulze R, Meehan KJ, Lopez A, et al. Low-fluence 1,064-nm laser hair reduction for pseudofolliculitis barbae in skin types IV, V, and VI. *Dermatol Surg.* 2009;35(1):98–107.

94. Attia A, El Noury A, Abd Alhafez M. Intense pulsed light hair removal in a patient with congenital hypertrichosis terminalis. *Pediatr Dermatol.* 2012;29(2):219–220.

95. Cheung ST, Lanigan SW. Naevoid hypertrichosis treated with alexandrite laser. *Clin Exp Dermatol.* 2004;29(4):435–436.

96. Highton L, Chan WY, Khwaja N, Laitung JK. Treatment of hidradenitis suppurativa with intense pulsed light: a prospective study. *Plast Reconstr Surg.* 2011;128(2):459–465.

97. Chui CT, Berger TG, Price VH, Zachary CB. Recalcitrant scarring follicular disorders treated by laser-assisted hair removal: a preliminary report. *Dermatol Surg.* 1999;25(1):34–37.

98. Parlette EC, Kroeger N, Ross EV. Nd:YAG laser treatment of recalcitrant folliculitis decalvans. *Dermatol Surg.* 2004;30(8):1152–1154.

99. Shim TN, Abdullah A, Lanigan S, Avery C. Hairy intraoral flap—an unusual indication for laser epilation: a series of 5 cases and review of the literature. *Br J Oral Maxillofac Surg.* 2011;49(7):e50–e52.

100. Moreno-Arias GA, Vilalta-Solsona A, Serra-Renom JM, Benito-Ruiz J, Ferrando J. Intense pulsed light for hairy grafts and flaps. *Dermatol Surg.* 2002;28(5):402–404.

101. Conroy FJ, Mahaffey PJ. Intraoral flap depilation using the long-pulsed alexandrite laser. *J Plast Reconstr Aesthet Surg.* 2009;62(11):e421–e423.

102. Lumley C. Intraoral hair removal on skin graft using Nd:YAG laser. *Br Dent J.* 2007;203(3):141–142.

103. Bernstein EF. Hair growth induced by diode laser treatment. *Dermatol Surg.* 2005;31(5):584–586.

104. Leavitt M, Charles G, Heyman E, Michaels D. HairMax LaserComb laser phototherapy device in the treatment of male androgenetic alopecia: a randomized, double-blind, sham device-controlled, multicentre trial. *Clin Drug Investig.* 2009;29(5):283–292.

105. Kim WS, Lee HI, Lee JW, et al. Fractional photothermolysis laser treatment of male pattern hair loss. *Dermatol Surg.* 2011;37(1):41–51.

106. Lee GY, Lee SJ, Kim WS. The effect of a 1550 nm fractional erbium-glass laser in female pattern hair loss. *J Eur Acad Dermatol Venereol.* 2011;25(12):1450–1454.

107. Haedersdal M, Beerwerth F, Nash JF. Laser and intense pulsed light hair removal technologies: from professional to home use. *Br J Dermatol.* 2011;165(suppl 3):31–36.

108. Town G, Ash C. Are home-use intense pulsed light (IPL) devices safe? *Lasers Med Sci.* 2010;25(6):773–780.

109. Alster TS, Tanzi EL. Effect of a novel low-energy pulsed-light device for home-use hair removal. *Dermatol Surg.* 2009;35(3):483–489.

CHAPTER 5

Laser and Radiofrequency Treatments for Cutaneous Resurfacing

Lori A. Brightman, Kavitha K. Reddy, Jeremy A. Brauer, and Robert T. Anolik

■ INTRODUCTION

Cutaneous resurfacing encompasses the use of varied technologies to smooth, tighten, even, or otherwise restore epidermal and dermal appearance. Changes resulting from extrinsic aging, including ultraviolet light photodamage and other environmental insults, from chronologic aging, and/or scars resulting from surgery, acne, or other causes of inflammation or trauma may each be treated and significantly reduced or resolved with the appropriate application of laser and/or radiofrequency technology. Given the prevalence of epidermal and dermal abnormalities in the population, demand for effective and safe resurfacing procedures is high. Fortunately, significant advances in the arena of laser and radiofrequency technology have provided effective and diverse options for cutaneous resurfacing (Table 5-1).

■ LASER RESURFACING

Patient Selection

Resurfacing using laser treatment may be performed cautiously in a variety of skin phototypes. Risks of resurfacing include potential hyperpigmentation and hypopigmentation. Delayed hypopigmentation presents particularly after nonfractional ablative treatment. Patients with lighter skin types display the lowest risks of dyspigmentation after ablative treatments, and the ideal candidates are of skin phototypes I to IV. Nonablative resurfacing displays lower but continued risks of dyspigmentation, and all skin colors may be considered for treatment. Risks of postinflammatory hyperpigmentation are dependent in part on skin type, sun exposure, history of melasma or prior postinflammatory hyperpigmentation, and the density and energy delivered during treatment.[1] Patients at risk of inadequate stem cell populations to provide rapid reepithelialization, as a result of radiation exposure, morphea, or other conditions, are at risk for prolonged and poor healing and are best not treated using resurfacing techniques. Patients who have received isotretinoin or systemic retinoid treatment 6 to 12 months prior to treatment may display tendency to scarring and are generally deferred treatment until 6 to 12 months after exposure, although literature suggests the risks of laser treatment after isotretinoin exposure may be exaggerated.[2-4] Post-face lift (rhytidectomy) and blepharoplasty patients should also generally defer ablative laser treatment for a few months postoperatively due to possible altered blood supply and increased scarring risks.[5] Treatment of scar-prone areas such as the neck and chest is often avoided with nonfractional ablative lasers or performed more conservatively with fractional ablative or nonablative lasers. Longer healing times and the need for meticulous postoperative care are also important considerations when selecting and counseling patients to produce optimal results and satisfaction.

Ablative Resurfacing

Ablative lasers are defined by the capacity to produce sufficient thermal damage to create areas of complete tissue ablation or destruction (Figure 5-1). To date, these lasers have targeted water and include the carbon dioxide (CO_2) and erbium-doped yttrium aluminum garnet (Er:YAG) lasers. Ablative lasers were popularized in the 1980s, when they were used widely for resurfacing. Nonfractional ablative lasers destroy the epidermis and superficial dermis, allowing ablation of epidermal or superficial dermal cells or deposits (Figure 5-1). Therefore, a wide variety of conditions may be targeted including photodamaged or aged skin, atrophic scarring, rhinophyma, xanthelasma, angiofibromas, adnexal tumors, epidermal nevi, and many other conditions. The subsequent

TABLE 5-1
Devices for Cutaneous Resurfacing[a]

Device	Manufacturer	Wavelength	Fluence	Pulse Width	Comments
Ablative lasers					
Fraxel Re:pair	Solta Medical	10,600 nm; fractional	≤70 mJ/MTZ	N/A	Roller tip with intelligent optical tracking system, built-in air evacuator
SmartSkin	Cynosure	10,600 nm; fractional	≤30 W	150–20,000 μs	Scanning patterns
SmartXide DOT	DEKA Medical	10,600 nm; fractional	150 W	200 μs to 80 ms	Three scanning modes
UltraPulse	Lumenis	10,600 nm; fractional	1–225 mJ	<1 ms	CoolScan and DeepFX handpieces
Icon, 2940	Palomar	2940 nm; fractional	2–5.5 mJ/0.1 mm	0.25–5 ms	
ProFractional	Sciton	2940 nm; fractional	≤400 J/cm²	Variable	Expandable module
Harmony Pixel 2940	Alma Lasers	2940 nm; fractional	300–2500 mJ/p	Short, medium, or long	
Xeo Pearl	Cutera	2790 nm; available pearl fractional	60–320 mJ/microspot	600 μs	Combination ablation and coagulation
Nonablative lasers					
Fraxel Dual	Solta Medical	1550/1927 nm	≤70/≤20 mJ/MTZ	N/A	Integrated Zimmer cooling; intelligent optical tracking system
Icon, 1540	Palomar	1540 nm; fractional	≤70 mJ/microbeam	10 and 15 ms	
ARAMIS	Quantel Derma	1540 nm	≤126 J/cm²	3.3 ms	Skin cooling
Affirm	Cynosure	1440, 1320 nm	≤14 J/cm²	3 ms	Air cooling
MOSAIC	Lutronic	1550 nm	4–70 mJ	N/A	Hair and skin treatment tips
Clear + Brilliant	Solta Medical	1440 nm	≤9 mJ/MTZ	N/A	Low, medium, and high settings; 1927 nm system under investigation
Portrait PSR	Energist Group	Plasma energy	1–10 W	N/A	
Radiofrequency devices					
ePrime	Syneron/Candela	Radiofrequency	Maximum voltage 84 VRMS	N/A	Bipolar paired microneedles
Aluma	Lumenis	Radiofrequency, bipolar	2–20 W	1–5 s	6 × 25 and 3 × 18 mm tips
eMatrix	Syneron/Candela	Radiofrequency, bipolar, fractional	≤62 mJ/pin	N/A	Spot size 12 × 12 mm, 64 or 144 pins
Thermage	Solta Medical	Radiofrequency, monopolar	≤400 W	200 ms	CPT and NXT systems

[a]List is not comprehensive. Individuals should verify all information with device manufacturer.

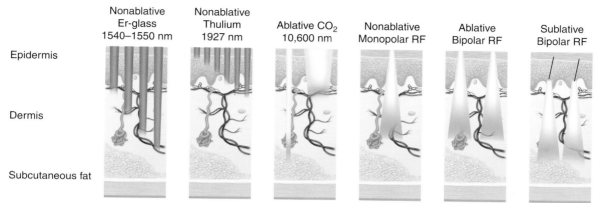

▲ **FIGURE 5-1** Ablative, sublative, and nonablative options for cutaneous resurfacing. Ablative treatments destroy or vaporize epidermal tissue. Sublative treatments destroy dermal tissue while sparing the overlying epidermis. Nonablative treatments produce thermal damage without tissue vaporization.

reepithelialization after nonfractional ablative laser treatment sometimes produces dramatic improvements in texture and tone, but also potential risks of hyperpigmentation or hypopigmentation (Figure 5-2), prolonged erythema and healing times, and scarring, especially when used over large surface areas.[4] These risks have been mitigated with the development of fractional photothermolysis (FP). Fractional ablative laser techniques are able to achieve significant efficacy with great improvements in safety compared with nonfractional laser treatments, and have become critical tools in the resurfacing armamentarium.

CARBON DIOXIDE LASER The CO_2 laser has a wavelength of 10,600 nm, which is absorbed by water. At fluences above the tissue vaporization threshold (5 J/cm^2), ablation occurs.[6-8] Below this threshold, coagulation and tissue dessication occurs.[9] Fluence is proportional to the beam diameter, such that larger beam diameters more common in the past can lead to charring effects.[4] At fluences of 5 J/cm^2 and pulse widths of less than 1 millisecond, optical penetration reaches 20 to 30 μm in depth with thermal damage extending to 100 to 150 μm.[6-8] Nonfractional CO_2 wavelengths may be delivered by 2 types of devices, 1 with high-power single pulses applied in specific modifiable patterns and another using a lower-energy scanning continuous wave laser.[4]

ERBIUM LASER Er:YAG lasers (2940 nm) represent another class of ablative lasers targeting water. Although clinical results are generally comparable to those of the CO_2 laser, the Er:YAG is better absorbed

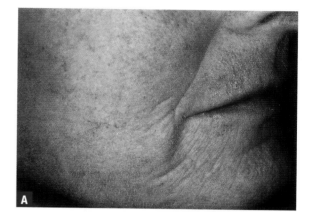

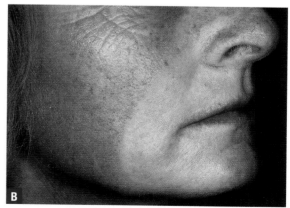

▲ **FIGURE 5-2 A.** A 50-year-old woman with significant facial rhytides and laxity. **B.** Eight months following perioral CO_2 laser resurfacing, there is marked hypopigmentation, improvement of rhytides and improvement of laxity.

by water allowing for limited ablation with less surrounding thermal damage. Variable pulse Er:YAG lasers permit modification of the pulse duration to allow for more ablation or more thermal damage depending on the operator preference.[10] The shorter wavelength also has a shorter penetration, reaching 1 to 3 μm per 1 J/cm^2 (10–40 μm).[4] Although the Er:YAG lasers retain many clinical uses, CO$_2$ lasers appear to be more often preferred based on comparative trials.[10,11]

FRACTIONAL ABLATIVE LASERS With the advent of fractional laser technology in 2004, resurfacing technology gained a significant advance in safety through the concept of FP, or treatment of small fractions of skin within a given area.[12] In doing so, FP allows untreated intervening skin to provide follicular stem cells for rapid reepithelialization of the nearby damaged skin, resulting in more rapid healing and reduced risks of hyperpigmentation or hypopigmentation and scarring. Histology of treated skin shows multiple microthermal zones composed of a tapered ablative zone, surrounded by an eschar and then zone of thermal coagulation[13] (Figure 5-1). Depths of 1 to 1.5 mm have been demonstrated with higher energy levels (70 mJ).[14] Reepithelialization occurs in a matter of 2 to 3 days, and extrusion of microepidermal necrotic debris produces small pepper-like flakes on the skin.[13]

CLINICAL EFFECTS Ablative lasers, both fractional and nonfractional, have demonstrated efficacy in a variety of clinical conditions. Aging skin and photodamage is a primary indication for treatment (Figures 5-3 and 5-4). Studies have shown reduced rhytides, and a mild degree of tightening of lax skin after fractional and nonfractional CO$_2$ laser treatments of photodamaged skin, with fractional treatments showing the greater safety profile.[15–20] Multiple scar types, including hypertrophic and atrophic scars, also have been observed to improve after fractional ablative laser treatment.[14] Atrophic scars, including acne scars, surgical, and traumatic scars, have shown significant improvement after fractional ablative treatments in multiple studies, including objective improvements in depth using 3-dimensional imaging[21–23] (Figure 5-5). One study of 15 subjects with skin phototypes I to IV and moderate to severe acne scarring showed a mean 67% improvement in acne scar depth and 26% to 50% improvement in texture, atrophy, and overall improvement after a series of 2 to 3 full-face fractional CO$_2$ laser treatments.[19] Scars often respond even when mature or long-standing; however, optimal results are often obtained when scars are treated early, at 6 to 10 weeks after the causative injury[4] (for complete review, please refer to Chapter 9). Actinic cheilitis and fibrofatty residuum after involution of infantile hemangiomas also improve with fractional ablative laser treatments.[14,24] Hypopigmentation from a variety of causes including prior nonfractional ablative treatments frequently improves using fractional ablative treatments.[14] Genetically based dermatoses including epidermal nevi,[25] and angiofibroma in the setting of tuberous sclerosis, are also successfully treated with fractional or nonfractional ablative lasers, although gradual recurrence over time is not infrequent due to the continued action of genetically mutated cells.

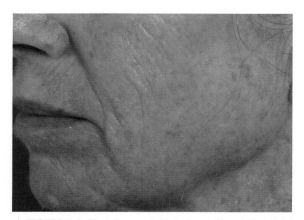 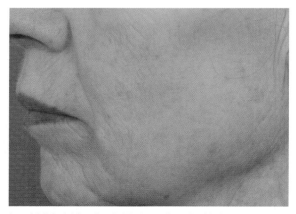

▲ **FIGURE 5-3** Photodamaged skin before (left) and after (right) a series of full facial fractional ablative carbon dioxide laser treatments demonstrates improvement in rhytides, lentigines, tone, and texture.

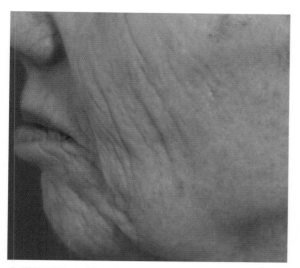
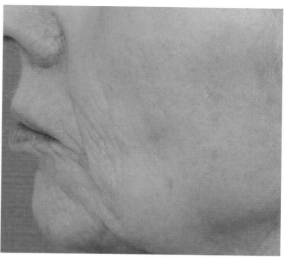

▲ **FIGURE 5-4** A female with photodamaged facial skin (left) shows improvement (right) in rhytides, lentigines, texture, and tone after fractional ablative carbon dioxide laser treatment.

Nonablative Resurfacing

Nonablative lasers produce limited thermal damage without causing ablation or vaporization of tissue. The epidermis remains intact during treatment. With the reduced damage, there is typically a reduced efficacy per treatment compared with ablative laser treatment, and most often a need for multiple treatments to achieve optimal results. In addition, while multiple nonablative treatments typically provide large cumulative improvements, results may not reach the same level of improvement as might be seen with 1 to multiple ablative treatments. However, side effects are reduced, healing is more rapid, wound care is more convenient, and complications are fewer.

Popular fractional nonablative lasers include a dual wavelength 1927 nm thulium and 1550 nm erbium-doped fiber laser (Fraxel Dual, Solta Medical), a 1540 nm laser (Lux1540 Handpiece, Palomar), and a 1440 nm laser (Clear + Brilliant, Solta Medical). Multiple other fractional nonablative resurfacing

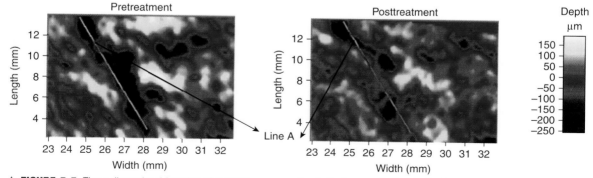

▲ **FIGURE 5-5** Three-dimensional imaging of atrophic acne scarring (left) shows reduction in depth of scars after fractional ablative carbon dioxide laser resurfacing (right). (Reproduced from Chapas AM, Brightman L, Sukal S, et al. Successful treatment of acneiform scarring with CO_2 ablative fractional resurfacing. *Lasers Surg Med.* 2008;40(6):381–386, copyright 2008.)

treatments are available, including a fractional 532 nm diode laser, 1350 nm infrared laser, 1064/2940 nm Er:YAG, 2790 nm yttrium scandium gallium garnet (YSSG), and fractional radiofrequency devices.

CLINICAL EFFECTS Nonablative laser resurfacing generally results in improvements that are often reduced in comparison to ablative resurfacing outcomes, and requires multiple treatment sessions for optimal effect. However, the reduced risks, more convenient and simple wound care, side effects, and duration of side effects (downtime) all make nonablative treatments a popular, effective, and safe option for improvement of a variety of cutaneous conditions. Nonablative resurfacing has produced significant improvement in photodamage, rhytides, skin texture, and scarring, with improvements generally increasing over series of multiple treatments (Figure 5-6). Manstein et al used nonablative FP in 30 patients and demonstrated 34% showed moderate or greater improvement in wrinkles and 47% moderate or greater improvements in texture 3 months after treatment.[12] Further improvements in texture, photodamage-associated hyperpigmentation, and rhytides have been demonstrated by Geronemus, with superficial to moderate rhytides responding more than deep rhytides.[26] Nonfacial sites have also shown substantial improvements in photodamage with an excellent safety profile after nonablative treatments[27,28] (Figure 5-7).

Treatment with lower-energy nonablative fractional devices has also resulted in improvements in texture and tone. While efficacy appears lower, side effects including erythema, edema, and risks of hyperpigmentation or hypopigmentation are also typically reduced in comparison, making these devices attractive options for those desiring reduced to no downtime, those seeking more frequent or adjunctive treatment options, and those seeking to minimize irritation or postinflammatory risks. A study of 20 patients with Fitzpatrick skin phototypes I to IV receiving full-face treatments (Clear + Brilliant laser, Solta Medical) consisting of 8 passes at high-energy setting, every 2 weeks for a total of 6 treatments, reported significant reduction in pore count and size with 95% of patients reporting improvement in pore appearance and 100% reporting improvement in skin texture and overall appearance.[29] A lower-energy device primarily for home use, a fractional nonablative 1410 nm diode laser (PaloVia Skin Renewing Laser, Palomar Medical Technologies, Burlington, Massachusetts), has been reported to produce microthermal zones of injury extending to 250 μm.[30] The manufacturer-recommended treatment regimen is daily use for 1 month, followed by twice-weekly maintenance treatments.[31] Two prospective studies, 1 with 34 patients and 1 with 90 patients (total of 124 patients), each showed 90% of patients demonstrated 1 grade of improvement in periorbital rhytides as assessed by a blinded investigator after the initial 4-week treatment phase.[30] In both studies, 79% of patients maintained this grade of improvement after another 4 to 12 weeks of twice-weekly maintenance treatments. Patient self-assessment showed similar efficacy, with 87% of patients reporting reduction in periorbital rhytides.

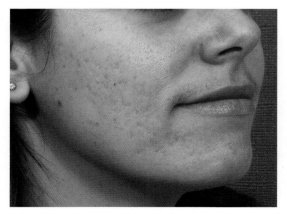 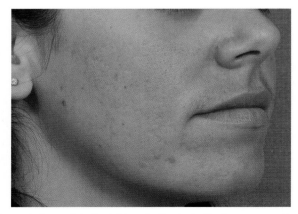

▲ **FIGURE 5-6** A young adult with atrophic acne scarring (left) demonstrates a clinically visible reduction in depth of acne scars after multiple nonablative 1550 nm laser treatments (right).

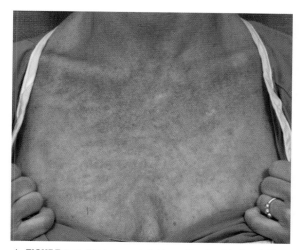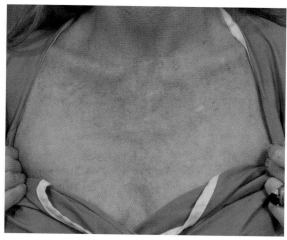

▲ **FIGURE 5-7** Photodamaged skin on the chest before (left) and after (right) multiple nonablative fractional 1927 nm laser treatments.

Actinic keratoses have also shown substantial improvements after a series of nonablative FP treatments (Figure 5-8). After 10 patients received 5 to 10 treatments every 4 to 6 weeks with a 1550 nm fractional laser and use of 0.025% tretinoin cream between treatments, 54% improvement in actinic keratoses was found to persist at 6 months posttreatment.[32] In 14 patients treated with five 1550 nm fractional laser treatments, a similar 55% clinical improvement was found at 6 months posttreatment, although histologic changes of actinic keratoses persisted in most of the posttreatment biopsy specimens.[33] In addition to cutaneous photodamage, actinic cheilitis has been treated successfully using the 1927 nm fractional nonablative laser.[34]

Melasma has shown dramatic improvements of 75% to 100% clearance in some reports[35] and moderate to poor response in others.[36,37] Responses appear to be variable, with darker skin types noted to often show less improvement and show greater risks of dyspigmentation after resurfacing treatments.[36] Hypopigmentation has also shown improvement

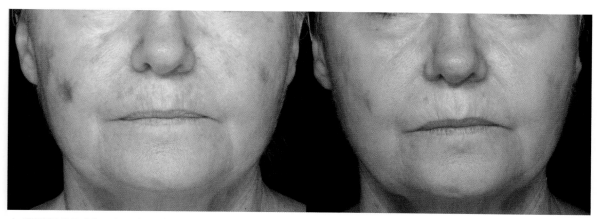

▲ **FIGURE 5-8** A female patient with several actinic keratoses (left) shows significant reduction in lesion count (right) 6 months after a series of 4 fractional nonablative 1927 nm laser treatments.

following both fractional ablative and nonablative laser treatments.

Acne scarring responds well to nonablative FP after a series of treatments in a variety of skin types, showing 22% to 75% improvement in depth in a variety of studies.[21,26,38] Surgical and several other scar types also improve utilizing laser resurfacing. For complete discussion, the reader is referred to Chapter 9.

RADIOFREQUENCY

Mechanism of Action

Radiofrequency is a form of electrical energy that produces thermal injury in the dermis as a result of tissue impedance of current flow.[39] Thermal injury results in subsequent neocollagenesis. Elastogenesis has also been demonstrated following fractional radiofrequency microneedle treatment.[39] These histologic changes result in clinical effects of lifting, tightening, and increased elasticity of treated skin.[40] The mechanism is chromophore-independent and does not rely on selective photothermolysis. Bulk heating may affect epidermal cells and several devices employ epidermal cooling technology and/or careful monitoring of dermal and of surface temperatures.[41] Monopolar, bipolar, and tripolar devices are available. The duration of the given pulse may be fixed or modified. The depth and pattern of injury depends on the position and distance of the treatment tip and/or needles, the amount of current applied, the tissue resistance, and the duration of current application.[41]

Plasma skin resurfacing results from the reaction of high-energy radiofrequency energy with nitrogen gas, producing nitrogen plasma (an ionized gas) that may be directed to produce thermal damage at various cutaneous levels, with effects varying from superficial sloughing to dermal heating with subsequent neocollagenesis.[42]

Patient Selection

All skin phototypes may be treated using radiofrequency technology for resurfacing. The desired depth(s) of injury should be considered when selecting the appropriate device and placement of the device. Patients having pacemakers or implantable cardiac defibrillators should not be treated or should receive cardiology clearance prior to treatment. A history of metal implants or other permanent implants (eg, permanent fillers or silicone) in the treatment area is also a contraindication.

Clinical Effects

Clinical studies of radiofrequency show significant improvements in rhytides and laxity (Figures 5-9 and 5-10) that increase over 3 to 6 months after treatment. Monopolar, bipolar, and tripolar RF devices each produce improvements,[43,44] with effects dependent largely on treatment settings and passes performed. Fifteen patients with facial skin laxity were treated with microneedle radiofrequency (Miratone, Primaeva Medical; Evolastin, Syneron/Candela) and 3- and 6-month photographic results were compared by blinded evaluators with photographs after surgical face-lifting.[39] Statistically significant improvements in facial laxity were found, at 16% for fractional microneedle radiofrequency treatment and 49% for surgical face-lift treatment, and patient satisfaction with RF was high (60% satisfied, 33% very satisfied, 0% dissatisfied). Patients returned to normal activities within 24 hours, had no scarring or adverse effects, and side effects persisted for 5 to 10 days, while the face-lift patients resumed normal activities at 7 to 10 days and all had surgical scarring. A study of 26 women in Korea treated with 3 fractional RF treatments at 4- to 6-week intervals (Matrix RF, Syneron/Candela) found moderate improvements 6 weeks after the third treatment in facial smoothness, tightness, brightness, and overall improvement, with a concomitant reduction in elastosis.[45]

The cheeks in particular appear to respond optimally to radiofrequency treatments, while the neck improves though not as significantly.[41,46] In a study of a nonablative monopolar radiofrequency device (ThermaCool TC, Thermage, Inc), 50 subjects of skin phototypes I to IV with mild to moderate cheek or neck laxity receiving a single treatment with the device demonstrated significant improvement for 28 of 30 patients in the nasolabial and melolabial folds, and in 17 of 20 patients in neck laxity, using a quartile grading scale.[41] Improvements in cheek laxity continued to increase at each visit over the 6-month follow-up period.[41] Ruiz-Esparza and Gomez reported 14 of 15 patients treated with a single monopolar or bipolar radiofrequency session (Thermage, Solta Medical) on the lower one third of the face showed improvement in laxity, with the cheeks responding more optimally than the neck.[47] Studies by Hsu and Kaminer, and Alster and Tanzi suggest younger patients respond more optimally, and that patients over the age of 62 with significant photodamage may not respond.[41,48] In addition, higher-energy treatments appear to produce more significant results.[41,48]

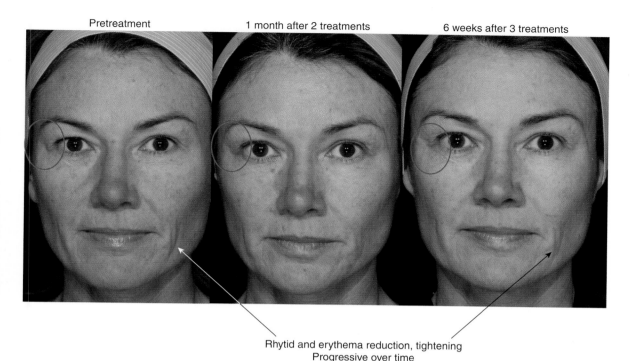

Pretreatment   1 month after 2 treatments   6 weeks after 3 treatments

Rhytid and erythema reduction, tightening
Progressive over time

▲ **FIGURE 5-9** A female patient with facial laxity before (left) demonstrates improvement in rhytides and laxity 1 month after 2 bipolar radiofrequency treatments (Matrix RF, Syneron/Candela) (middle), with continued improvement at 6 weeks after 3 treatments.

Multiple-pass, lower-fluence treatments appear to be less effective but also produce measurable improvements. A study of 66 subjects with moderate facial laxity treated with a maximum of 5 monopolar RF passes (ThermaCool device, average 83 J/cm², 556 pulses) to the lower face and neck showed 84% had independently judged photographic improvement at 6 months after treatment.[49]

Periorbital skin has also shown improvements in laxity following superficial radiofrequency treatments, again often improving over 4 to 6 months after treatment (ThermaCool, Thermage, Solta Medical).[50] A multicenter study of 86 patients treated with radiofrequency (ThermaCool, Thermage, Solta Medical) found that 80% showed modest improvement in periorbital laxity and brow elevation.[51] A prospective multicenter study of 72 patients with eyelid laxity treated with a single treatment using a 0.25 cm² monopolar RF tip (ThermaCool, Thermage, Solta Medical) and specialized large-area polycarbonate protective eye shields showed 88% of subjects demonstrated upper eyelid tightening, 86% showed reduction of hooding,

and 71% to 74% showed lower eyelid tightening.[50,52] It was noted that as with other RF studies performed at various anatomic sites, results were somewhat variable with some patients not showing improvement.[50]

Plasma skin resurfacing can affect the epidermis or dermis depending on the device and settings used. Multiple low- and mid-energy-level treatments have shown improvement in superficial rhytides, skin texture, and discoloration; however, single or few high-energy treatments have been found to be most effective, and more effective in particular at producing skin tightening.[53] In addition, scars have shown improvement after treatment.[54] A study by Kilmer et al reported a single full-face treatment at high energies (3.0–4.0 J) produced a mean improvement of 50% in overall facial rejuvenation at 1 month, with continuing improvements at 9 months after treatment.[53,55] Another study using a single high-energy full-face treatment showed a 30% decrease in rhytid depth at 6 months after treatment, using silicone molding of rhytides.[56] Multiple lower-energy treatments have been studied. In 1 series of 3 treatments, a 37% improvement in

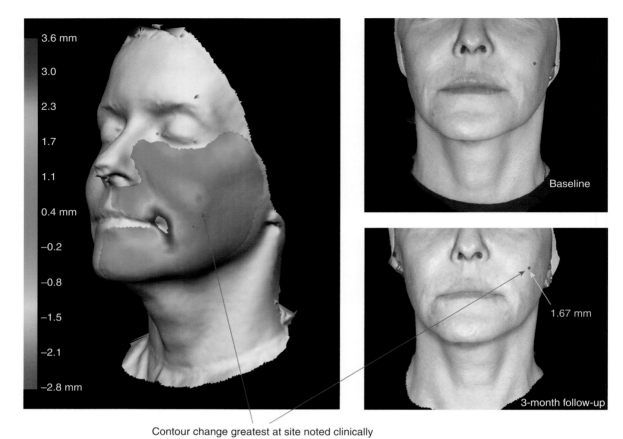

Contour change greatest at site noted clinically

▲ **FIGURE 5-10** A female patient demonstrates improvement in laxity of the cheek 3 months after microneedle radiofrequency treatment (Evolastin, Syneron/Candela). Lifting of the cheek by 1.67 mm and increased volume are demonstrated by 3-dimensional imaging (blue and green areas represent areas of increased volume).

rhytides was found at 3-month follow-up and histology showed reduced solar damage and increased new collagen formation.[57] Lower-energy treatments are also recommended for improvement of nonfacial body sites, and Alster and Konda have shown improvement of moderate photodamage after treatment (1.0–1.8 J) of the neck, chest, and hands.[42]

Preoperative and Postoperative Care

Ablative treatments breach the skin barrier, allowing entry of pathogens and resulting in potential for serious and widespread infection, scarring, and even sepsis that is increased if inadequate care taken. Oral antiherpetic prophylaxis is advised for all patients undergoing full-face or perioral ablative or nonablative resurfacing regardless of clinical HSV history beginning 1 day preoperatively and continuing for 7 to 10 days or until reepithelialization is complete.[58] Patients who cannot take or refuse antiviral prophylaxis should be treated with extreme caution or not treated. Oral antibiotic prophylaxis against common skin flora using cephalosporins, penicillin derivatives, or macrolides is advised during the same time period.[58] Antifungals are generally not prescribed, although they may be considered.[59] Ocular protection is critical during ablative laser treatment and should be provided using external goggles, or, if the periorbital area is to be treated, intraocular shields. After ablative procedures, the patient is treated with distilled water soaks, application of petrolatum ointment, and placement of a sterile protective face mask to protect against infection and maintain a moist environment. The mask may be removed when recovering in a clean home environment. Most topicals containing active ingredients such as glycolic acids or scrubs should be discontinued a few weeks prior to the procedure, although topical tretinoin may be continued and may even improve outcomes.[4,60] Postoperative gentle cleansing with frequent soaks using distilled water and moist wound care using a petrolatum-based ointment are critical to optimal reepithelialization and minimized risk of scarring. After reepithelialization is complete, light moisturizers are recommended and makeup may generally be applied. Photoprotection for at least several weeks is critical to reducing risks of further erythema and risks of dyspigmentation.

Nonablative treatments also require oral antiherpetic prophylaxis regardless of clinical HSV history beginning 1 day prior to resurfacing and continuing for 3 to 5 days or until superficial healing is complete. Oral antibiotics are generally not required. Ocular protection appropriate to the energy source being utilized should be provided. Patients treated with nonablative treatments should gently cleanse the skin twice daily and apply a light moisturizer. Petrolatum-based ointments should be applied on areas of any scabbing until resolved. Photoprotection remains important to preoperative and postoperative care and reduced risks of dyspigmentation.

Anesthesia

Nonablative laser treatments most often can be performed with use of topical anesthesia alone, although injected local anesthesia or other measures may be considered as needed. Ablative treatment is likely to produce significant pain without adequate injected local anesthesia. Injection of local anesthesia either into the treatment areas or as a nerve block is recommended for optimal prevention of pain. For microneedle-based radiofrequency devices, topical anesthesia is sometimes adequate, and injected or tumescent local anesthesia is often recommended. In addition, for full-face ablative or large-area ablative laser treatments, adjunctive agents such as anxiolytics, mild sedatives, or nonsteroidal anti-inflammatory agents are frequently helpful. General anesthesia is rarely required for any resurfacing treatment unless the patient is unable to tolerate treatment under local anesthesia due to age or other concerns or prefers to be treated under general anesthesia. Cold air cooling during the laser procedure also aids in improving patient comfort.[4]

Side Effects

Ablative treatments produce immediate erythema, crusting, oozing, and bleeding. Reepithelialization typically occurs over several weeks in nonfractional ablation, and in 2 to 3 days for fractional ablative treatments. Erythema wanes over 1 to 3 months in fractional ablative treatment and may persist for several months after nonfractional ablative treatment.

Immediately after nonablative laser resurfacing treatments, erythema and edema generally appear and last 2 to 3 days. The erythema is often followed by areas of desquamation for 1 to 2 days. After radiofrequency treatments, erythema is generally short-lived, lasting 2 to 12 hours.[41] Slight scaling may appear for 3 to 5 days posttreatment.

For all resurfacing treatments, intensity and duration of side effects are often dependent on the type of energy, density, fluence, and number of passes delivered. Postoperative 590 nm yellow light LED treatment has been shown to reduce the duration of erythema following fractional nonablative laser treatment.[61] Edema may be mitigated by use of postoperative oral or topical corticosteroids. Petechiae or purpura is not an uncommon event. Crusting should be avoided by use of frequent soaks and moist wound care. Typically pain is minimal to none postoperatively and significant posttreatment pain should prompt evaluation for possible infection or other cause. Acneiform eruptions are common for a self-limited period after nonablative and ablative laser treatments and best managed through use of minimally to noncomedogenic products and topical agents for the treatment of acne such as 2.5% benzoyl peroxide.

Complications

All laser and radiofrequency resurfacing treatments carry some risks of hyperpigmentation, hypopigmentation, and/or scarring. Scarring is an uncommon complication with radiofrequency treatments and nonablative or fractional ablative laser treatments, but can occur, usually as a result of high fluences, excessive passes or pulse stacking, inadequate preoperative or postoperative care, aggressive treatment of scar-prone sites, or other factors.[4,62,63] Scarring risks are higher after nonfractional ablative treatments. Patients should be evaluated at regular intervals in particular following ablative treatment to assess for an incipient scarring or complications. Scarring or impending scarring should be promptly treated using appropriate skin care, possible laser treatment for the scar type, and, in the case of hypertrophic scars, consideration of intralesional 5-FU and/or triamcinolone, pulsed dye laser, silicone gel sheeting, or other treatments.

Hyperpigmentation is best treated with aggressive photoprotection and use of topical antipigmentation agents. Hypopigmentation may be relative, appearing as a result of reduced dyspigmentation in the treated area compared with photodamaged surrounding skin, or localized. Fractional laser treatment, excimer laser treatment, and/or use of topical repigmentation-promoting drugs (eg, bimatoprost) may be considered for treatment of hypopigmentation. Infection with bacteria, fungi, atypical mycobacterium, and/or herpes simplex virus has been reported and is best managed by appropriate culture and treatment course with close evaluations.

In addition to risks of scarring and dyspigmentation, radiofrequency treatments heat the deep dermis and may affect nerves. Temporary dysesthesias have been rarely reported.[41] Subcutaneous fat atrophy has also been reported rarely and typically resolves over the course of several months.[64]

CONCLUSIONS

Cutaneous resurfacing techniques continue to evolve, providing increasing options for treatment of a myriad of epidermal and dermal conditions. Signs of photodamage including epidermal atrophy, dyspigmentation, solar elastosis, reduced collagen levels, and actinic keratoses can all be improved with appropriate treatment. In addition, scars from nearly any cause have the potential for improvement using resurfacing techniques. These noninvasive ablative and nonablative resurfacing methods allow for improvements in skin quality, texture, and tone for a wide variety of patients.

REFERENCES

1. Chan HH, Manstein D, Yu CS, Shek S, Kono T, Wei WI. The prevalence and risk factors of post-inflammatory hyperpigmentation after fractional resurfacing in Asians. *Lasers Surg Med.* 2007;39(5):381–385.
2. Zachariae H. Delayed wound healing and keloid formation following argon laser treatment or dermabrasion during isotretinoin treatment. *Br J Dermatol.* 1988; 118(5):703–706.
3. Bernestein LJ, Geronemus RG. Keloid formation with the 585-nm pulsed dye laser during isotretinoin treatment. *Arch Dermatol.* 1997;133(1):111–112.
4. Brightman LA, Brauer JA, Anolik R, et al. Ablative and fractional ablative lasers. *Dermatol Clin.* 2009;27(4): 479–489, vi–vii.
5. Hayes DK, Berkland ME, Stambaugh KI. Dermal healing after local skin flaps and chemical peel. *Arch Otolaryngol Head Neck Surg.* 1990;116(7):794–797.
6. Walsh JT Jr, Flotte TJ, Anderson RR, Deutsch TF. Pulsed CO_2 laser tissue ablation: effect of tissue type and pulse duration on thermal damage. *Lasers Surg Med.* 1988; 8(2):108–118.
7. Kauvar AN, Waldorf HA, Geronemus RG. A histopathological comparison of "char-free" carbon dioxide lasers. *Dermatol Surg.* 1996;22(4):343–348.
8. Green HA, Domankevitz Y, Nishioka NS. Pulsed carbon dioxide laser ablation of burned skin: in vitro and in vivo analysis. *Lasers Surg Med.* 1990;10(5):476–484.
9. Kauvar AN, Geronemus RG. Histology of laser resurfacing. *Dermatol Clin.* 1997;15(3):459–467.
10. Newman JB, Lord JL, Ash K, McDaniel DH. Variable pulse erbium:YAG laser skin resurfacing of perioral rhytides and side-by-side comparison with carbon dioxide laser. *Lasers Surg Med.* 2000;26(2):208–214.
11. Khatri KA, Ross V, Grevelink JM, Magro CM, Anderson RR. Comparison of erbium:YAG and carbon dioxide lasers in resurfacing of facial rhytides. *Arch Dermatol.* 1999; 135(4):391–397.
12. Manstein D, Herron GS, Sink RK, Tanner H, Anderson RR. Fractional photothermolysis: a new concept for cutaneous remodeling using microscopic patterns of thermal injury. *Lasers Surg Med.* 2004;34(5):426–438.
13. Hantash BM, Bedi VP, Kapadia B, et al. In vivo histological evaluation of a novel ablative fractional resurfacing device. *Lasers Surg Med.* 2007;39(2):96–107.
14. Hunzeker CM, Weiss ET, Geronemus RG. Fractionated CO_2 laser resurfacing: our experience with more than 2000 treatments. *Aesthet Surg J.* 2009;29(4):317–322.
15. Alexiades-Armenaka M, Sarnoff D, Gotkin R, Sadick N. Multi-center clinical study and review of fractional ablative CO_2 laser resurfacing for the treatment of rhytides, photoaging, scars and striae. *J Drugs Dermatol.* 2011; 10(4):352–362.
16. Haedersdal M, Moreau KE, Beyer DM, Nymann P, Alsbjorn B. Fractional nonablative 1540 nm laser resurfacing for thermal burn scars: a randomized controlled trial. *Lasers Surg Med.* 2009;41(3):189–195.
17. Waldorf HA, Kauvar AN, Geronemus RG. Skin resurfacing of fine to deep rhytides using a char-free carbon dioxide laser in 47 patients. *Dermatol Surg.* 1995;21(11): 940–946.
18. Fitzpatrick RE, Goldman MP, Satur NM, Tope WD. Pulsed carbon dioxide laser resurfacing of photo-aged facial skin. *Arch Dermatol.* 1996;132(4):395–402.
19. Chapas AM, Brightman L, Sukal S, et al. Successful treatment of acneiform scarring with CO_2 ablative fractional resurfacing. *Lasers Surg Med.* 2008;40(6): 381–386.
20. Gotkin RH, Sarnoff DS, Cannarozzo G, Sadick NS, Alexiades-Armenakas M. Ablative skin resurfacing with a novel microablative CO_2 laser. *J Drugs Dermatol.* 2009;8(2):138–144.
21. Alster TS, Tanzi EL, Lazarus M. The use of fractional laser photothermolysis for the treatment of atrophic scars. *Dermatol Surg.* 2007;33(3):295–299.
22. Alster TS, West TB. Resurfacing of atrophic facial acne scars with a high-energy, pulsed carbon dioxide laser. *Dermatol Surg.* 1996;22(2):151–154 [discussion 4–5].

23. Weiss ET, Chapas A, Brightman L, et al. Successful treatment of atrophic postoperative and traumatic scarring with carbon dioxide ablative fractional resurfacing: quantitative volumetric scar improvement. *Arch Dermatol.* 2010;146(2):133–140.

24. Brightman LA, Brauer JA, Terushkin V, et al. Ablative fractional resurfacing for involuted hemangioma residuum. *Arch Dermatol.* 2012 Aug 20:1–5 [Epub ahead of print].

25. Michel JL, Has C, Has V. Resurfacing CO_2 laser treatment of linear verrucous epidermal nevus. *Eur J Dermatol.* 2001;11(5):436–439.

26. Geronemus RG. Fractional photothermolysis: current and future applications. *Lasers Surg Med.* 2006;38(3):169–176.

27. Jih MH, Goldberg LH, Kimyai-Asadi A. Fractional photothermolysis for photoaging of hands. *Dermatol Surg.* 2008;34(1):73–78.

28. Wanner M, Tanzi EL, Alster TS. Fractional photothermolysis: treatment of facial and nonfacial cutaneous photodamage with a 1,550-nm erbium-doped fiber laser. *Dermatol Surg.* 2007;33(1):23–28.

29. Saedi ND, Green JB, Dover JS, Arndt KA. Presented at: American Society for Laser Medicine and Surgery Annual Meeting; April 2012; Kissimmee, FL. Available at: http://www.solta.com/press/129.

30. Metelitsa AI, Green JB. Home-use laser and light devices for the skin: an update. *Semin Cutan Med Surg.* 2011;30(3):144–147.

31. Palomar Medical Technologies. Manufacturer Web site. Available at: http://www.palovia.com. Accessed 1/4/12.

32. Prens SP, Vries KD, Neumann MH, Prens EP. Nonablative fractional resurfacing in combination with topical tretinoin cream as a field treatment modality for multiple actinic keratosis: a pilot study and a review of other field treatment modalities. *J Dermatol Treat.* 2012 [Epub ahead of print].

33. Katz TM, Goldberg LH, Marquez D, et al. Nonablative fractional photothermolysis for facial actinic keratoses: 6-month follow-up with histologic evaluation. *J Am Acad Dermatol.* 2011;65(2):349–356.

34. Ghasri P, Admani S, Petelin A, Zachary CB. Treatment of actinic cheilitis using a 1,927-nm thulium fractional laser. *Dermatol Surg.* 2012;38(3):504–507.

35. Rokhsar CK, Fitzpatrick RE. The treatment of melasma with fractional photothermolysis: a pilot study. *Dermatol Surg.* 2005;31(12):1645–1650.

36. Goldberg DJ, Berlin AL, Phelps R. Histologic and ultrastructural analysis of melasma after fractional resurfacing. *Lasers Surg Med.* 2008;40(2):134–138.

37. Naito SK. Fractional photothermolysis treatment for resistant melasma in Chinese females. *J Cosmet Laser Ther.* 2007;9(3):161–163.

38. Lee HS, Lee JH, Ahn GY, et al. Fractional photothermolysis for the treatment of acne scars: a report of 27 Korean patients. *J Dermatol Treat.* 2008;19(1):45–49.

39. Alexiades-Armenakas M, Rosenberg D, Renton B, Dover J, Arndt K. Blinded, randomized, quantitative grading comparison of minimally invasive, fractional radiofrequency and surgical face-lift to treat skin laxity. *Arch Dermatol.* 2010;146(4):396–405.

40. Willey A, Kilmer S, Newman J, et al. Elastometry and clinical results after bipolar radiofrequency treatment of skin. *Dermatol Surg.* 2010;36(6):877–884.

41. Alster TS, Tanzi E. Improvement of neck and cheek laxity with a nonablative radiofrequency device: a lifting experience. *Dermatol Surg.* 2004;30(4 pt 1):503–507 [discussion 7].

42. Alster TS, Konda S. Plasma skin resurfacing for regeneration of neck, chest, and hands: investigation of a novel device. *Dermatol Surg.* 2007;33(11):1315–1321.

43. Alexiades-Armenakas M, Dover JS, Arndt KA. Unipolar versus bipolar radiofrequency treatment of rhytides and laxity using a mobile painless delivery method. *Lasers Surg Med.* 2008;40(7):446–453.

44. Levenberg A. Clinical experience with a TriPollar radiofrequency system for facial and body aesthetic treatments. *Eur J Dermatol.* 2010;20(5):615–619.

45. Lee HS, Lee DH, Won CH, et al. Fractional rejuvenation using a novel bipolar radiofrequency system in Asian skin. *Dermatol Surg.* 2011;37(11):1611–1619.

46. Yu CS, Yeung CK, Shek SY, Tse RK, Kono T, Chan HH. Combined infrared light and bipolar radiofrequency for skin tightening in Asians. *Lasers Surg Med.* 2007;39(6):471–475.

47. Ruiz-Esparza J, Gomez JB. The medical face lift: a noninvasive, nonsurgical approach to tissue tightening in facial skin using nonablative radiofrequency. *Dermatol Surg.* 2003;29(4):325–332 [discussion 32].

48. Hsu TS, Kaminer MS. The use of nonablative radiofrequency technology to tighten the lower face and neck. *Semin Cutan Med Surg.* 2003;22(2):115–123.

49. Bogle MA, Ubelhoer N, Weiss RA, Mayoral F, Kaminer MS. Evaluation of the multiple pass, low fluence algorithm for radiofrequency tightening of the lower face. *Lasers Surg Med.* 2007;39(3):210–217.

50. Biesman BS, Baker SS, Carruthers J, Silva HL, Holloman EL. Monopolar radiofrequency treatment of human eyelids: a prospective, multicenter, efficacy trial. *Lasers Surg Med.* 2006;38(10):890–898.

51. Fitzpatrick R, Geronemus R, Goldberg D, Kaminer M, Kilmer S, Ruiz-Esparza J. Multicenter study of noninvasive radiofrequency for periorbital tissue tightening. *Lasers Surg Med.* 2003;33(4):232–242.

52. Carruthers J, Carruthers A. Shrinking upper and lower eyelid skin with a novel radiofrequency tip. *Dermatol Surg.* 2007;33(7):802–809.

53. Bogle MA, Arndt KA, Dover JS. Plasma skin regeneration technology. *J Drugs Dermatol.* 2007;6(11):1110–1112.

54. Kono T, Groff WF, Sakurai H, Yamaki T, Soejima K, Nozaki M. Treatment of traumatic scars using plasma skin regeneration (PSR) system. *Lasers Surg Med.* 2009;41(2):128–130.

55. Kilmer S, Semchyshyn N, Shah G, Fitzpatrick R. A pilot study on the use of a plasma skin regeneration device (Portrait PSR3) in full facial rejuvenation procedures. *Lasers Med Sci.* 2007;22(2):101–109.

56. Potter MJ, Harrison R, Ramsden A, Bryan B, Andrews P, Gault D. Facial acne and fine lines: transforming patient outcomes with plasma skin regeneration. *Ann Plast Surg.* 2007;58(6):608–613.

57. Bogle MA, Arndt KA, Dover JS. Evaluation of plasma skin regeneration technology in low-energy full-facial rejuvenation. *Arch Dermatol.* 2007;143(2):168–174.

58. Nestor MS. Prophylaxis for and treatment of uncomplicated skin and skin structure infections in laser and cosmetic surgery. *J Drugs Dermatol.* 2005;4(6 suppl):S20–S25.

59. Conn H, Nanda VS. Prophylactic fluconazole promotes reepithelialization in full-face carbon dioxide laser skin resurfacing. *Lasers Surg Med.* 2000;26(2):201–207.

60. Alt TH. Technical aids for dermabrasion. *J Dermatol Surg Oncol.* 1987;13(6):638–648.

61. Alster TS, Wanitphakdeedecha R. Improvement of post-fractional laser erythema with light-emitting diode photomodulation. *Dermatol Surg.* 2009;35(5):813–815.

62. Ross RB, Spencer J. Scarring and persistent erythema after fractionated ablative CO_2 laser resurfacing. *J Drugs Dermatol.* 2008;7(11):1072–1073.

63. Fife DJ, Fitzpatrick RE, Zachary CB. Complications of fractional CO_2 laser resurfacing: four cases. *Lasers Surg Med.* 2009;41(3):179–184.

64. Weiss RA, Weiss MA, Munavalli G, Beasley KL. Monopolar radiofrequency facial tightening: a retrospective analysis of efficacy and safety in over 600 treatments. *J Drugs Dermatol.* 2006;5(8):707–712.

CHAPTER 6

Devices for the Improvement of Body Contour

Lori A. Brightman, Kavitha K. Reddy, and Robert T. Anolik

INTRODUCTION

With an increase in both sedentary activities and cosmetic consciousness, demand for treatments that improve body contour continues to grow.[1] Several invasive and noninvasive options for body contouring exist. While liposuction and other surgical corrections remain the gold standard for invasive body contouring, patient demand for noninvasive methods of contouring has grown significantly. American Society for Plastic Surgery 2011 survey data found noninvasive treatments for cellulite have grown by 21% from 2010 to 2011 and 58% from 2000 to 2011, while liposuction has decreased by 42% from 2000 to 2011, and invasive surgical body contouring procedures after massive weight loss decreased by 8% from 2010 to 2011.[2] Risks and undesirable side effects of invasive treatments, including significant pain, swelling, recovery time, infection, and surgical scars, may be avoided with many noninvasive treatment options. The field has expanded tremendously in recent years, growing to include treatments that have been reported to reduce fat and promote adjuvant skin tightening, with subsequent reduction in circumference. Devices currently producing these effects use technology that targets fat through infrared heat, radio frequency (RF), ultrasound, and/or cryolipolysis.

PATIENT SELECTION

Current noninvasive body contouring options most often have the potential to provide mild-to-moderate reductions in fat and/or mild improvements in skin laxity, with resultant reduction in circumference (Table 6-1). Typically these changes occur over a period of weeks to months and for many devices may require multiple treatments. Therefore, the ideal candidates are patients with normal to slightly increased, stable body weight with mild-to-moderate excess fat who will demonstrate improvement in contour with proportionate mild-to-moderate fat

reduction.[3] Good general health, exercise, and nutrition are important factors that likely influence results and particularly maintenance of results. Proper candidate selection, patient education, and management of expectations are important to achieving the goal of patient satisfaction. Patients demonstrating unrealistic expectations, or signs of body dysmorphic disorder, are unlikely to achieve optimal satisfaction. Patient preference for surgical or noninvasive options is an important factor in treatment choice. Individual patient factors including the location of excess fat, depth of fat, presence and severity of cellulite, size of the affected area, overlying skin elasticity, proximity to bone or underlying structures, history of previous surgeries, and desired speed, recovery time, and cost of treatment each influences treatment choice (Table 6-2).

PATIENT EXAMINATION

Accurate and consistent patient evaluation allows for assessment and monitoring of treatment efficacy and of changes in body contour. Ideally, evaluations should be performed prior to, during the series of, and after body contouring treatments. Initial evaluation begins with a thorough history and physical examination on consultation. A complete medical history including age, past medical history, medication list, allergy list, history of prior surgeries, and any history of poor or abnormal wound healing or scarring is obtained. The patient's height and weight should be documented, along with the body mass index (BMI). The patient should be examined in a well-lit area, wearing a gown free of garments over the examined areas, in the upright position. The examination focuses on shape of the affected area, location and quantity of excess fat, and overlying skin quality and elasticity. Any scars or abnormalities should be documented. Surrounding cosmetic units should be examined for a possible contribution to the

TABLE 6-1
Devices for the Improvement of Body Contour

Device Name	Category	Manufacturer	Regulatory Agency Clearance
Exilis	Radio frequency (monopolar)	BTL	FDA, CE
Acoustic Wave Therapy	Acoustic wave	BTL	FDA, CE
Accent 980	Diode laser	Alma Lasers	FDA, CE
SmoothShapes	Diode laser	Cynosure	FDA, CE
Lipotherme	Diode laser	Energist/Osyris	FDA, CE
SlimLipo	Diode laser	Palomar	FDA
Duolipo	Diode laser and radio frequency	Ilooda Co Ltd	Pending
LuxDeepIR Fractional Handpiece	Infrared	Palomar	FDA, CE
SkinTyte SP	Infrared	Sciton	FDA, CE
TriActive	Laser plus suction massage	Cynosure	FDA, CE
Omnimax	Laser, radio frequency, infrared, IPL	SharpLight	CE
Smartlipo TriPlex	Nd:YAG laser	Cynosure	FDA, CE
ProLipo Plus	Nd:YAG laser	Sciton	FDA, CE
Soprano XL NIR	Near-infrared	Alma Lasers	FDA, CE
Harmony XL ST	Near-infrared	Alma Lasers	FDA, CE
Maximus	Radio frequency	Pollogen	CE
truSculpt	Radio frequency	Cutera	FDA, CE
Accent XL and Elite	Radio frequency (bipolar and monopolar forms)	Alma Lasers	FDA, CE
New MIDAS	Radio frequency (bipolar, monopolar)	Hironic Ltd	CE
VelaShape	Radio frequency (bipolar), infrared, massage	Syneron/Candela	FDA, CE
Reaction	Radio frequency (bipolar), suction	Viora	FDA, CE
Thermage CPT	Radio frequency (monopolar)	Solta Medical	FDA
Apollo	Radio frequency (tripolar)	Pollogen	CE
Formax Plus	Radio frequency, infrared, IPL	SharpLight	CE
VASER Shape (MC1)	Ultrasound and suction massage	Sound Surgical Technologies	FDA, CE
VASER Shape, MedSculpt	Ultrasound and suction massage	Sound Surgical Technologies	FDA, CE
VASER Lipo	Ultrasound-assisted liposuction	Sound Surgical Technologies	FDA, CE
Body Jet	Water-jet-assisted liposuction	Human Med	FDA, CE
UltraShape	Ultrasound, radio frequency	UltraShape Ltd	CE
Ultherapy	Ultrasound	Ulthera Inc	FDA, CE
LipoSonix	Ultrasound	Solta Medical	FDA, CE
Zeltiq	Cryolipolysis	Zeltiq Ltd	FDA, CE
Zerona	Low-level laser therapy	Erchonia	FDA, CE

contour abnormality. Bilateral examination should be performed and any areas of asymmetry should be noted. Baseline and follow-up standardized assessments using 2-dimensional images along with circumference measurements, laser levels, foot placement mats, fixed lighting, black backgrounds, and consistent physician-provided disposable garments, and/or ideally 3-dimensional imaging, allow optimal monitoring of changes in body contour.[4]

LIPOSUCTION

Liposuction and other surgical corrections were the original first-line choice for body contouring for many years.[3] Benefits include an ability to remove significant volumes of fat, rapid reduction of fat, and an ability often to target more precise areas for improvement. However, the resulting scars, recovery time, and the risks, including infection and occasional

TABLE 6-2
Treatment Options Based on Patient Concerns

Excess Fat Volume	Skin Laxity	Cellulite
Invasive		
Liposuction	Laser lipolysis	Laser lipolysis
Laser lipolysis		Subcision
Mesotherapy/drug treatment		Carboxytherapy
		Mesotherapy
Noninvasive		
Cryolipolysis	Infrared heat	Suction/massage
Radio frequency	Radio frequency	Infrared
Ultrasound		Radio frequency
		Ultrasound

unsatisfactory cosmetic outcome, are of concern to many patients. As noninvasive options improve in both safety and efficacy and many patients favor these laser-, light-, or other energy-based treatments, demand for nonsurgical options has increased.[1] Noninvasive options often permit liposuction to be avoided entirely. The patient should be informed of available noninvasive and invasive options, and the patient's particular goals should be clearly established. When patients elect to undergo liposuction procedures, liposuction (including traditional suction-assisted liposuction, and more recent energy-based liposuction techniques such as ultrasound-, laser-, and RF-assisted liposuction) may be used before or after other body contouring treatments.

LASER LIPOLYSIS

Laser lipolysis, or laser-assisted liposuction (LAL), utilizes a laser fiber to emulsify and thermocoagulate adipose tissue, while promoting collagenesis and tissue tightening. The combination of these effects promotes reduction in circumference and improvement in contour of the treated area (Figures 6-1 to 6-3). The emulsified fat is removed more easily using small cannulas, which appears to reduce associated edema, purpura, and recovery times. Nd:YAG lasers have been most often used, although other lasers also may be utilized to perform the technique. A study by Kim and Geronemus of 29 patients treated with laser lipolysis reported 17% fat reduction as demonstrated on MRI, along with 37% subject-assessed clinical improvement at 3 months with quick recovery times and good skin retraction observed.[5] With proper operator technique,

the procedure is generally safe. A study of 537 cases performed under tumescent anesthesia reported no systemic adverse events, 1 case of local infection treated with oral antibiotics, and 4 burns.[6] Burns may be generally prevented by continuous movement of the laser fiber and use of adequate temperature monitoring. Nineteen of the 537 (3.5%) patients required revisions or touch-ups, a rate which is lower than the 12% to 13% liposuction touch-up rate reported in the literature.[6]

RADIO-FREQUENCY DEVICES

RF devices were initially employed in aesthetic medicine to treat skin laxity of the head and neck.[7-11] Subsequently RF was investigated as a tool in body contouring.[12] RF energy represents a subset of the electromagnetic spectrum, and unlike lasers, which rely on chromophore absorption, RF effects are based on electrical properties of the target tissue. RF devices generate heat through resistance to electric current flow in tissue. The heat is generally uniformly distributed, in a manner referred to as volumetric bulk heating. The epidermis is generally spared when appropriate settings and temperatures are utilized, making RF treatment an option for patients of any skin color.[1]

Devices typically include a generator and handheld tip. Some devices include cryogen or other cooling to protect the epidermis. Coupling fluid is applied to treatment areas. Treatment tip size and geometry can be varied to accommodate different anatomic locations and target depths.[13] A number of polarities are used in these devices.[1] Monopolar devices utilize an electrode with a grounding pad, and bipolar RF devices incorporate 2 electrodes. For monopolar systems (Thermage, Solta Medical; Accent, Alma Lasers; truSculpt, Cutera), a delivery electrode is placed over the target tissue and a return electrode is placed at a distant site. Bipolar systems (VelaShape, Syneron Medical) combine a delivery and a return electrode into the same handpiece, producing conductive RF energy. Lastly, a tripolar system (TriPollar, Pollogen) incorporates 1 positive and 2 negative electrodes. In addition to polarity, frequencies vary between RF devices. Thermage (Solta Medical, Hayward, California) delivers RF at 6 MHz, while VelaShape products (Syneron/Candela, Yokneam Illit, Israel) use 1 MHz, and Alma products (Alma Lasers, Buffalo Grove, Illinois) use 40 MHz. Some variable-frequency devices are in development that can be changed based on tissue impedance.[14]

10.45 kJ
Total aspirate = 50 cm^3

Pretreatment   3 months posttreatment

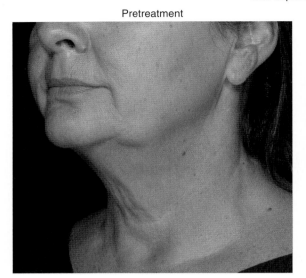 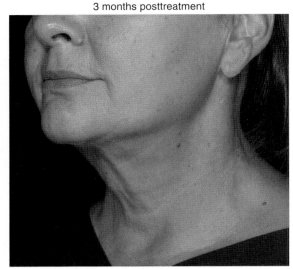

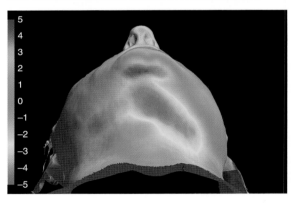

▲ **FIGURE 6-1** Reduced submental volume 3 months after laser-assisted liposuction using a 924/975-nm device (SlimLipo, Palomar) with 10.45 kJ of energy delivered and 50 mL of aspirate removed. Improvement is visible both clinically and by 3-dimensional imaging (red and orange areas represent sites of greatest volume loss).

17.0 J
Total aspirate = 50 cm^3

Pretreatment   1 week posttreatment   12 weeks posttreatment

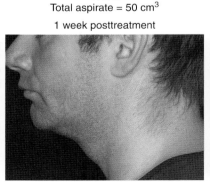 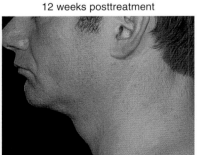

▲ **FIGURE 6-2** Submental contour improvement observed at 1 week and at 3 months after use of 1064-nm Nd:YAG laser–assisted liposuction (LipoLite, Syneron/Candela).

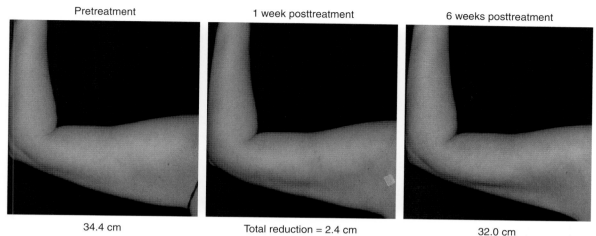

Pretreatment — 34.4 cm

1 week posttreatment — Total reduction = 2.4 cm

6 weeks posttreatment — 32.0 cm

▲ **FIGURE 6-3** Posterior upper arm treated using 1064-nm Nd:YAG laser-assisted liposuction (LipoLite, Syneron/Candela) with 14.0 J energy delivered and 375 mL of aspirate removed. Six weeks after treatment the upper arm circumference was reduced by 2.4 cm.

Clinical RF studies have shown mild-to-moderate improvements in circumferential reduction of various body sites. Treatment with monopolar RF devices has been reported to improve circumferences and skin laxity in a number of studies (Figures 6-4 and 6-5). A study of 12 subjects treated with monopolar RF (ThermaCool TC, Thermage, Solta Medical) showed an average 0.9 cm decrease in waist circumference at 6 months after a single treatment.[12] In studies using bipolar RF with infrared heat and massage, reported reductions of circumference have typically ranged from 1.7 to 2.45 cm for the thigh, 0.9 to 3.5 cm for the abdomen,[12,15–17] 0.60 to 0.71 cm for the arm, and 1.43 to 1.82 cm for the abdomen[1] (Figures 6-6 and 6-7). The mechanism for reduction includes improvements in skin laxity after collagen fibril shortening and neocollagenesis.[1,7] Heat induces collagen fibers to undergo some degree of denaturation, which has been seen on

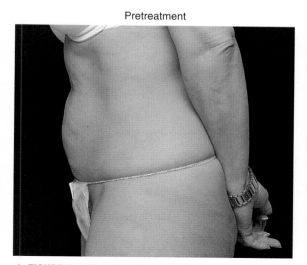

Pretreatment

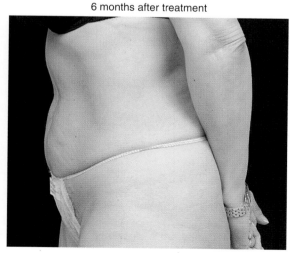

6 months after treatment

▲ **FIGURE 6-4** Reduction of abdominal circumference and improvement of skin laxity 6 months after a single treatment with monopolar radio frequency (ThermaCool TC, Thermage, Solta Medical).

Pretreatment

4 months posttreatment

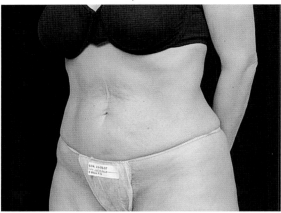

▲ **FIGURE 6-5** Reduced abdominal circumference 4 months after treatment of the abdomen with monopolar radio frequency (Thermage, Solta Medical).

Baseline mean circumference = 57 cm   2 cm reduction   3-month mean circumference = 55 cm

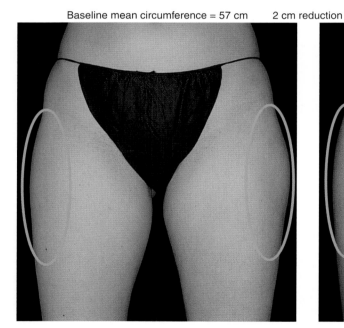

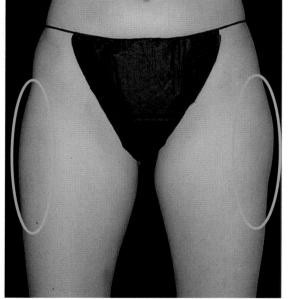

▲ **FIGURE 6-6** Improved lateral thigh ("saddlebag") contour and reduced thigh circumference (2.0 cm decrease) 3 months after treatment with bipolar radio frequency, infrared heat, and mechanical massage (VelaShape, Syneron/Candela). Three-dimensional imaging 3 months after treatment confirms the greatest improvement was seen in the "saddlebag" lateral thigh areas (red areas represent sites of greatest volume loss).

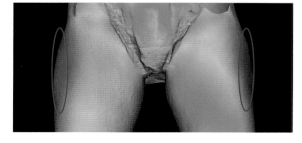

Baseline

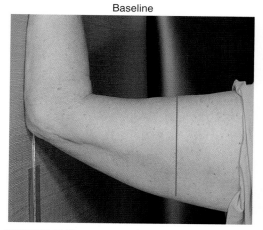

Posttreatment #4: 1.8 cm loss

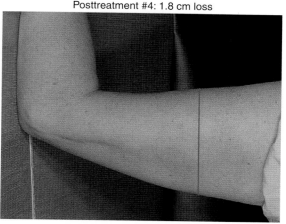

▲ **FIGURE 6-7** The upper arm shows 1.8 cm reduction in circumference after 4 treatments with bipolar radio frequency, infrared heat, and mechanical massage (VelaShape, Syneron/Candela).

electron microscopy, and may recover with subsequent collagen shortening.[18] The ensuing inflammatory cascade is also believed to increase neocollagenesis, evidenced by collagen type 1 messenger RNA found in treated tissue.[18] Histology generally shows edema, perivascular infiltrate, and vessel ectasia shortly after treatment, while dermal thickening or fibrosis follows in the weeks to months thereafter.[14,15,19] One study reported a 49% increase in dermal thickness when comparing treated with control dermis.[19] Some studies have additionally shown subcutaneous adipocyte reduction and lysis after RF treatments.[14,20] Depth of clinical effect reaches several millimeters in depth. On electron microscopy, collagen fibril changes were noted to peak at 3 to 4 mm, yet reach depths of 5 mm.[18] One device (TiteFX, Invasix) combines RF energy with a high-voltage electroporation pulse delivered at the goal peak epidermal temperature, potentially increasing adipocyte destruction and improving longevity of results.[3] Several body contouring devices introduce infrared energy into the skin and subcutaneous fat in order to promote adipocyte volume reduction, as well as skin tightening. In particular, RF devices frequently combine IR and RF energies along with mechanical massage (VelaShape, Syneron/Candela). Surface temperature monitoring in many of these devices promotes safe treatment and helps to avoid potential overheating and/or superficial epidermal burns.

RF treatment generally carries low risk. Patients with pacemakers should not be treated. In general, temporary and mild erythema and edema occur after treatment. Transient crusting, depressions, dysesthesias, anesthesias, and other effects have been summarized in past reviews, though are infrequent in our experience using appropriate treatment parameters and performance.[13]

ULTRASOUND

Standard ultrasound devices have been in existence for many decades and utilize echogenic waves to produce subsurface tissue imaging as well as therapeutic effects. Nonfocused ultrasound has little influence on tissue and has not produced effective body contouring improvements.[3] Focused ultrasound (UltraShape Contour, UltraShape Ltd; LipoSonix, Solta Medical) delivers energy to a precise depth, mechanically disrupting adipocyte membranes and providing fat reductions.[21] Cavitation-induced zones of adipocyte injury have been visualized after treatment with sparing of nerves and vascular structures in the skin with appropriate treatment.[22] An inflammatory response follows with clearance of lipids and cellular debris and subsequent reduction in local adipose tissue volume.[23] Good tissue contact is important to safe and effective ultrasound energy delivery and therefore a coupling gel is used, and a contact sensor and/or imaging system is typically integrated to allow operator confirmation of good skin contact. All skin phototypes may be treated utilizing ultrasound technology.

Clinical studies evaluating focused ultrasound for body contouring have shown reductions in circumference and improvements in skin laxity. A study of 30 patients who underwent 3 focused ultrasound treatments (UltraShape Contour I, UltraShape Ltd) at 1-month intervals, with varying sites treated including the abdomen, thighs, flanks, inner knees, and male breasts, showed 3.95 cm mean circumferential reduction and 2.28 cm mean fat thickness reduction.[21] However, when a similar study was performed in Asia, with 53 patients treated also with 3 treatments at 1-month intervals (UltraShape Contour I, UltraShape Ltd), no significant improvements were seen in abdominal contour.[24] The reasons for the difference in findings are not clear, and may be related to body frame differences or other as yet unclear factors. Another study of 164 patients (137 treated, 27 controls) receiving a single focused ultrasound treatment (UltraShape Contour I, UltraShape Ltd) showed 2 cm mean circumferential reduction and 2.9 mm mean fat thickness reduction.[25] Mild blistering was noted in 2 patients, and 1 patient experienced a mild dermal erosion that was reported to have resolved in the follow-up period. No significant changes in serum triglycerides or in liver ultrasound findings were seen in these studies. Early clinical studies of a more recent high-intensity focused ultrasound device (LipoSonix, Solta Medical), using energies of 140 J/cm^2 or higher and focal depths of 1.1 to 1.8 cm with at least 2 passes delivered, have shown reductions in circumference of 2 to 5 cm after a single treatment session, though often with patient pain and discomfort, and investigation into optimal treatment settings continues[3,26] (Figure 6-8).

CRYOLIPOLYSIS

Cryolipolysis is the selective damage of fat following cold exposure, a concept based on adipocyte vulnerability observed at these temperatures.[27,28] The goal is to target subcutaneous fat while preserving less susceptible surrounding tissue. Melanocytes are not affected at appropriate cooling rates and temperatures and therefore all skin phototypes may be treated. The exact mechanism of fat reduction is poorly understood. The commercially available cryolipolysis system (Zeltiq) consists of a control unit and cup-shaped applicator. Skin is prepared with a coupling gel pad. The cup is positioned over the area to be treated, and a vacuum within the applicator pulls the tissue up between 2 cooling plates. The tissue is maintained between the plates by the applicator where it is cooled gradually. The major treatment variables are duration (up to 60 minutes) and the cooling intensity factor (CIF). The CIF reflects the rate of heat efflux out of the tissue and translates to milliwatts per square centimeter.

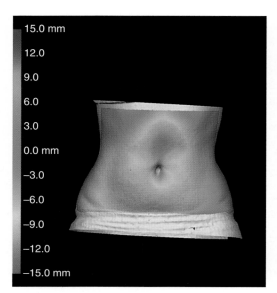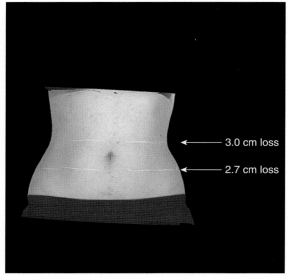

▲ **FIGURE 6-8** Abdomen after a single treatment with high-intensity focused ultrasound (LipoSonix, Solta Medical) demonstrates reduced circumference using 3-dimensional imaging (red areas represent sites of greatest volume loss).

Pretreatment

2 months after single treatment

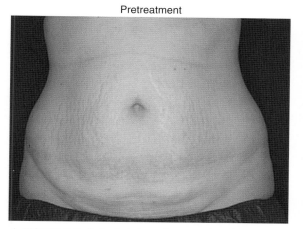
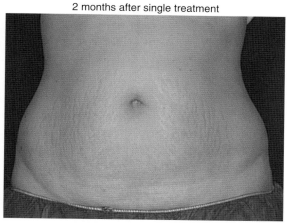

▲ **FIGURE 6-9** Abdominal circumference reduced by 6.3 cm 2 months after a single cryolipolysis treatment using a large applicator (Zeltiq, Zeltiq Ltd). At 4 months after treatment, circumference was reduced by 11 cm.

Pig studies preceded human clinical trials. Porcine adipocytes have been cultured, cooled, and examined to better understand the cryolipolysis process.[29] Although some cells in published studies showed apoptotic changes, those cultured at the coldest temperatures showed necrotic death. In an early study, a cooling device was applied to numerous body sites on 1 pig for 5 to 21 minutes at −7°C.[29] After 3.5 months, subcutaneous fat layer reduction reached 40% compared with untreated areas. Dosimetry evaluation in 4 pigs revealed increased and more long-lasting adipocyte inflammation on histology at relatively colder exposures. Another pig study reaffirmed the fat reduction effects, and also included histologic data over time.[30] Immediately after treatment, no changes were observed; however, in the days and weeks posttreatment, an inflammatory infiltrate appeared, lipids were phagocytosed, interlobular septae became thickened, and adipocytes were reduced. The histology correlates with the clinical finding that cryolipolysis effects are not immediate, but rather develop over months. Human studies followed animal preclinical trials. Clinical improvements have been demonstrated in common areas of excess fat, including areas on the abdomen (Figures 6-9 and 6-10), back and the so-called lower back, and flank "love handles." Reductions in the

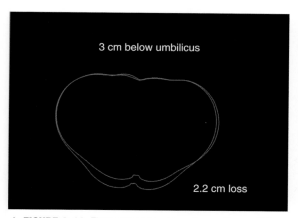

3 cm below umbilicus

2.2 cm loss

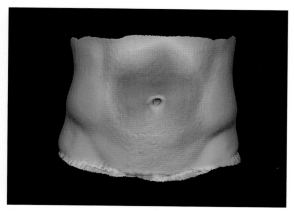

▲ **FIGURE 6-10** Three-dimensional imaging confirms a 2.2 cm reduction in abdominal circumference after a single cryolipolysis treatment of the lower abdomen (Zeltiq, Zeltiq Ltd) using a large applicator. Concentric circles represent pretreatment and posttreatment abdominal circumference as measured from axial view. Areas of greatest volume loss are colored red.

fat layer, assessed by ultrasound at follow-up treatments, are reported in ranges of 18.2% to 25.5%.[31-33]

Cryolipolysis appears generally safe. Minor bruising, erythema, and numbness have been reported, while long-term adverse effects are likely rare.[33] Since adipocytes are targeted, some have looked for effects on serum lipids and liver values over time. Among the pig studies, in which 15% to 30% body surface areas were treated, 1 reported a statistically significant change, namely, a fall in triglycerides, immediately after treatment.[29] This change was minor and attributed to preanesthesia fasting. Another pig study reports all lipid levels remained within normal limits.[30] In human studies, both lipid and liver levels have been measured without significant changes, except for 1 report of a fall in high-density lipoprotein (HDL) cholesterol that later returned to baseline.[33]

Cryolipolysis studies have also expressly looked for effects on peripheral nerves.[34] Transient sensory reduction, as determined by a neurologist, was found in 6 of 9 assessed, but sensation returned in fewer than 7 weeks. Histologic evaluation showed no lasting effects on nerve fibers. A careful medical history is needed to maintain safety. In particular, temperature-related conditions such as cryoglobulinemia, cold urticaria, and paroxysmal cold hemoglobinuria should be avoided. When the proper candidate is selected, cryolipolysis represents a generally safe, effective, and simple option for body contouring.

LOW-LEVEL LIGHT THERAPY (LLLT)

LLLT is a category of treatment utilizing low-energy laser or light energy with the goal of prevention or treatment of a variety of diseases. LLLT by definition does not cause any gross visual or temperature changes in the tissue during treatment and falls within parameters of a power of 10^{-3} to 10^{-1} W, wavelength of 300 to 10,600 nm, pulse rate of 0 to 5000 Hz, pulse duration of 1 to 500 milliseconds, total irradiation time of 10 to 3000 seconds, intensity (power/area) of 10^{-2} to 10^{0} W/cm^2, and dose (power × irradiation time/area) of 10^{-2} to 10^{2} J/cm^2.[35,36] All skin phototypes may be treated. LLLT utilizes extremely low doses of energy and has to date most often shown minimal-to-mild and variable efficacy in many studies, leading many to question the efficacy and/or cost-benefit ratio. Some investigators have reported cellular changes following LLLT, and a small number of studies have reported positive effects in body contouring.

One LLLT device (Zerona, Erchonia Medical), a 635-nm diode array device positioned within 6 in of the body for a 20-minute treatment to each side of the body, has been marketed for body contouring. The treatments are recommended by the company to be performed every 48 hours for a total of 6 to 12 treatments, and patients are also advised to walk 30 minutes daily, drink at least 1 L of water, and take a supplement containing niacin and other compounds.[3] The mechanism of action is reported to be through cytochrome oxidase modulation, leading to creation of a temporary adipocyte membrane pore with possible egress of intracellular fat.[3] A study reported LLLT improved skin retraction and postoperative recovery after liposuction.[3] Some LLLT studies have reported reductions in circumference of treated areas. One study giving 8 LLLT treatments over 4 weeks reported a 2.15 cm waist circumference reduction by the completion of the eighth treatment.[37] Another study of 689 subjects treated 3 times per week for 2 weeks reported a mean circumferential reduction of 3.27 in in the waist, hips, and thighs.[38] A clinical trial of the Zerona device reported a 2.8 cm circumferential reduction compared with the sham treatment group and improvement in patient satisfaction (70% in treatment group vs 26% satisfied in sham group).[3] However, a split-body study of 5 subjects failed to show any statistically significant difference as a result of the Zerona device.[39] The device appears very safe, with LLLT showing little to no risk in published studies, although the results remain minimal or highly variable in published studies.

SUCTION AND/OR MASSAGE DEVICES

Suction and massage devices were introduced more than 20 years ago for the purpose of body contouring. Mechanical stress may stimulate dermal fibroblasts to increase neocollagenesis, and is theorized to also help to flush lipoproteins from adipocytes or to promote more complete destruction and clearance of injured adipocytes into lymphatic channels.[3] Suction and massage have shown minimal-to-mild benefits in circumferential reduction, with significantly lower efficacy than most of the above-described energy-based devices. In addition, these devices often recommend lengthy and multiple treatment sessions. For these reasons, they have generally not been the preferred method of body contouring treatment and have been used more frequently as an adjunctive method before, during, or after other energy-based body contouring treatments.

For example, suction is a component of some popular RF-based treatments (VelaShape, Syneron/Candela; SmoothShapes, Cynosure; Reaction, Viora Ltd). In addition, massage is frequently performed after cryolipolysis to reduce the temporary tissue hardening and studies are being performed to evaluate whether this improves efficacy of the treatment.

BODY CONTOURING DRUGS

The introduction of evidence-based systemic or local drug treatments represents an important area of therapeutic advancement in body contouring. Several fat-reducing drugs are under investigation. A synthetic injectable form of sodium deoxycholate (ATX-101, Kythera Biopharmaceuticals), a biologic detergent, is being evaluated for the reduction of submental fat deposits. Another injectable agent under investigation for the reduction of local fat deposits (LIPO-102, Lithera Inc) is a combination of the β_2-adrenergic agonist salmeterol xinafoate, believed to induce lipolysis in adipocytes, and the glucocorticoid fluticasone proprionate that likely enhances the action of salmeterol. Clinical trials of LIPO-102 have shown weekly injections for 4 to 8 weeks resulted in significant reductions in abdominal circumference and volume by 3-dimensional imaging.[40] Drug therapy presents a developing alternative or adjuvant treatment option for patients seeking body contouring. FDA-approved drugs should be distinguished from many unregulated, incompletely characterized, or unsafe substances marketed for the purpose of body contouring that unfortunately have resulted in serious adverse events in a number of cases.[41]

CONCLUSIONS

Focused ultrasound, RF, cryolipolysis, and other noninvasive body contouring treatments continue to improve in efficacy and represent excellent options for the improvement of body contour. Safety is generally excellent, although appropriate training, parameters, and patient selection remain important prerequisites. Drugs influencing fat storage and volume represent an important developing treatment option. Adjuvant or alternative therapies such as massage, suction, and infrared heat may provide additional benefits. With the development of successful body contouring treatments, patients suffering from excess fat or contour changes can now benefit from noninvasive mild-to-moderate reductions of fat, resulting in a more healthy appearance and ultimately greater patient satisfaction.

REFERENCES

1. Brightman L, Weiss E, Chapas AM, et al. Improvement in arm and post-partum abdominal and flank subcutaneous fat deposits and skin laxity using a bipolar radiofrequency, infrared, vacuum and mechanical massage device. *Lasers Surg Med.* 2009;41(10):791–798.
2. American Society of Plastic Surgeons. 2011 plastic surgery procedural statistics. <http://www.plasticsurgery.org/news-and-resources/2011-statistics-.html>.
3. Mulholland RS, Paul MD, Chalfoun C. Noninvasive body contouring with radiofrequency, ultrasound, cryolipolysis, and low-level laser therapy. *Clin Plast Surg.* 2011;38(3):503–520, vii-iii.
4. Weiss ET, Barzilai O, Brightman L, et al. Three-dimensional surface imaging for clinical trials: improved precision and reproducibility in circumference measurements of thighs and abdomens. *Lasers Surg Med.* 2009;41(10):767–773.
5. Kim KH, Geronemus RG. Laser lipolysis using a novel 1,064 nm Nd:YAG laser. *Dermatol Surg.* 2006;32(2):241–248 [discussion 7].
6. McBean JC, Katz BE. A pilot study of the efficacy of a 1,064 and 1,320 nm sequentially firing Nd:YAG laser device for lipolysis and skin tightening. *Lasers Surg Med.* 2009;41(10):779–784.
7. Fitzpatrick R, Geronemus R, Goldberg D, Kaminer M, Kilmer S, Ruiz-Esparza J. Multicenter study of noninvasive radiofrequency for periorbital tissue tightening. *Lasers Surg Med.* 2003;33(4):232–242.
8. Nahm WK, Su TT, Rotunda AM, Moy RL. Objective changes in brow position, superior palpebral crease, peak angle of the eyebrow, and jowl surface area after volumetric radiofrequency treatments to half of the face. *Dermatol Surg.* 2004;30(6):922–928 [discussion 8].
9. Alster TS, Tanzi E. Improvement of neck and cheek laxity with a nonablative radiofrequency device: a lifting experience. *Dermatol Surg.* 2004;30(4 pt 1):503–507 [discussion 7].
10. Fritz M, Counters JT, Zelickson BD. Radiofrequency treatment for middle and lower face laxity. *Arch Facial Plast Surg.* 2004;6(6):370–373.
11. Bogle MA, Ubelhoer N, Weiss RA, Mayoral F, Kaminer MS. Evaluation of the multiple pass, low fluence algorithm for radiofrequency tightening of the lower face. *Lasers Surg Med.* 2007;39(3):210–217.
12. Anolik R, Chapas AM, Brightman LA, Geronemus RG. Radiofrequency devices for body shaping: a review and study of 12 patients. *Semin Cutan Med Surg.* 2009;28(4):236–243.
13. Sukal SA, Geronemus RG. Thermage: the nonablative radiofrequency for rejuvenation. *Clin Dermatol.* 2008;26(6):602–607.
14. van der Lugt C, Romero C, Ancona D, Al-Zarouni M, Perera J, Trelles MA. A multicenter study of cellulite treatment with a variable emission radio frequency system. *Dermatol Ther.* 2009;22(1):74–84.
15. Goldberg DJ, Fazeli A, Berlin AL. Clinical, laboratory, and MRI analysis of cellulite treatment with a unipolar radiofrequency device. *Dermatol Surg.* 2008;34(2):204–209 [discussion 9].
16. Manuskiatti W, Wachirakaphan C, Lektrakul N, Varothai S. Circumference reduction and cellulite treatment with a TriPollar radiofrequency device: a pilot study. *J Eur Acad Dermatol Venereol.* 2009;23(7):820–827.

17. Alster TS, Tanzi EL. Cellulite treatment using a novel combination radiofrequency, infrared light, and mechanical tissue manipulation device. *J Cosmet Laser Ther.* 2005; 7(2):81–85.

18. Zelickson BD, Kist D, Bernstein E, et al. Histological and ultrastructural evaluation of the effects of a radiofrequency-based nonablative dermal remodeling device: a pilot study. *Arch Dermatol.* 2004;140(2): 204–209.

19. Kaplan H, Gat A. Clinical and histopathological results following TriPollar radiofrequency skin treatments. *J Cosmet Laser Ther.* 2009;11(2):78–84.

20. Trelles MA, Mordon SR. Adipocyte membrane lysis observed after cellulite treatment is performed with radiofrequency. *Aesthetic Plast Surg.* 2009;33(1):125–128.

21. Moreno-Moraga J, Valero-Altes T, Riquelme AM, Isarria-Marcosy MI, de la Torre JR. Body contouring by noninvasive transdermal focused ultrasound. *Lasers Surg Med.* 2007;39(4):315–323.

22. Brown SA, Greenbaum L, Shtukmaster S, Zadok Y, Ben-Ezra S, Kushkuley L. Characterization of nonthermal focused ultrasound for noninvasive selective fat cell disruption (lysis): technical and preclinical assessment. *Plast Reconstr Surg.* 2009;124(1):92–101.

23. Haar GT, Coussios C. High intensity focused ultrasound: physical principles and devices. *Int J Hyperthermia.* 2007; 23(2):89–104.

24. Shek S, Yu C, Yeung CK, Kono T, Chan HH. The use of focused ultrasound for non-invasive body contouring in Asians. *Lasers Surg Med.* 2009;41(10):751–759.

25. Teitelbaum SA, Burns JL, Kubota J, et al. Noninvasive body contouring by focused ultrasound: safety and efficacy of the Contour I device in a multicenter, controlled, clinical study. *Plast Reconstr Surg.* 2007;120(3):779–789 [discussion 90].

26. Fatemi A. High-intensity focused ultrasound effectively reduces adipose tissue. *Semin Cutan Med Surg.* 2009; 28(4):257–262.

27. Epstein EH Jr, Oren ME. Popsicle panniculitis. *N Engl J Med.* 1970;282(17):966–967.

28. Diamantis S, Bastek T, Groben P, Morrell D. Subcutaneous fat necrosis in a newborn following icebag application for treatment of supraventricular tachycardia. *J Perinatol.* 2006;26(8):518–520.

29. Manstein D, Laubach H, Watanabe K, Farinelli W, Zurakowski D, Anderson RR. Selective cryolysis: a novel method of non-invasive fat removal. *Lasers Surg Med.* 2008;40(9):595–604.

30. Zelickson B, Egbert BM, Preciado J, et al. Cryolipolysis for noninvasive fat cell destruction: initial results from a pig model. *Dermatol Surg.* 2009;35(10):1462–1470.

31. Riopelle JG, Tsai M, Kovach B. Lipid and liver function effects of the cryolipolysis procedure in a study of male love handle reduction. Annual Meeting of the American Society for Laser Medicine and Surgery; 2009; National Harbor, MD.

32. Dover J, Burns J, Coleman S, et al. A prospective clinical study of non-invasive cryolipolysis for subcutaneous fat layer reduction—interim report of available subject data. Annual Meeting of the American Society for Laser Medicine and Surgery; 2009; National Harbor, MD.

33. Klein KB, Zelickson B, Riopelle JG, et al. Non-invasive cryolipolysis for subcutaneous fat reduction does not affect serum lipid levels or liver function tests. *Lasers Surg Med.* 2009;41(10):785–790.

34. Coleman SR, Sachdeva K, Egbert BM, Preciado J, Allison J. Clinical efficacy of noninvasive cryolipolysis and its effects on peripheral nerves. *Aesthetic Plast Surg.* 2009; 33(4):482–488.

35. Posten W, Wrone DA, Dover JS, Arndt KA, Silapunt S, Alam M. Low-level laser therapy for wound healing: mechanism and efficacy. *Dermatol Surg.* 2005;31(3): 334–340.

36. Schindl A, Schindl M, Pernerstorfer-Schon H, Schindl L. Low-intensity laser therapy: a review. *J Investig Med.* 2000;48(5):312–326.

37. Caruso-Davis MK, Guillot TS, Podichetty VK, et al. Efficacy of low-level laser therapy for body contouring and spot fat reduction. *Obes Surg.* 2011;21(6):722–729.

38. Jackson RF, Stern FA, Neira R, Ortiz-Neira CL, Maloney J. Application of low-level laser therapy for noninvasive body contouring. *Lasers Surg Med.* 2012;44(3):211–217.

39. Elm CM, Wallander ID, Endrizzi B, Zelickson BD. Efficacy of a multiple diode laser system for body contouring. *Lasers Surg Med.* 2011;43(2):114–121.

40. Duncan D, Rotunda AM. Injectable therapies for localized fat loss: state of the art. *Clin Plast Surg.* 2011;38(3): 489–501, vii.

41. Atiyeh BS, Ibrahim AE, Dibo SA. Cosmetic mesotherapy: between scientific evidence, science fiction, and lucrative business. *Aesthetic Plast Surg.* 2008;32(6): 842–849.

CHAPTER 7

Laser and Light Therapies for the Treatment of Acne Vulgaris

Christine A. Liang, Julie K. Karen, and Elizabeth K. Hale

■ OVERVIEW

Acne vulgaris is a common, often chronic disease affecting 85% of teenagers and persisting in up to 50% of adults.[1-3] The psychosocial impact of acne is significant and has been shown to cause low self-esteem, depression, and decreased quality of life.[4,5] The estimated annual cost of acne treatment is over $1 billion in the United States.[6] Conventional medical treatments for acne, both topical and oral, have side effects making them inconvenient and sometimes intolerable for patients. Thus, a search for other treatments has led to investigations on the effectiveness and tolerability of laser- and light-based therapies. In recent years usage of these devices has gained in popularity among dermatologists.[7]

Laser- and light-based treatments can be used to improve comedonal and inflammatory acne, oily skin, and acne scarring. Like the medical treatment of acne, laser and light therapies attempt to target key pathogenic factors producing acne lesions: sebum production by sebaceous glands, *Propionibacterium acnes* proliferation and inflammation, and follicular hyperproliferation.[8] Depending on the wavelength and technique used, these devices are thought to work by directly killing *P. acnes*, damaging sebaceous glands, or both.[9] *P. acnes* produce endogenous porphyrins within sebaceous glands. These porphyrins are activated by light energy to form reactive oxygen species that kill bacteria.[10] Peak porphyrin absorptions lie in the visible light range, with maximal absorption in the blue light wavelength at 415 nm.[11] Blue, red, and green light individually decrease *P. acnes* counts without damaging sebaceous glands.[10] It is thought that direct thermal damage to sebaceous glands occurs with the use of nonablative infrared lasers (1320, 1450, 1540 nm), as they have greater depth of penetration.[12] More recently, photopneumatic therapy combining vacuum suction and broadband light has been used to treat comedonal and inflammatory lesions.[13]

■ CHOOSING THE RIGHT LASER OR LIGHT SOURCE FOR THE LESION

It is important to choose the right laser or light source for the type of acne. Table 7-1 lists all the laser/light sources that have been studied for the treatment of acne vulgaris. Depending on the patient's skin, a combination of these devices can be used, as well as combining these treatments with medical therapy. The following sections of this chapter will detail methods for using selected lasers that we use most commonly for the treatment of acne vulgaris.

TABLE 7-1
Devices for the Treatment of Acne Vulgaris

ACNE TARGET	LASER OR LIGHT SOURCE
Inflammatory	Visible light lasers
	Red light
	Blue light
	532-nm KTP laser
	585- and 595-nm pulsed dye laser
	Intense pulsed light
	Photodynamic therapy
	Photopneumatic therapy
Sebaceous gland activity	Infrared lasers
	1450-nm diode
	1320-nm Nd:YAG
	1540-nm erbium glass
	Photodynamic therapy
	Radio frequency
Comedonal	Photopneumatic therapy

Targeting Inflammatory Lesions

BLUE LIGHT Maximal porphyrin absorption lies in the blue light range (415 nm); accordingly, irradiation of *P. acnes* with blue light leads to bacterial destruction.[14] Multiple studies have looked at the use of blue light for acne vulgaris, reporting 60% to 70% mean reduction in inflammatory lesions.[15-19] The studies had a relatively small number of patients and used different durations of light exposure and number of treatments, making it difficult to determine the optimal regimen. The ClearLight device (Lumenis Ltd, Santa Clara, California) has shown the best results in studies, although no head-to-head study comparing blue light devices has been performed. A small study ($n = 12$) using Blu-U (Dusa Pharmaceuticals, Inc, Wilmington, Massachusetts) showed a 34% average reduction in inflammatory acne counts after 4 weeks of twice-weekly blue light therapy.[11]

ClearLight uses a high-intensity (fluence 90 mW/cm^2), narrow-band (405–420 nm) blue light and can be safely used on all Fitzpatrick skin types. It can easily be used to treat the face, chest, and back. No topical anesthetic is required. Time of exposure varies from 8 to 15 minutes in the studies and was repeated twice weekly for 4 to 5 weeks. An air-cooling device (Zimmer; MedizinSystems, Irvine, California) can be utilized if desired by the patient, but most patients do not feel significant pain or excessive heat during the treatments, in contrast to topical photodynamic therapy (PDT) using the blue light. In addition, therapy-induced side effects such as erythema or irritation are not usually seen. In the 8 studies examining blue light for mild-to-moderate acne vulgaris, most reported no side effects at all; however, 2 patients reported dryness and 1 study reported worsening of nodulocystic acne in 20% of the study patients.[16,17] ClearLight is well tolerated by patients and easy to use; however, acne clearing can be variable and relapse rates are high after discontinuation of therapy.

COMBINATION OF BLUE AND RED LIGHT Although the strongest porphyrin photoexcitation coefficient lies in the 407- to 420-nm band, a limitation of blue light is its poor penetration to reach the poryphrins in the sebaceous follicles. Red light (660 nm) has increased depth of penetration into the skin and may also have anti-inflammatory effects. One randomized, open-label study ($n = 107$) of mild-to-moderate acne compared mixed blue-red light with blue light alone or 5% benzoyl peroxide. Study patients received 15 minutes of daily irradiation (cumulative dose

320 J/cm^2 for blue light and 202 J/cm^2 for red light) over a 12-week treatment period. The results showed a 76% improvement in inflammatory lesions with mixed blue-red light and 58% improvement in comedones, which was statistically superior compared with blue light or benzoyl peroxide.[18] The authors conclude that phototherapy with mixed blue-red light, probably by combining antibacterial and anti-inflammatory action, is an effective means of treating mild-to-moderate acne vulgaris with no significant short-term adverse effects. However, the tedious nature of a regimen requiring daily treatments limits the utility of this treatment.

KTP LASER The potassium titanyl phosphate (KTP) 532-nm green light pulsed laser also activates bacterial porphyrins while penetrating more deeply than blue light modalities. It has been shown to improve short-term acne severity with no side effects. In a split-face study, the laser (Laserscope, San Jose, California) was applied in a paintbrush technique with continuous contact cooling across the entire surface to deliver a cumulative laser fluence of 16,000 J/cm^2 to the treatment side by applying individual pulses of 12 J/cm^2 with a 30- to 40-millisecond pulse width and a 1 to 5 Hz frequency repetition rate.[20] Each patient received 2 treatments per week for 2 weeks. There was a 34.9% and 20.7% reduction in acne severity score at 1- and 4-week posttreatments, a modest short-term improvement. Of note, no side effects were seen, making this a very well-tolerated treatment. Another study showed no difference between once- and twice-weekly applications.[21] Randomized controlled trials are lacking for KTP lasers in acne treatment.

PULSED DYE LASER The flashlamp-pumped pulsed dye laser (PDL) is used for selective photothermolysis of the vascular component of acne inflammation, and is also believed to act by directly killing bacteria.[8] The 585- or 595-nm PDL penetrates deeper into the dermis than blue light. Results are mixed on the efficacy of this laser in acne vulgaris. A randomized, blinded, placebo-controlled trial ($n = 41$) using a 585-nm PDL (5 mm spot size, 1.5–3.0 J/cm^2, and 350 microseconds pulse, NLite System, ICN Pharmaceuticals, Inc, Costa Mesa, California) showed 49% reduction in inflammatory lesion counts versus 10% in controls at 12-week follow-up after 1 treatment.[22] However, another study using the same device did not show statistically significant changes in acne lesion counts.[23] Furthermore, PDL used as adjuvant therapy to topical treatment showed no superior benefit than using topicals alone.[24] An uncontrolled study employing the long-pulsed 595-nm PDL (7 mm spot size, 9.5–11 J/cm^2, 10 milliseconds pulse) with 2 successive treatments at 4-week intervals found significant acne clearance.[25] Side effects with PDL include transient purpura, erythema, and potential for postinflammatory hyperpigmentation.[23,26]

PHOTODYNAMIC THERAPY PDT treats both inflammation and sebaceous gland activity and will be discussed in detail later in this chapter.

Targeting Sebaceous Gland Activity

For patients who have increased sebaceous gland activity (facial or truncal acne lesions and oily skin), nonablative infrared lasers that penetrate deeper into the dermis are useful. These wavelengths are long enough to target sebaceous glands while epidermal cooling systems protect the surface. Three wavelengths (1320, 1450, and 1540 nm) have been utilized in clinical trials for acne vulgaris.[8]

1450-nm LASER Of the infrared lasers, the 1450-nm laser has been the best studied for the treatment of acne vulgaris and in small uncontrolled studies shows efficacy maintained over a 12-month period.[27] In a study of patients ($n = 19$) with inflammatory facial acne vulgaris, all patients had a reduction in acne lesions, and mean counts decreased by 83% after 3 treatments.[28] Notably, a recent randomized split-face, investigator-blinded clinical trial did not show the treated side to be superior to the control side. However, both sides of the face showed improvement in acne, and the authors postulate a possible systemic effect of the laser.[29]

The 1450-nm laser (Smoothbeam™, Candela Corp, Wayland, Massachusetts) is most commonly used to treat acne on the face, neck, and back. All Fitzpatrick skin types can be treated. Topical anesthetic applied 30 to 60 minutes prior to treatment is highly recommended as the treatment can be painful.

With Fitzpatrick skin types I to III, settings are commonly a 6 mm spot size at energy fluences from 11 to 14 J/cm^2, and the dynamic cooling device (DCD) at 30 to 40 milliseconds. When treating skin types IV to VI, the cryogen is decreased to avoid cryogen-induced hyperpigmentation. A lower energy fluence (11 J/cm^2) and DCD setting (30 milliseconds) can be used when treating acne on the neck or other thin-skinned areas. Most commonly, a single-pass technique is used over

the treatment area with double passes to areas of increased breakouts. Because of the pain often associated with higher energy levels, 1 split-face study examined using lower fluences (11 J/cm^2 or lower) with stacked double pulses or double-pass treatment of single pulses.[30] Stacking pulses resulted in slightly higher efficacy (57.6% vs 49.8% reduction of lesions); however, 2 patients in the stacked pulse group experienced cryogen-induced transient hyperpigmentation. Thus, in patients who cannot tolerate the pain at higher energy levels, one should consider reducing energy levels and using a single-pulse, multiple-pass technique. Intervals between treatments are 3 to 4 weeks, typically requiring 3 to 5 treatments for best results.

The most common side effects are pain, erythema, and edema at treatment sites, lasting from 30 minutes to up to 24 hours after the procedure. Some patients report transient worsening of their acne lasting about 1 week, and patients should be warned about this possibility. Posttreatment, apply ice or cool packs followed by a moisturizer with sunscreen. Patients should be counseled on careful photoprotection following the procedure.

Patients can expect a decrease in lesion counts and less oily skin. In a study using the 1450-nm laser, lesion counts were reduced by 75% with lasting results at 12-month follow-up.[27] Another study using the 1450-nm laser with cryogen spray cooling on inflammatory acne lesions of the back reported 98% decrease in lesion counts, compared with 6% with cryogen spray alone.[31] In both of these studies, side effects were minimal and transient. Infrared lasers also promote collagen remodeling that may improve the appearance of acne scars. This makes the infrared lasers an excellent choice in patients who have active acne vulgaris and acne scarring.

PHOTODYNAMIC THERAPY PDT involves the application of a photosensitizer followed by irradiation with a light source. This results in a photo-oxidative reaction and cytotoxic effect on *P. acnes* and sebaceous glands.[14] Three photosensitizers have been studied for PDT of acne: aminolevulinic acid (ALA), methyl aminolevulinate (MAL), and indocyanin green (ICG). Irradiation with blue or red light, IPL, diode, and PDL has been used for acne. Of these, activation with red light has shown the best long-term results in acne.[32,33] Red light penetrates more deeply into the dermis reaching the level of the sebaceous glands. Multiple studies have shown significant reductions in acne lesion counts and decreased sebum production.[32–37]

The optimal treatment regimen using PDT is unclear, as the various studies performed have used different incubation and irradiation times. Clinical outcomes will vary depending on skin preparation, drug applied and incubation time, light source, and treatment parameters. Various skin preparations have been used for PDT. Degreasing the skin should increase drug penetration, although no comparative studies of pretreatment preparations have been performed. Pretreatment cleansing with 70% isopropyl alcohol, 2% salicylic acid, mild skin cleansers, acetone scrub, and microdermabrasion has been used.[38] Over half of the studies apply the drug under occlusion for increased penetration. Care should be taken to apply the medication uniformly to the treatment area.

For ALA and MAL, studies use incubation times ranging from 15 minutes to 4 hours, with the majority using a 3-hour incubation.[32–34] These long incubations (3–4 hours) followed by red light exposure have shown acne remissions in long-term follow-up. Short-contact PDT (10- to 30-minute incubation) with lower fluences or other light sources (IPL, blue light, PDL) has been tried in an effort to make PDT more tolerable to patients with regard to time and cutaneous side effects. However, the results of these regimens are less efficacious than long incubation times with red light.[38] MAL and ALA appear to have similar efficacy (only studied with long incubation time plus red light), supported by 1 head-to-head comparison study.[32,33]

A wide range of fluences has been used in PDT for acne vulgaris. When high-fluence (150 J/cm^2) red light treatment is employed over several treatment sessions, significant and long-term improvement in acne is seen with a decrease in sebum production (Figure 7-1). Alternatively, treatment of inflammatory acne with superficial PDT can be performed at low fluences and activation with IPL, PDL, or blue light. Relative to red light PDT, these treatments are less painful with fewer side effects; however, lesion reduction is modest and temporary.[38]

Adverse effects are the main disadvantage of PDT. Common reactions include moderate-to-severe pain, erythema (lasting 3–5 days but up to 4 weeks), edema (1–4 days), and transient skin tanning. Less common are a sterile pustular eruption, crusts (starting in 2–4 days), acute transient acne flare (3–4 weeks posttreatment), exfoliation (4–10 days), and postinflammatory hyperpigmentation. Rarely, blisters or contact hypersensitivity may occur.[38] Antiviral prophylaxis is recommended in those with a history of recurrent mucocutaneous herpes simplex. Reactions to PDT are often severe enough to require discontinuation of treatment or absence from work/school. Pain during PDT can be minimized by spritzing cool water and using fan ventilation, or with use of a forced-air

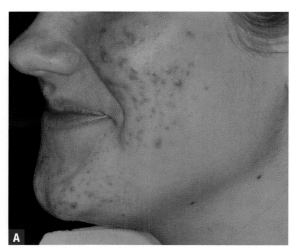 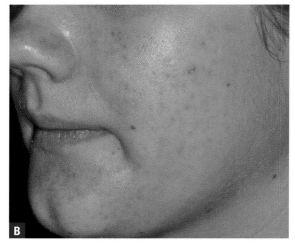

▲ **FIGURE 7-1** A young female patient with noninflammatory and inflammatory acne (**A**) demonstrates significant improvement (**B**) one month following two monthly PDT treatments (ALA incubation for 90 minutes followed by photo-illumination with pulsed dye laser (V-beam, Candela, Wayland, MA) (10 mm, 10 ms, 8 J/cm^2) followed by red light (Omnilux LED, 633 nm) (GlobalMed Technologies Co., Glenn Ellen, CA). Photos courtesy of Dr. Vic Ross.

skin cooling device (Zimmer; MedizinSystems).[38] Patients should be advised to avoid bright light exposure for 48 hours, including UV and indoor visible light. Patients should be aware that sunscreens do not effectively block all visible light wavelengths; thus, avoidance is preferred. Normally, complete skin healing is seen at 1 week, although skin erythema and hyperpigmentation has been reported to last up to 4 weeks posttreatment, particularly in darker-skinned patients.

RADIO FREQUENCY Nonablative radio-frequency devices have primarily been studied for acne scar remodeling but have also been utilized for inflammatory acne vulgaris. The postulated mechanism of action is a reduction of sebaceous gland activity and dermal remodeling by heating of the dermis, or thermotherapy. In an uncontrolled trial of 22 patients with moderate-to-severe inflammatory acne (average fluence per energy delivery was 72 J/cm^2, ThermaCool TC; Thermage, Inc, Hayward, California), an "excellent" response was found in 82% with no side effects.[39] A combination device of pulsed light and radio-frequency energy (Aurora AC, Syneron Medical Ltd, Yokneam, Israel)

was evaluated in an uncontrolled trial of patients with moderate acne and led to a mean lesion count reduction of 47% and histologic evidence of decreased sebaceous gland size.[40] Further controlled trials with longer follow-up times are needed to better define the benefit of this modality.

Comedonal Acne

PHOTOPNEUMATIC THERAPY Photopneumatic technology (Isolaz and PPx, Aesthera Corp, Pleasanton, California) uses a gentle vacuum to draw target tissue into the treatment tip and delivers intense pulsed light (400–1200 nm) to dermal targets. The vacuum tip elevates the sebaceous gland, opens the pore, and evacuates sebaceous blockage. This is the only current device that treats comedonal lesions and reduces acne lesions by directly removing trapped sebum.[13,41] Broadband light is then delivered through the tip and thought to provide antibacterial and anti-inflammatory effect.[13] In a retrospective review (*n* = 56), the median physician-rated clearance was 50% after a single treatment and 90% after 4 treatments[42] (Figure 7-2). No long-term follow-up has been performed.

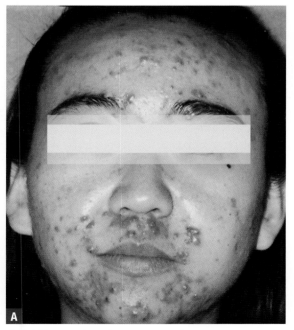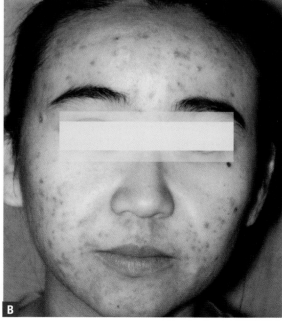

▲ **FIGURE 7-2** Pre- (**A**) and post- (**B**) five treatments with photopneumatic therapy (Isolaz, Aesthera Inc, Pleasanton, CA) with notable improvement. Photos courtesy of Dr. Vic Narurkar.

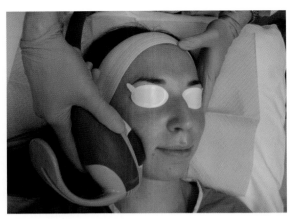

▲ **FIGURE 7-3** A female patient appears comfortable while undergoing treatment with photopneumatic therapy (Isolaz, Aesthera Inc, Pleasanton, CA).

Photopneumatic therapy can be used in all Fitzpatrick skin types. Skin is cleansed with mild soap and water to remove debris prior to treatment. No topical anesthetic is required, as the procedure is well tolerated (Figure 7-3). Thus, this treatment is a good option for pregnant or lactating patients, for whom avoidance of a topical anesthetic is often desired. To reduce discomfort, a cryogen spray (TipSpray, Aesthera Corp) can be used to cool the treatment tip before skin irradiation and after every 3 to 5 pulses. Filter tips of 400 nm can be used for skin types I to III and a filter of 580 nm for type IV skin. Pneumatic energy of 3 psi is applied with recommended delivery of fluences ranging from 3.6 to 4.2 J/cm^2. A single pass to the entire face is performed, followed by a second pass to more severely affected areas as indicated. A gentle skin moisturizer and sunscreen are recommended for post-skin care.

The most common side effects are temporary erythema, resolving several hours after treatment, and mild pain during the procedure.[13,42] Worsening of acne can be seen during the first week after treatment and patients should be made aware of this. However, adverse events such as scarring, dyspigmentation, and persistent erythema are not seen.

At-home over-the-counter anti-acne devices. In recent years, there has been an explosion in the development of devices designed for at-home treatment of acne. These small, user-friendly, low-energy devices employ heat, light, or a combination of both. Several light-emitting diode (LED) devices emitting blue and/or red light, as well as a few heat-based (infrared) devices, are now available. A comprehensive overview of these devices can be found in Chapter 10.

CONCLUSION

Laser- and light-based treatments are another option in the armamentarium for acne vulgaris. They can be used as monotherapy or in conjunction with other medications. For patients who are noncompliant, cannot tolerate long-term antibiotic therapy or isotretinoin use, or have failed conventional therapies, treatment with a laser/light-based source offers a promising alternative. However, patients should understand that while these devices are convenient and minimally invasive, the downsides are often cost and the requirement of multiple office visits, as well as pain and erythema. Realistic expectations should be set, as there are some patients who show only modest benefit, and most individuals will require several treatments.

We consider laser- and light-based therapies to be a useful complement to oral and topical treatments, or as an alternative option when patients have failed or cannot tolerate conventional therapies. They are particularly useful as an adjunct when a patient has reached 40% to 50% clearance with topical therapies. In our practice, infrared laser treatments are sometimes considered as part of first-line treatment, in addition to topical and oral medications, in patients who have active scarring and are looking for treatment for both acne and scars. The reader should refer to Chapter 5, detailing fractional resurfacing which is the preferred treatment for patients with acne scarring, without active acne lesions. Although further studies need to be performed to determine optimal treatment regimens and long-term follow-up, laser- and light-based therapies show promising results in the treatment of acne vulgaris.

REFERENCES

1. Webster GF. Acne vulgaris. *BMJ*. 2002;325(7362):475–479.
2. Goulden V, McGeown CH, Cunliffe WJ. The familial risk of adult acne: a comparison between first-degree relatives of affected and unaffected individuals. *Br J Dermatol*. 1999;141(2):297–300.
3. Goulden V, Stables GI, Cunliffe WJ. Prevalence of facial acne in adults. *J Am Acad Dermatol*. 1999;41(4):577–580.
4. Thomas DR. Psychosocial effects of acne. *J Cutan Med Surg*. 2004;8(suppl 4):3–5.
5. Layton AM. Psychosocial aspects of acne vulgaris. *J Cutan Med Surg*. 1998;2(suppl 3):19–23.

6. James WD. Clinical practice. Acne. *N Engl J Med*. 2005; 352(14):1463–1472.

7. Thiboutot D, Gollnick H, Bettoli V, et al. New insights into the management of acne: an update from the Global Alliance to Improve Outcomes in Acne group. *J Am Acad Dermatol*. 2009;60(5 suppl):S1–S50.

8. Kim GK, Del Rosso JQ. Laser and light-based therapies for acne vulgaris: a current guide based on available data. *J Drugs Dermatol*. 2010;9(6):614–621.

9. Hamilton FL, Car J, Lyons C, Car M, Layton A, Majeed A. Laser and other light therapies for the treatment of acne vulgaris: systematic review. *Br J Dermatol*. 2009;160(6): 1273–1285.

10. Sigurdsson V, Knulst AC, van Weelden H. Phototherapy of acne vulgaris with visible light. *Dermatology*. 1997; 194(3):256–260.

11. Gold MH, Rao J, Goldman MP, et al. A multicenter clinical evaluation of the treatment of mild to moderate inflammatory acne vulgaris of the face with visible blue light in comparison to topical 1% clindamycin antibiotic solution. *J Drugs Dermatol*. 2005;4(1):64–70.

12. Lloyd JR, Mirkov M. Selective photothermolysis of the sebaceous glands for acne treatment. *Lasers Surg Med*. 2002;31(2):115–120.

13. Shamban AT, Enokibori M, Narurkar V, Wilson D. Photopneumatic technology for the treatment of acne vulgaris. *J Drugs Dermatol*. 2008;7(2):139–145.

14. Mariwalla K, Rohrer TE. Use of lasers and light-based therapies for treatment of acne vulgaris. *Lasers Surg Med*. 2005;37(5):333–342.

15. Elman M, Slatkine M, Harth Y. The effective treatment of acne vulgaris by a high-intensity, narrow band 405–420 nm light source. *J Cosmet Laser Ther*. 2003;5(2): 111–117.

16. Kawada A, Aragane Y, Kameyama H, Sangen Y, Tezuka T. Acne phototherapy with a high-intensity, enhanced, narrow-band, blue light source: an open study and in vitro investigation. *J Dermatol Sci*. 2002;30(2): 129–135.

17. Tzung TY, Wu KH, Huang ML. Blue light phototherapy in the treatment of acne. *Photodermatol Photoimmunol Photomed*. 2004;20(5):266–269.

18. Papageorgiou P, Katsambas A, Chu A. Phototherapy with blue (415 nm) and red (660 nm) light in the treatment of acne vulgaris. *Br J Dermatol*. 2000;142(5):973–978.

19. Morton CA, Scholefield RD, Whitehurst C, Birch J. An open study to determine the efficacy of blue light in the treatment of mild to moderate acne. *J Dermatolog Treat*. 2005;16(4):219–223.

20. Baugh WP, Kucaba WD. Nonablative phototherapy for acne vulgaris using the KTP 532 nm laser. *Dermatol Surg*. 2005;31(10):1290–1296.

21. Yilmaz O, Senturk N, Yuksel EP, et al. Evaluation of 532-nm KTP laser treatment efficacy on acne vulgaris with once and twice weekly applications. *J Cosmet Laser Ther*. 2011;13(6):303–307.

22. Seaton ED, Charakida A, Mouser PE, Grace I, Clement RM, Chu AC. Pulsed-dye laser treatment for inflammatory acne vulgaris: randomised controlled trial. *Lancet*. 2003;362(9393):1347–1352.

23. Orringer JS, Kang S, Hamilton T, et al. Treatment of acne vulgaris with a pulsed dye laser: a randomized controlled trial. *JAMA*. 2004;291(23):2834–2839.

24. Karsai S, Schmitt L, Raulin C. The pulsed-dye laser as an adjuvant treatment modality in acne vulgaris: a randomized controlled single-blinded trial. *Br J Dermatol*. 2010;163(2):395–401.

25. Yoon HJ, Lee DH, Kim SK, et al. Acne erythema improvement by long-pulsed 595-nm pulsed-dye laser treatment: a pilot study. *J Dermatolog Treat*. 2008;19(1):38.

26. Seaton ED, Mouser PE, Charakida A, Alam S, Seldon PM, Chu AC. Investigation of the mechanism of action of nonablative pulsed-dye laser therapy in photorejuvenation and inflammatory acne vulgaris. *Br J Dermatol*. 2006;155(4):748–755.

27. Jih MH, Friedman PM, Goldberg LH, Robles M, Glaich AS, Kimyai-Asadi A. The 1450-nm diode laser for facial inflammatory acne vulgaris: dose-response and 12-month follow-up study. *J Am Acad Dermatol*. 2006; 55(1):80–87.

28. Friedman PM, Jih MH, Kimyai-Asadi A, Goldberg LH. Treatment of inflammatory facial acne vulgaris with the 1450-nm diode laser: a pilot study. *Dermatol Surg*. 2004; 30(2 pt 1):147–151.

29. Darne S, Hiscutt EL, Seukeran DC. Evaluation of the clinical efficacy of the 1,450 nm laser in acne vulgaris: a randomized split-face, investigator-blinded clinical trial. *Br J Dermatol*. 2011;165(6):1256–1262.

30. Uebelhoer NS, Bogle MA, Dover JS, Arndt KA, Rohrer TE. Comparison of stacked pulses versus double-pass treatments of facial acne with a 1,450-nm laser. *Dermatol Surg*. 2007;33(5):552–559.

31. Paithankar DY, Ross EV, Saleh BA, Blair MA, Graham BS. Acne treatment with a 1,450 nm wavelength laser and cryogen spray cooling. *Lasers Surg Med*. 2002;31(2): 106–114.

32. Wiegell SR, Wulf HC. Photodynamic therapy of acne vulgaris using methyl aminolaevulinate: a blinded, randomized, controlled trial. *Br J Dermatol*. 2006;154(5): 969–976.

33. Wiegell SR, Wulf HC. Photodynamic therapy of acne vulgaris using 5-aminolevulinic acid versus methyl aminolevulinate. *J Am Acad Dermatol*. 2006;54(4): 647–651.

34. Hongcharu W, Taylor CR, Chang Y, Aghassi D, Suthamjariya K, Anderson RR. Topical ALA-photodynamic therapy for the treatment of acne vulgaris. *J Invest Dermatol*. 2000;115(2):183–192.

35. Taub AF. A comparison of intense pulsed light, combination radiofrequency and intense pulsed light, and blue light in photodynamic therapy for acne vulgaris. *J Drugs Dermatol*. 2007;6(10):1010–1016.

36. Horfelt C, Stenquist B, Larko O, Faergemann J, Wennberg AM. Photodynamic therapy for acne vulgaris: a pilot study of the dose-response and mechanism of action. *Acta Derm Venereol*. 2007;87(4):325–329.

37. Gold MH, Biron JA, Boring M, Bridges TM, Bradshaw VL. Treatment of moderate to severe inflammatory acne vulgaris: photodynamic therapy with 5-aminolevulinic acid and a novel advanced fluorescence technology pulsed light source. *J Drugs Dermatol*. 2007;6(3):319–322.

38. Sakamoto FH, Lopes JD, Anderson RR. Photodynamic therapy for acne vulgaris: a critical review from basics to clinical practice: part I. Acne vulgaris: when and why consider photodynamic therapy? *J Am Acad Dermatol*. 2010;63(2):183–193 [quiz 193–194].

39. Ruiz-Esparza J, Gomez JB. Nonablative radiofrequency for active acne vulgaris: the use of deep dermal heat in the treatment of moderate to severe active acne vulgaris (thermotherapy): a report of 22 patients. *Dermatol Surg.* 2003;29(4):333–339 [discussion 339].

40. Prieto VG, Zhang PS, Sadick NS. Evaluation of pulsed light and radiofrequency combined for the treatment of acne vulgaris with histologic analysis of facial skin biopsies. *J Cosmet Laser Ther.* 2005;7(2):63–68.

41. Omi T, Munavalli GS, Kawana S, Sato S. Ultrastructural evidence for thermal injury to pilosebaceous units during the treatment of acne using photopneumatic (PPX) therapy. *J Cosmet Laser Ther.* 2008;10(1):7–11.

42. Wanitphakdeedecha R, Tanzi EL, Alster TS. Photopneumatic therapy for the treatment of acne. *J Drugs Dermatol.* 2009;8(3):239–241.

CHAPTER 8

Photodynamic Therapy

Tracey Newlove and Robert T. Anolik

▮ BACKGROUND

Throughout the 20th century, scientists explored the use of photodynamic therapy (PDT) in medicine. PDT is a photochemical reaction in which a photosensitizing molecule, a light source, and tissue oxygen interact to produce targeted tissue destruction. Although PDT was initially thought to have great potential, its clinical use was postponed by worries of prolonged retention of the photosensitizer. By the late 20th century, 5-aminolevulinic acid (ALA) was shown to convert itself into an effective photosensitizing molecule, namely, protophorphyrin IX, in targeted tissue while also having a reasonable period of tissue retention.[1] This work paved the way for dermatologic applications. Topical PDT lends itself well to cutaneous disease because of the ease of application of a photosensitizer and delivery of light. In 1999, the Food and Drug Administration (FDA) approved the use of topical ALA and blue light for the treatment of actinic keratoses (AK), and its list of on- and off-label indications has since continued to expand.

▮ MECHANISM AND OVERVIEW OF TREATMENT

In PDT, the photosensitizing molecule absorbs photon energy from a light source. That energy bumps a stably orbiting electron into an excited state. The excited states are transient, but during this state tissue interaction is possible. Excited porphyrins are known to interact with tissue oxygen, producing singlet oxygen species and, in turn, intense oxidative damage. Ultimately, there is cell death, vascular injury, inflammation, and immunologic responses. Porphyrins are commonly used photosensitizers in dermatologic practice because of this interaction with oxygen.

PDT photosensitizers can be delivered systemically (oral or intravenous), topically, and intralesionally.

Systemic delivery is necessary when large-molecular-weight photosensitizers are used that do not penetrate the stratum corneum. They are often transported throughout the body bound to low-density lipoprotein (LDL) and gain entry into target tissue via LDL receptors. Photosensitizers, such as the commonly used ALA and methyl-esterified ALA (MAL), can be delivered topically because of their relatively low molecular weight and ability to penetrate into the epidermis. ALA and MAL subsequently convert into the photosensitive protoporphyrin IX (PpIX) as part of the porphyrin biosynthetic pathway. MAL represents an esterified form of ALA that is more lipophilic and therefore may penetrate more deeply into the skin. In addition, MAL has been shown to have greater selectivity than ALA for cells in lesional skin of AK[2] and acne.[3] As the cellular uptake mechanisms for these agents differ, the intensity of pain may be lower during PDT using MAL than that using ALA.

Both light- and laser-based systems can be used to activate PDT. Whatever source is selected, the chosen wavelength or wavelengths are between 400 and 800 nm for several reasons. These wavelengths avoid the carcinogenic effect of ultraviolet (UV) light (<400 nm), can deliver enough photon energy, and cover the absorption peaks of the porphyrin photosensitizers.

The treatment parameters in PDT notably include light dose. The light dose is reported as fluence, defined as the photons delivered per unit area, or joules per centimeter squared. Two of the other important parameters mentioned with PDT are power and irradiance. Power is defined as the photons delivered per unit time, or joules per second, and is reported as watts. Additionally, irradiance is defined as power per unit area, or watts per centimeter squared. The duration of light exposure to achieve a targeted light dose (ie, fluence) can be calculated by the following relationship: irradiance (W/cm^2) × exposure time (seconds) = fluence (J/cm^2).

At the time of writing this chapter, the FDA-approved uses of PDT for dermatologic conditions include ALA and MAL for topical PDT of nonhyperkeratotic AK. Protocols vary among physicians, and many off-label uses are being studied and integrated into practice. A variety of protocols and indications will be discussed in greater detail later in this chapter.

Generally speaking, for topical PDT, the first step is to remove all makeup, dirt, and skin oils. In our practice, this is performed with an alcohol cleanse followed by an acetone scrub. We encourage the patient to be in a well-ventilated room and breathe through the mouth to limit pungent nasal inhalation of the acetone. A topical photosensitizer is then applied thoroughly to the targeted skin surfaces. Once applied, time is allowed for the topical agents to be absorbed and converted into the photosensitizing agent PpIX. During this period of time, known as the incubation period, careful protection from light should be followed. In our practice, the incubation period occurs in a dimly lit exam room. After the incubation period, we apply light or laser at predetermined doses (Figure 8-1). Because of the burning and itching sensation during treatment, our patients are given the hose of a Zimmer (information available at www.zimmercoolers.com) air cooling device to pass over the skin. After treatment, the patient washes the affected skin with soap and water, and then covers the treated area with sunscreen. A variety of sun protective clothing and hats are worn depending on the areas treated, and the patient can

go home. The patient is instructed to protect the treated area from light exposure for at least the next 48 to 72 hours.

INDICATIONS

The most widely studied use for topical PDT is in the management of neoplastic and preneoplastic conditions such as AK, Bowen disease, and basal cell carcinoma (BCC). More recently, protocols have been developed for inflammatory dermatoses such as psoriasis, acne, and hidradenitis suppurativa (HS) as well as infectious diseases caused by viruses, bacteria, and parasites. Protocols continue to be explored, sometimes harnessing newer light sources, such as combining topical PDT with nonablative laser therapy. In 2008, a workshop of the British Photodermatology Group helped coalesce the available data into published guidelines for the use of topical PDT[4] that are shown in Table 8-1.

NONMELANOMA SKIN CANCER

Actinic Keratosis/Actinic Cheilitis

AK both serve as a marker for a person at risk for squamous cell carcinoma (SCC) and represent premalignant lesions thought to be part of a continuum along the path to the development of SCC. Gene profiling of human skin reveals similar differentially expressed genes in AK and SCC when compared with normal sun-exposed and non-sun-exposed skin, supporting the fact that these are closely linked lesions.[5] It is estimated that 0.1% to 10% of untreated AK will develop into SCC[6,7] with an estimated 60% to 100% of cutaneous SCCs arising in conjunction with an AK.[8–11] Importantly there is no reliable clinical or histological method to predict which individual lesion will progress to an invasive SCC.[12] The reported rate of spontaneous remission of AK varies widely, but may be as high as 25%.[13] Current accepted modalities for the treatment of AK include cryotherapy,[14,15] electrodessication and curettage,[16] chemical peels,[17] topical therapies such as 5-fluorouracil (5-FU),[18] imiquimod,[19–21] or diclofenac,[22] and PDT.[23–25] An example of a patient's AK resolving with PDT is shown in Figure 8-2.

In December 1999, the US FDA approved PDT with Levulan® Kerastick® (ALA) and the BLU-U® Blue Light Photodynamic Therapy Illuminator (DUSA Pharmaceuticals, Wilmington, Massachusetts), for the treatment of nonhyperkeratotic AK on the face and scalp.

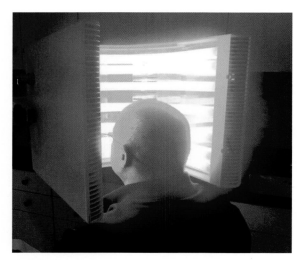

▲ **FIGURE 8-1** This patient is undergoing photodynamic therapy with blue light one hour after aminolevulinic acid was applied to his face.

TABLE 8-1

Clinical Indications for Topical Photodynamic Therapy in Dermatology: Recommendations and Evidence Assessment

STRENGTH OF RECOMMENDATION	QUALITY OF EVIDENCE	INDICATION
A	I	Actinic keratoses
		Bowen disease
		Superficial basal cell carcinoma
B	I	Thin nodular basal cell carcinoma
		Inflammatory acne
		Viral warts
		Genital warts
		Cutaneous leishmaniasis
B	II-iii	Photorejuvenation
C	II-iii	Localized cutaneous T-cell lymphoma (CTCL)
		Vaginal intraepithelial neoplasia
C	III	Extramammary Paget disease
C	IV	Skin cancer prevention
D	I	Psoriasis
D	II-iii	Invasive squamous cell carcinoma

Reproduced from Morton CA, McKenna KE, Rhodes LE. Guidelines for topical photodynamic therapy: update. *Br J Dermatol.* 2008; 159:1245–1266.

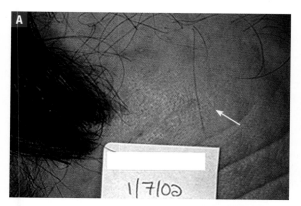

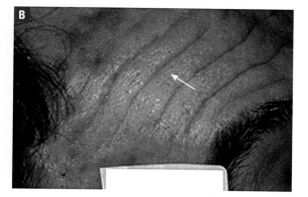

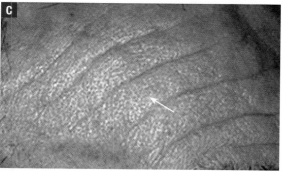

▲ **FIGURE 8-2 A.** Multiple actinic keratoses (AKs) on the right forehead in a man with type II skin are shown prior to treatment (arrow). **B.** Following topical 5-aminolevulinic acid and laser treatment, mild erythema was noted at the previously identified AK sites (arrow), as well as at sites of subclinical AKs. **C.** The AKs were clear at the 2-month follow-up interval (arrow).

In June 2008, the US FDA approved PDT with Metvixia® (methyl aminolevulinate hydrochloride) (Penn Pharmaceutical Services Ltd, Tafarnaubach Industrial Estate, Tredegar, Gwent, MP22, 3AA, UK) and the Aktilite® CL128 lamp, based on red light-emitting diode (LED), for the treatment of thin and moderately thick, nonhyperkeratotic, nonpigmented AK of the face and scalp.

FDA approval was bolstered by invaluable studies into PDT, and further studies continue to emerge that may optimize on- and off-label therapies. The results of selected trials for topical PDT for AK are shown in Table 8-2. The initial dose-finding studies in 40 patients with AK found no significant difference in clinical responses with 10%, 20%, or 30% ALA combined with red light.[26] Notably, face and scalp were more effectively treated than lesions on the trunk and extremities and the presence of hyperkeratosis inhibited uptake of photosensitizer. Subsequently, a phase 2, multicenter, investigator-blinded, light-dose study with 20% ALA and blue light found that a maximal response (88% Clearance rate [CR]) requires more than 2 J/cm^2 and is maximal at 10 J/cm^2.[27] In 2004, a phase 3 multicenter, investigator-blinded, randomized controlled trial (RCT) in 243 patients with ALA and blue light found clearance rates of 77% at 8 weeks after a single treatment; clearance rates increased to 89% at 12 weeks after a second treatment was performed at 8 weeks.[28] Clearance rates for MAL-PDT are similar to those shown for ALA-PDT, ranging from 69% to 91% for complete clinical clearance of individual lesions. Further studies have endorsed these doses and high clearance rates. Incubation times have ranged from 4 hours under occlusion to 18 hours without occlusion, and light sources include argon-pumped dye laser,[26] intense pulsed light,[36] red light,[29] and blue light.[27]

Relative to standard therapies for AK, such as cryotherapy[31,35] or topical 5-FU,[29] topical PDT of the face and scalp has shown equivalence or superiority along with superior cosmetic outcomes. Both MAL-PDT and ALA-PDT have been proven inferior to cryotherapy for AK on the extremities.[26,34]

For the treatment of actinic cheilitis, the absence of a stratum corneum on mucosal surfaces theoretically facilitates uptake of topical photosensitizers. In a comparative trial of 20% ALA-PDT versus pulsed dye laser (PDL) without the use of a topical photosensitizer, 19 patients who had failed prior treatment of biopsy-proven actinic cheilitis received topical 20% ALA with long-pulsed PDL (595 nm) at monthly intervals for 1 to 3 treatments.[37] Long-pulsed PDL refers to the use of longer pulse durations that leads to only transient purpura. Complete clearance was achieved in 68% of

TABLE 8-2

Results of Selected Trials for Topical PDT for Actinic Keratoses

Reference ALA	Study Design	No. of Patients	Treatment Parameters	Results	Comment
Jeffes et al[26]	Prospective vehicle-controlled, phase 1	40 (240 AKs)	ALA (10%, 20%, 30%); 3-h incubation; argon-pumped dye laser (630 nm); 10–150 J/cm^2	91% CR rate for face, scalp; 43% CR rate for trunk, extremities; 8-week follow-up	No difference in clinical response for 10%, 20%, and 30% ALA
Jeffes et al[27]	Multicenter double-blind RCT, phase 2	36 (144 AKs)	ALA (20%); 14- to 18-h incubation; blue light (417 nm); 2–10 J/cm^2; 3–10 mW/cm^2	66% CR; 8-week follow-up	CR increased to 88% if second treatment at week 8
Piacquadio et al[28]	Multicenter double-blind RCT, phase 3	243 (1258 AKs)	ALA (20%); 14- to 18-h incubation; blue light (417 nm); 10 mW/cm^2	83% CR; 8-week follow-up	CR increased to 91% if second treatment at week 8
Kurwa et al[29]	Prospective, paired comparison trial of ALA-PDT vs 5-FU on dorsal hands	17	ALA (20%); 4-h incubation; red light (580–740 nm); 150 J/cm^2; 86 mW/cm^2	Reduction in total surface area of AKs of 70% (ALA-PDT) vs 73% (5-FU)	Single treatment of ALA-PDT vs 5-FU twice daily for 3 weeks

(continued)

TABLE 8-2

Results of Selected Trials for Topical PDT for Actinic Keratoses *(Continued)*

REFERENCE	STUDY DESIGN	NO. OF PATIENTS	TREATMENT PARAMETERS	RESULTS	COMMENT
Alexiades Armenakas and Geronemus[30]	Prospective, open label	41 (3622 AKs)	ALA (20%); 3-h incubation; long-pulsed PDL (595 nm); 4–7.5 J/cm^2	Mean lesion clearance at 4 months of 93% for head; 71% for extremities and 65% for trunk	
MAL					
Ruiz-Rodriguez et al[36]	Multicenter double-blind RCT	77 (502 AKs)	MAL; 3-h incubation; red light (570–670 nm); 75 J/cm^2; 50–200 mW/cm^2	CR 82% (patient response); 89% (lesion response) at 3 months	MAL superior to placebo ($P > .001$)
Pariser et al[32]	Multicenter double-blind RCT	49 (363 AKs) for MAL; 47 (360 AKs) for placebo	MAL; 3-h incubation; red light (630 nm); 37 J/cm^2 with 2 treatments at 1-week intervals	CR 86% (lesion response); 59% (patient response) at 3 months	MAL superior to placebo ($P < .0001$)
Freeman et al[33]	Multicenter placebo-controlled open-label RCT of MAL-PDT vs placebo-PDT vs cryotherapy	200 (855 AKs)	MAL; 3-h incubation; red light (570–670 nm); 75 J/cm^2; 50–250 mW/cm^2 with 2 treatments at 1-week intervals	CR (lesion response) of 91% for MAL-PDT vs 68% for cryotherapy vs 30% for placebo-PDT at 3 months	MAL superior to cryotherapy and placebo-PDT in terms of response rates and cosmetic outcome
Szeimies et al	Multicenter open-label RCT of MAL-PDT vs cryotherapy	193 (699 AKs)	MAL; 3-h incubation; red light (570–670 nm); 75 J/cm^2; 70–200 mW/cm^2, second treatment at 1 week for lesions not located on face or scalp	CR (lesion response) of 69% for MAL-PDT vs 75% for cryotherapy at 3 months	MAL-PDT superior to cryotherapy in terms of cosmetic outcome ($P = .035$)
Kaufmann et al[34]	Multicenter intraindividual RCT of PDT vs cryotherapy for AKs on extremities	121 (1343 AKs)	MAL; 3-h incubation; red light (630 nm); 37 J/cm^2; re-treatment at week 12 if no clinical response	CR (lesion response) of 78% for MAL-PDT vs 88% for cryotherapy ($P = .002$) at 6 months	MAL-PDT superior to cryotherapy for cosmetic outcome ($P < .001$) and patient preference ($P < .001$)
Morton et al[35]	Multicenter intraindividual RCT of MAL-PDT vs cryotherapy on face/scalp	119 (1501 AKs)	MAL; 3-h incubation; red light (630 nm); 37 J/cm^2; re-treatment at week 12 if no clinical response	CR (lesion response) of 83% for MAL-PDT vs 72% for cryotherapy at week 12; 86% vs 83% at week 24	MAL-PDT superior to cryotherapy in terms of subjective patient and investigator preference ($P < .001$)

AK, actinic keratosis; ALA, aminolevulinic acid; MAL, methyl aminolevulinic acid; PDL, pulsed dye laser; CR, clearance rate; RCT, randomized controlled trial.

ALA-PDT patients, while clearance was not observed in either of the 2 control patients.

The current guidelines recommend topical PDT for AKs with a strong recommendation (A) and high quality of evidence (level 1).[4] Hyperkeratotic lesions and lesions located on the extremities may not respond as well to treatment.

Squamous Cell Carcinoma In Situ/Bowen Disease

Bowen disease is a form of intraepithelial neoplasia with a risk of transformation into SCC ranging from 3% to 5% for cutaneous lesions and possibly as high as 10% for mucosal variants.[38] Reported clearance rates of squamous cell carcinoma in situ (SCCIS) with topical PDT range from 86% to 94% with either ALA-PDT or MAL-PDT with rates of recurrence of 10% to 24% at 1 year.[35,38,39] Short-term clearance rates and long-term recurrence rates are similar to cryotherapy[40] or 5-FU[41] in comparison trials; however, recurrence rates are, in general, higher compared with surgical excision. Cosmetic results and patient-reported pain scores for PDT are superior to cryotherapy or 5-FU.

Morton et al compared ALA-PDT versus a single freeze–thaw cycle of cryotherapy for the management of 40 lesions of SCCIS in 19 patients; treatments were repeated until complete clinical response was observed in all lesions.[40] ALA-PDT was noninferior to cryotherapy in terms of overall lesion response rates, but associated with significantly less pain, lower recurrence rates, and higher chance of responding to a single treatment session. Lesion size was a significant predictor of initial treatment response. When compared with topical fluorouracil, Salim et al found initial and 1-year response rates of 88% and 82% for ALA-PDT versus 67% and 48% for topical fluorouracil, respectively.[41] In a direct comparison trial of several treatment modalities, complete clinical response for SCCIS at 3 months was 93% (103/111) in the MAL-PDT group, 21% (4/19) in the placebo-PDT group, 86% (73/85) in the cryotherapy group, and 83% (24/29) in the fluorouracil group.[42] The estimated sustained complete response rate of lesions at 12 months was 80% in the MAL-PDT group, 67% in the cryotherapy group, and 69% in the fluorouracil group with a statistically significant difference between MAL-PDT and the combined standard therapy group.

Studies have included various illumination sources (eg, filtered xenon arc, diode, halogen, laser), wavelengths (red, green, blue/violet light), topical photosensitizers (ALA, MAL), and dosing schedules; hence, comparisons between studies may be difficult to interpret. Morton et al determined that red light (630 nm) was superior to green light (540 nm) with initial clearance rates of 94% and 88% and 1-year clearance rates of 72% and 48% for the 2 different wavelengths, respectively.[43] Dijkstra et al found similar initial clearance rates of 90% to 100% with a violet light source (400–450 nm).[44] In the largest study of MAL-PDT, Truchuelo et al included 51 lesions treated with gentle curettage followed by illumination with a red light source and reported clearance rates of 76% at a median of 16 months after 2 treatments.[45] In general, longer wavelengths are preferred as they offer the advantage of deeper penetration.

Topical PDT offers a potential advantage to standard therapy in the management of SCCIS in unusual sites such as the nipple, subungual areas, or digits[46–49] as well as sites of poor wound healing such as the lower leg, areas of prior radiation exposure, and in patients with epidermolysis bullosa.[50–52] Complete resolution of localized Bowenoid papulosis was seen in 2 patients[53] and partial or complete resolution was seen in 2 of 4 patients with erythroplasia of Queyrat treated with ALA-PDT.[54,55]

Invasive Squamous Cell Carcinoma

There are limited published data to support the use of PDT for treatment of invasive cutaneous SCC. The limited depth of penetration of topical photosensitizers as well as illumination sources prohibits widespread implementation of topical PDT for management of invasive SCC.

In the largest study of invasive SCC as of the time of writing this chapter, histopathologic response was seen in only 2 of 6 nodular SCCs (33%) and 10 of 12 superficial SCCs with MAL-PDT.[56] Isolated case reports demonstrate efficacy of a single session of intralesional ALA-PDT for an invasive SCC on the cheek with histological cure confirmed at 3 months and prolonged clinical cure at 16 months.[57] The protocol used was injection of 0.8 cm^2 of a 10% ALA solution prepared by mixing the ALA powder (Medac GmbH, Hamburg, Germany) with normal saline; this was incubated for 4 hours, and then irradiated with noncoherent red light (570–670 nm). Based on currently available data, there is fair evidence to reject the use of topical PDT for invasive SCC (strength of evidence D).[4]

Basal Cell Carcinoma

BCC is the most common nonmelanoma cancer. It has an indolent clinical course with a low potential for metastasis; however, it can be locally aggressive with extensive tissue destruction. Published cure rates for BCC with PDT have ranged from 62% to 91% for superficial BCCs and 50% to 92% for the nodular subtype with both 5-ALA and MAL being employed as photosensitizers. Selected studies are shown in Table 8-3. In a review of 12 published trials, the weighted complete response rates were 87% for superficial BCCs and 53% for nodular BCCs.[67] Clearance rates and recurrence rates are similar when compared with cryotherapy; however, they are proven inferior to standard surgical excision in comparison trials.[61,68]

In a longitudinal study of 60 BCCs of various histological subtypes (superficial, nodular, morpheaform, micronodular, and infiltrative), the authors found 10-year complete response rates of 60% after 1 treatment session and 87% after 2 treatment sessions with dimethylsulfoxide (DMSO)-supported ALA-PDT with red light and pretreatment curettage.[59] Predictors of treatment failure included male gender, recurrent tumor, and a single treatment session. In contrast to

other published studies, no significant difference was found in response rates among the various histological subtypes. In the largest study of MAL-PDT to date, Fantini et al included 194 BCCs in 135 patients treated with gentle curettage followed by illumination with a red light source with either 1 or 2 cycles.[58] Complete response rates of 89% and 33% for superficial and nodular BCC were observed. Several predictors of better clinical response included location on the trunk, depth ≤0.5 mm, and absence of ulceration.

In a study of MAL-PDT versus cryotherapy, similar response rates of 97% and 95% at 3 months and 87% and 74% at 5 years, respectively, were seen.[65] Wang et al similarly showed no difference in efficacy for 88 superficial and nodular BCCs randomized to either ALA-PDT or standard cryotherapy, but superior cosmesis was achieved with PDT.[60] In a multicenter randomized trial of MAL-PDT versus standard surgical excision in 101 patients with nodular BCC, there was no difference in clinical response at 3 months with 98% complete response for surgery

TABLE 8-3

Select Studies Evaluating the Efficacy of Photodynamic Therapy for Basal Cell Carcinoma

REFERENCE	STUDY DESIGN	NO. OF PATIENTS (LESIONS)	TREATMENT PARAMETERS	RESULTS	COMMENT
Fantini et al[58]	Multicenter, prospective, single-intervention trial	135 patients (194 BCCs; 116 sBCCS, 78 nBCCs)	MAL; 3-h incubation; red light (630 nm); 37 J/cm²; second treatment at 1 week (n = 142); third treatment at 2–3 months (n = 6)	CR of 62% (121/194); 82% for sBCCs; 44 vs nBCCs; 37% for infiltrative BCCs with a mean of 23.5-month follow-up time (6–84 months)	Factors associated with treatment failure included nodular and infiltrative subtype, location on lower limbs, ulceration, tumor thickness
Christensen et al[59]	Prospective, open-label, longitudinal study	44 patients (60 nBCCs)	DMSO + 20% ALA-PDT; 1–2 treatment sessions, halogen light source (550–700 nm); 150–230 mW/cm²	CR of 75% (45/60); 60% after 1 treatment session and 87% after 2 treatment sessions at 10 years	Factors associated with treatment failure included male gender, recurrent tumor, single treatment session
Wang et al[60]	Prospective, open-label, randomized trial of ALA-PDT vs cryotherapy	88 patients; 47 (PDT), 41 (cryotherapy)	ALA; 6-h incubation; frequency-doubled Nd:YAG (635 nm); 100 ms; 60 J/cm²; 60–100 mW/cm²; repeat treatment at 4 weeks, 8 weeks, 3 months as necessary	Similar clinical and histological recurrence rates of 25% and 5% (PDT) vs 15% and 13% (cryosurgery) at 12 months	Shorter healing time, superior cosmetic outcome with PDT

(continued)

TABLE 8-3
Select Studies Evaluating the Efficacy of Photodynamic Therapy for Basal Cell Carcinoma *(Continued)*

REFERENCE	STUDY DESIGN	NO. OF PATIENTS (LESIONS)	TREATMENT PARAMETERS	RESULTS	COMMENT
Rhodes et al[61,62]	Multicenter, prospective, randomized trial of MAL-PDT vs surgery for nodular BCC	97 patients (105 lesions); 53 (MAL-PDT); 52 (surgery)	MAL; 3-h incubation; red light (570–670 nm); 75 J/cm^2; 50–200 mW/cm^2; 2 treatments at weekly intervals; third treatment at 3 months if no CR	No significant difference in CR between surgery (51/52 lesions; 98%) and MAL-PDT (48/53 lesions; 91%) 5-Year sustained lesion complete response rates were 96% (surgery) and 76% (MAL-PDT) ($P = .01$)	Better cosmetic outcome with MAL-PDT at all time points from 3 to 60 months
Calzavara Pinton[63]	Retrospective case series	$N = 23$ sBCCs, 30 nBCCs, 4 pBCCs	20% ALA; 6- to 8-h under occlusion; argon-pumped dye laser (630 nm); treatments repeated every other day until complete response	For sBCCs, 100% initial CR; 84% long-term CR; mean number of treatments of 2.0 (range 1–3) For nBCCs, 80% initial CR; 50% long-term CR; mean number of treatments of 4.0 (range 2–8) No pigmented BCC responded after mean of 4 treatments (range 2–8)	
Foley et al[64]	Two multicenter, randomized, double-blind studies	$N = 65$ patients (75 nBCCs)	MAL; 3-h incubation; broad-spectrum red light (75 J/cm^2, 570–670 nm); 2 weekly treatments, and then re-treated at 3 months if nonresponsive	Histologically verified CR in 55/75 lesions (73%) vs 20/75 (27%) placebo at 6 months Most effective for facial lesions (89% complete response)	Cosmetic outcome was good or excellent in 98% of responding lesions
Basset-Seguin et al[65]	Multicenter, prospective, randomized trial of MAL-PDT vs cryotherapy	$N = 118$ patients (219 sBCCs); $n = 60$ (114) MAL-PDT; $n = 58$ (105)	MAL; 3-h incubation; broad-spectrum red light (570–670 nm); 75 J/cm^2; 150 mW/cm^2; single treatment with re-treatment at 3-month intervals if nonresponsive	Similar 5-year recurrence rates of 20% (cryotherapy) vs 22% (MAL-PDT) ($P = .86$)	More patients with excellent cosmetic outcome with MAL-PDT (60%) vs cryotherapy (16%) ($P < .0001$)
Soler et al[66]	Retrospective	$N = 350$ lesions	MAL; gentle curettage; 3–24 h under occlusion; broadband halogen light (570–670 nm); 100 ± 180 mW/cm^2; 50 ± 200 J/cm^2	CR in 310/350 (89%) at 6 months; CR in 277/350 (79%) at 35 months	

versus 91% for MAL-PDT.[62] A 5-year follow-up however showed significantly higher estimated sustained lesion response rate for surgery at 96% compared with 76% for MAL-PDT.[61]

Measures that have been attempted in order to improve the cure rate of BCCs with topical PDT include curettage to debulk tumor tissue, pretreatment or admixture with DMSO to enhance penetration, admixture of photosensitizer with ethylenediaminetetraacetic acid (EDTA) or desferroxamine to enhance PpIX formation through iron chelation, prolonged incubation times (up to 48 hours), repeated illumination,[69] and intralesional infiltration of photosensitizer.

Authors of this text presented preliminary data regarding the effectiveness of noncoherent blue light in the intralesional PDT of BCC.[70] In this prospective, IRB-approved study of 20 BCCs, each BCC was injected with 20% ALA, incubated for 1 hour, and exposed to noncoherent blue light for 1000 seconds (10 J/cm^2). If without clinical clearance at 8 weeks, a second treatment was performed. Clinical and punch biopsy evaluations were performed at 16 weeks, 1 year, and 2 years after PDT. At the time of the presented data, all 20 BCCs had been evaluated at 16 weeks, showing recurrence at 2 sites on histology. For those 18 sites still negative at 16 weeks, 13 had been reevaluated at 1 year, with 4 additional sites of recurrence. Seven had returned for their 2-year exam, and another site showed recurrence. Overall, the recurrence rate in the 2-year study window was 35% (7 of 20 sites) at the time of the presentation. Notably, physicians graded cosmetic outcome as good to excellent in two thirds or more of the treatment sites at all follow-up exams. No unusual adverse event was appreciated. At the time of writing this chapter, all sites have been evaluated by histology at 1 year and no additional recurrences were found over the 4 cited above. As for histology at 2 years, all but 2 of the still negative BCC sites have been reevaluated and no additional recurrences were found over the 1 cited above. One patient refused rebiopsy at 2 years and the other could not be performed because the patient moved out of state. Therefore, the overall recurrence rate in the 2-year study window remains 35% (7 of 20 sites) with the available data.

PDT may offer an advantage in the management of difficult-to-treat clinical scenarios such as the management of multiple BCCs in patients with basal cell nevus syndrome. Several case reports have highlighted the reduction in tumor burden and superior clinical outcome with broad application topical PDT in these patients.[71-75] A dramatic response to systemic PDT in a patient with basal cell nevus syndrome is demonstrated in Figure 8-3.

Current evidence indicates topical PDT to be an effective therapy for superficial (<2 mm thick) BCC, at least as effective as cryotherapy, but with superior healing and cosmesis, and with particular advantages in large and multiple lesions. Topical PDT is less effective for nodular BCC, and although adjunctive therapy with prior curettage or with penetration enhancers, or fractionated treatment may improve results, there is no published randomized evidence of its benefit.

Use of PDT in Organ Transplant Recipients

Skin cancer constitutes the most common posttransplant malignancy in solid organ transplant recipients (OTR).[76-79] In particular, these patients suffer from high rates of nonmelanoma skin cancers (NMSC) with a dramatic 65-fold increase of SCCs over the general population.[80-83] NMSC are therefore a major source of morbidity and mortality in this specialized population. As such, there have been multiple prospective trials evaluating the efficacy of PDT in the prevention and treatment of NMSC in this population, as shown in Table 8-4.

In a RCT of ALA-PDT in OTR versus healthy controls, the response rate was not significantly different at 4 weeks but clinical clearance was lower in OTR at 12 weeks.[84] This either suggests the key role of the immune response in tumor clearance after PDT or simply reflects the high rate of new lesion formation in OTR during this time period. Evaluating whether prophylactic PDT reduced frequency of new SCC formation, de Graaf et al showed no significant reduction in invasive SCC at 24 months with 1 or 2 PDT treatments,[85] whereas Willey et al reported a significant median reduction during the same time frame with cyclic PDT every 4 or 8 weeks.[86]

In contrast, all published studies investigating the use of MAL-PDT in OTR have shown significant improvement in AK with complete response rates of 64%[87] and 76%,[88] respectively, in 2 different trials. Another study by Wulf et al focused on prevention of new cutaneous lesions such as warts, AK, SCC, and BCC after a single MAL-PDT treatment combined with curettage. The authors report both a significantly increased time to first lesion and a 3-fold reduction in new lesions at 1 year in the treatment group.[89]

In conclusion, PDT appears to be safe and effective in the management of premalignant lesions in OTR;

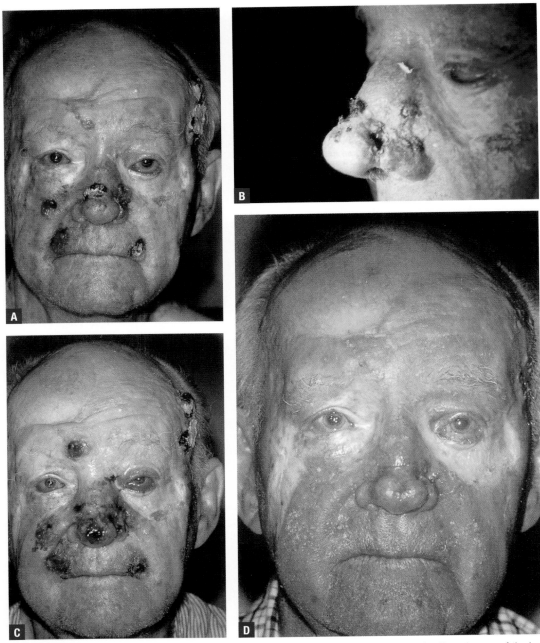

▲ **FIGURE 8-3 A.** A patient with nevoid basal cell carcinoma syndrome and multiple recurrent basal cell carcinomas of the head and neck. **B.** At 72 hours after intravenous injection of 3 mg/kg of HPD, tumor fluorescence can be observed. **C.** At 48 hours after light exposure with 38 J/cm² of light produced by an argon-pumped 63-nm dye laser, there is edema and erythema of the treated lesions. **D.** One month after treatment, the eschars and necrotic debris have sloughed off the treated areas. Residual tumor cells, as demonstrated by biopsy of the ala of the nose and the left nasolabial fold, were successfully retreated in a similar manner. (Reprinted with permission from Tse DT, Kersten RC, Anderson RL. Hematoporphyrin derivative photoradiation therapy in managing nevoid basal cell carcinoma syndrome. *Arch Ophthalmol.* 1984;102:990–994.)

TABLE 8-4

Select Trials Evaluating the Efficacy of Photodynamic Therapy in the Prevention and Treatment of NMSC in Organ Transplant Recipients

Author	Study Design	Results
Dragieva et al[84]	20 OTRs vs 20 immunocompetent controls treated once or twice with PDT with visible light and 5-ALA × 5 h; 12-week follow-up	No difference at 4 weeks but significantly lower rate of complete clearance at 12 weeks in OTR. Complete response of 86% at 1 month and 68% at 3 months in OTRs vs 94% and 89% for controls
Dragieva et al[87]	17 OTR in double-blinded, randomized design treated twice with curettage, and then PDT with visible light and MAL × 3 h; 16-week follow-up	Significant improvement over placebo with 56/62 individual lesions responding to MAL vs 0/67 lesions responding to placebo. MAL patients with complete response in 13/17, partial response in 3/17
de Graaf et al[85]	40 OTR in left/right design treated once or twice with PDT with 400–450 nm light source and ALA × 4 h; 2-year follow-up	Occurrence of new SCC not significantly different between PDT-treated arm and control arm. Fifteen SCCs in PDT arms and 10 SCCs in control arms. Trend toward decreased number of keratoses in PDT group
Wulf et al[89]	28 RTR in left/right design treated in open-label study of curettage, and then PDT with 570–670 nm red light source and MAL × 3 h; 12-month follow-up	Mean time to occurrence of new skin lesion (AK, BCC, keratoacanthoma, SCC, or warts) significantly longer in treated PDT area than that in control (9.6 months vs 6.8 months). Absolute number of new lesions was 3 times higher in control areas than in treated areas
Piaserico et al[88]	15 RTR with treatment-resistant AK in open-label study of curettage, and then PDT with 533 nm red light source and MAL × 3 h; 3-month follow-up	Complete response in 64% of lesions and good response in 24%. Overall AK response rate of 71%. Overall response rate significantly higher on the scalp/face compared with that on dorsal hands (72% vs 40%)
Willey et al[86]	12 high-risk OTR in open-label pilot study of cyclic PDT with 417 nm blue light source and 5-ALA × 1 h, treated every 4 or 8 weeks × 2 years	Median reductions for the 12- and 24-month posttreatment SCCIS and SCC lesion counts from the 12-month pretreatment counts were 79.0% and 95.0%, statistically significant difference

OTR, organ transplant recipient; RTR, renal transplant recipient; PDT, photodynamic therapy; ALA, aminolevulinic acid; MAL, nethyl minolevulinic acid; AK, actinic keratosis; SCC, squamous cell carcinoma; BCC, basal cell.

however, it is still controversial whether this treatment plays a significant role in reducing the formation of SCC in this population.

Cutaneous T-cell Lymphoma

PpIX accumulation is inversely dependent on levels of intracellular iron, as iron is required for the conversion of PpIX to heme. Activated and malignant T lymphocytes express the transferrin receptor (CD71), which correlates with low intracellular iron levels. Given their low iron levels, CD71+ malignant T cells in mycosis fungoides (MF) are predicted to preferentially respond to topical PDT.[90] When malignant T lymphocytes from patients with MF and Sezary syndrome were cultured with a photosensitizing agent (silicon phthalocyanine

Pc 4) and exposed to LED light (670–675 nm), a marked dose-dependent increase in apoptosis of the malignant CD4+CD7- T lymphocytes was appreciated compared with normal lymphocytes.[91] Notably, photodamage to apoptosis regulator protein Bcl-2 plays a critical component in the mechanism of Pc 4-PDT-mediated cell killing of malignant lymphocytes in vitro.

One study showed complete clinical response in 7 of 9 plaque-stage MF lesions with MAL-PDT and a red light source.[92] Subsequently, the same group published long-term follow-up with 3 of 4 evaluable lesions showing long-term clinical and histological remission at 5 to 8 years without additional treatment.[93] Recently, 7 lesions in 4 patients with classic patch and tumor stage MF, anaplastic large-cell lymphoma, and CD8+ CTCL showed 100% clinical response with ALA-PDT with no remission at 18 months when combined with standard therapies.[94]

Presently, the role of PDT in the treatment of CTCL is not clearly established, but the limited data available indicate that it is a promising new alternative treatment of CTCL that warrants further exploration.

Extramammary Paget Disease

Extramammary Paget disease (EMPD) is a rare intraepithelial adenocarcinoma with a predilection for apocrine-bearing skin. A recent systematic review identified 21 case reports and 2 prospective case series reporting the utility of topical PDT for EMPD. Of 99 patients with a total of 133 extramammary lesions, 77 (58%) of the lesions showed a complete response, 52 (39%) a partial response, and 4 (3%) a minimal or no response to PDT.[95] Of note, however, is the fact that the majority of reports are limited by lack of long-term outcomes. Topical PDT may offer benefits of improved cosmetic outcomes, better patient tolerance, and less functional impairments over standard therapies.

INFLAMMATORY AND INFECTIOUS DERMATOSES

Warts

Antiviral PDT dates back to the 1930s when Schultz and Krueger reported the ability of photosensitizers to inactivate viruses or bacteriophages.[96] Most of the initial work was done with enveloped viruses that are rapidly inactivated when irradiated in the presence of photoactive dyes. The mechanisms of ALA-induced virucidal activity on nonenveloped viruses such as HPV are not as well studied. Most likely, ALA-PDT clears HPV by destruction of the infected cells via PpIX-generated photoproducts leading to damage of mitochondria[97] and cell membranes.[98] Topically applied ALA has been shown to selectively accumulate in virally infected cells with peak porphyrin concentrations at 5 hours after application and maximal ratio of virally infected to normal skin at 2 hours indicating maximum selectivity.[99] It has been proposed that this selectivity for virally infected skin is due to alterations in the stratum corneum overlying the lesion.

Clearance rates for warts with PDT have ranged from 56% to 100% with most studies performed on recalcitrant palmoplantar warts for which standard therapies had failed. In a study of ALA-PDT in 31 patients with 48 plantar warts, an overall clearance of 88% was achieved at 3 months, with better clearance seen in younger patients and larger warts and with longer treatment times.[100] A larger study of 264 verrucae compared PDL ALA-PDT versus LED ALA-PDT versus PDL alone with clearance rates of 100%, 96%, and 81%, respectively.[101] In another RCT of placebo-PDT versus ALA-PDT for 232 recalcitrant palmoplantar warts in 45 patients, higher total clearance and decreased mean size of warts were found at 14 and 18 weeks but not at 7 weeks.[102] Complete clearance of periungual hand warts in 18 of 20 patients (36 of 40 warts) was achieved in a pilot study of ALA-PDT after a mean of 4.7 biweekly treatments.[103]

In a RCT comparing use of ALA-PDT with red light for 1 to 3 treatments versus CO_2 ablation for treatment of condyloma, 100% clearance was seen in both groups but a higher recurrence rate of 19% was observed in the control group compared with 6% in the treatment group at 12 weeks.[104] Wang et al performed an open-label trial of 10% ALA incubated for 4 hours, and then irradiated with a 635-nm laser at 2-week intervals for treatment of HPV-associated cervical condylomata in 56 patients.[105] Clinical resolution and HPV viral clearance were obtained in 98% and 84%, respectively.

In conclusion, topical PDT offers high clearance rates and low recurrence rates for the management of cutaneous and genital warts, although it may be associated with higher pain when compared with standard therapies.

Acne

Acne is a chronic inflammatory disease of the pilosebaceous unit characterized by high sebum production and abnormal keratinization of follicular epithelium leading to comedone formation. Overgrowth of *Proprionobacterium acnes* in pilosebaceous units contributes to the development of inflammatory lesions. Lasers and light sources, including blue light, red light, pulsed dye laser, and diode laser, are increasingly being studied as therapeutic options in the treatment of acne.

The proposed mechanisms of ALA-PDT in acne include the suppression of *P. acnes*, direct injury to the sebaceous glands, and alteration of follicular keratinocyte shedding. *P. acnes* produces porphyrins, especially coproporphyrin III, which absorb light energy at the near UV and blue light spectrum.[106,107] These naturally occurring porphyrins can be activated with the use of combined red-blue light-based therapies that show mean improvements of 76% and 58% in inflammatory and comedonal lesions, respectively.[108]

Two recent systematic reviews have validated the use of PDT for acne[109,110] with the majority of included trials showing greater benefit from PDT when compared with light therapy alone. Results of these trials are summarized in Table 8-5. Due to the small size of the trials and poor quality of reported statistical variables, only 3 of the 8 published controlled trials could be included in the meta-analysis. The only trial that compared PDT with conventional acne therapies actually found a significant improvement in inflammatory lesions at 12 weeks for the adapalene-treated control group when compared with adapalene-IPL or adapalene IPL-MAL groups with mean reductions of 88%, 23%, and 65%, respectively.[117] When comparing ALA versus MAL-PDT, Wiegell and Wulf demonstrated equivalent reductions in inflammatory and noninflammatory lesion counts as well as

TABLE 8-5

Select Trials Utilizing Photodynamic Therapy for the Treatment of Acne Vulgaris

REFERENCE	NO. OF PATIENTS; LOCATION	STUDY PROTOCOL	KEY RESULTS
Genina (2004)[111]	$N = 12$; face or back	803 nm low-intensity diode ± ICG, single vs multiple treatment groups	23% improvement at 4 weeks for single treatment; 80% improvement at 4 weeks for multiple treatments; more improvement with severe acne
Haedersdal et al[112]	$N = 15$; face	Split-face with nonpurpuric long pulsed PDL 595 nm full-face treatment with MAL to randomized side; 3 treatments at 2-week intervals	Greater reduction in inflammatory lesion with MAL-LPDL at 4 weeks ($P = .03$) and 12 weeks ($P = .004$) with 80% reduction in lesion counts
Hongcharu et al[113]	$N = 22$; back	550–700 nm; ALA-light, ALA alone, light alone, untreated control. Single vs multiple treatment groups	Improvements of 50%–75% at 20 weeks with single and multiple treatments; single treatment significantly better than multiple treatments ($P < .01$)
Hörfelt et al[114]	$N = 30$; face	653 nm light plus MAL vs placebo-light; split-face trial; 2 biweekly treatments	MAL-PDT more effective than light alone at 4 and 10 weeks ($P < .05$); >50% improvement
Pollock et al[115]	$N = 10$; back	635 nm light-ALA vs light alone vs untreated; weekly for 3 weeks	Reduction in lesion counts with ALA-PDT only ($P < .0005$); 69% reduction in acne at 21-day follow-up
Rojanamatin and Choawawanich[116]	$N = 14$; face	550–700 nm light-ALA vs light alone; split-face trial; 3 treatments at 3- or 4-week intervals	87.7% reduction in mean acne lesion count at 12 weeks with ALA-PDT vs 67% reduction with light alone ($P < .05$)
Yeung et al[117]	$N = 30$; face	Topical adapalene in all treatment arms; split-face 530–750 nm light plus MAL vs light only; 4 treatments at 3-week intervals	Significant mean reduction in inflammatory lesion counts in control group only ($P = .01$). Significant reduction in comedones in MAL-PDT ($P = .05$) and light-only ($P = .01$) groups at 12 weeks
Wiegell and Wulf[3]	$N = 15$, face	Split-face single treatment MAL vs ALA; red light; 37 J/cm^2; 34 mW/cm^2	Median 59% reduction in inflammatory lesions from baseline; no significant difference between ALA- and MAL-treated arms in terms of efficacy or pain
Tuchin et al[118]	$N = 22$; face or back	Split-face or split-back; 803 nm light-ICG vs ICG alone; weekly or twice-weekly treatments depending on severity	No statistical analysis given. "Significant" improvement only in light-ICG group; better with multiple treatments, more severe acne; 67%–83% reduction in lesions

PDT, photodynamic therapy; ALA, aminolevulinic acid; MAL, nethyl minolevulinic acid; ICG, indocyanine-green; PDL, pulsed dye laser.

similar treatment-related pain and erythema.[3] In general, current data are limited by short follow-up times, small size, and lack of comparison to conventional therapies.

Hidradenitis Suppurativa

HS is a chronic, often recalcitrant condition that primarily affects apocrine gland–bearing skin in the axillae, groin, and buttocks. Follicular occlusion is presumed to lead to development of tender, inflamed abscesses and sinus tract formation. Clinical studies on the use of topical PDT for the treatment of HS are limited to isolated case reports with conflicting results. Gold et al noted a 75% to 100% clinical improvement in 4 patients treated with short-contact ALA-PDT and blue light,[119] and Schweiger et al showed 19% improvement in subjective patient quality-of-life improvement scores and 30% reduction in mean lesion counts in an open-label trial of ALA-PDT with a combination of blue light and IPL.[120] In contrast, minimal improvement has been noted with ALA-PDT with red light,[121] MAL-PDT with PDL,[122] or ALA-PDT with either red light or broadband.[123] Therefore, while PDT may be an option for treatment-resistant, recalcitrant HS, its use as a first-line therapy cannot be recommended.

Psoriasis

Psoriasis is a chronic inflammatory skin disease with a worldwide prevalence of 0.6% to 4.8%.[124] Once thought to be a disease of keratinocyte hyperproliferation and loss of differentiation, psoriasis has now been established to be a T-cell-mediated disease in which epidermal hyperplasia occurs as a result of immune system activation. Histologically psoriasis is characterized by a predominance of CD4+ T cells in the dermis and CD8+ T cells in the epidermis.[125] Many of the most efficacious therapies for psoriasis specifically lead to depletion of T cells in psoriatic lesions.

The purported mechanism of action of ALA-PDT in psoriasis includes inhibition of TNF-α, IL-1, and IL-6[126] and apoptosis of CD3+ T cells with systemic PDT.[127] Topical PDT of psoriatic plaques has been associated with a decreased expression of Ki-67 (a marker of epidermal proliferation) and increased expression of keratin 10 (a marker of terminal differentiation of keratinocytes). Analysis of the post-treatment T-cell infiltrate also reveals decreases in epidermal CD8+ cytotoxic T cells and CD45RO+ memory T cells with no change in quantity of epidermal CD4+ helper T cells suggesting an effect on T-cell influx into the skin.[128]

PpIX has been shown to preferentially accumulate in psoriatic plaques after topical application of 5-ALA with a steady increase in fluorescence over 5 hours and evidence of continued emission at 4 days.[129] The intensity of PpIX fluorescence is independent of the quantity of topical photosensitizer applied or presence of occlusion. In addition, at 4 days postapplication, PpIX has been shown to accumulate in psoriatic plaques remote from the treatment area.

The use of photodynamic therapy to treat psoriasis was first reported in 1937 using systemic administration of hematoporphyrin in combination with UV radiation[130]; however, this was associated with significantly prolonged photosensitivity, which limited its widespread use. In 1994, Boehncke et al first described the use of topical ALA combined with visible light irradiation (600–700 nm) for psoriasis showing efficacy equivalent to dithranol in 3 patients.[131] However, subsequent case reports and small, uncontrolled trials have shown conflicting results.[132–135] A randomized, double-blind phase I/II study in 12 patients of PDT with 3 different ALA concentrations of 0.1%, 1%, or 5% showed limited mean improvement of 38%, 46%, and 51%, respectively, with 20% improvement in control group.[135] In addition, 3 patients dropped out of the study due to treatment-induced pain and there were many times that irradiation had to be interrupted because of severe burning and pain in the remaining patients. Collins et al treated 22 patients with large plaque psoriasis; each patient had 4 squares treated within the area of psoriasis and 1 square served as a control.[136] Twenty percent ALA was applied for 4 hours and then irradiated with a modified slide projector (400–650 nm). Of the 80 treatment sites, 14 (18%) cleared, 6 (8%) showed a partial response, and 60 (75%) showed no improvement and relapse was seen within 2 weeks in some patients.

According to recently published guidelines for topical PDT by a workshop of the British Photodermatology Group, there is fair evidence to reject the use of the procedure (grade D) and it cannot be recommended for use in clinical practice.[4]

Photoaging and Photorejuvenation

Photoaging secondary to chronic actinic damage manifests as fine lines, sallowness, dyschromia, lentigines, and telangiectasias that frequently coexist with AK. With the implementation of topical PDT for the management of AK, improvements in clinical signs of photoaging have been noted and a growing body of evidence supports the efficacy of topical PDT for rejuvenation of photoaged skin. The mechanism of action is highly dependent on the various molecular targets. ALA-PDT on photodamaged skin of the forearm has been shown to stimulate epidermal proliferation, increase epidermal thickness, and upregulate collagen production.[137]

In a study of 14 patients treated with 2 sessions of MAL-PDT and irradiated with red light, 5 patients experienced improvement in skin texture, wrinkles, and firmness 3 months after treatment with 5 more patients experiencing marked improvement at 6 months.[138] Statistically significant increases in collagen fiber and decreases in elastic fibers were observed at 6 months as measured by morphometry and histopathology and correlated with clinical findings. A randomized, controlled, split-face study in 20 patients using ALA-PDT with IPL versus IPL showed that IPL-PDT could improve global photodamage, mottled pigmentation, and fine lines better than IPL alone.[139] Additional studies have also supported the superiority of combination ALA-PDT plus IPL over IPL alone.[140,141] A split-face, randomized trial of 9 patients treated with 3 biweekly treatments of MAL-PDT and a red light source compared 1-hour versus 3-hour incubation time.[36] A moderate improvement was seen in fine lines, tactile roughness, and skin tightness with more improvement in the 3-hour side, but no improvement in mottled hyperpigmentation or telangiectasias was observed in either group.

Additional Indications

Both ALA and MAL combined with PDT have been reported to be effective in the management of cutaneous leishmaniasis. The mechanism is likely a nonspecific tissue destruction rather than selective destruction of amastigotes. In a randomized investigator-blinded trial of 57 patients (97 lesions), receiving weekly ALA-PDT with red light, twice-daily topical paromycin, or placebo over 4 weeks, lesion clearance at 8 weeks was seen in 94%, 41%, and 13%, respectively.[142]

Case series have suggested efficacy of topical PDT for multiple other indications, including, but not limited to, lichen sclerosus, rosacea, perioral dermatitis, radiodermatitis, molluscum contagiosum, and erythrasma.

■ COMPLICATIONS AND LIMITATIONS

Pain is the most frequently reported side effect of PDT and is described as a burning or stinging sensation during light exposure. In a large retrospective review of patients treated with either ALA or MAL-PDT for a variety of indications (AK, BCC, SCCIS, Paget, lichen sclerosus), the strongest predictor of pain was size of treatment area.[143] Additional variables included diagnosis of AK and location of pain on face/scalp or genitalia. While Grapengiesser et al concluded that men experienced more pain during PDT than did women,[144] several subsequent studies have found that gender[145] and age[146] are poor predictors of pain.

In comparison trials of MAL-PDT versus ALA-PDT, MAL-PDT was associated with less pain during and after the procedure and fewer treatment interruptions due to pain.[147,148] The differences in pain between MAL and ALA have been attributed to the different methods of cellular uptake and transport of these compounds.[149] Finally, blue and green light sources are less painful compared with red light, but these light sources do not penetrate the tissue as deeply as the red light.[150] Methods employed to reduce pain include topical anesthesia, cold air analgesia, transcutaneous nerve stimulation, and local or regional nerve blocks.[151–153]

REFERENCES

1. Pottier RH, Chow YF, LaPlante JP, Truscott TG, Kennedy JC, Beiner LA. Non-invasive technique for obtaining fluorescence excitation and emission spectra in vivo. *Photochem Photobiol.* 1986;44:679–687.
2. Fritsch C, Homey B, Stahl W, Lehmann P, Ruzicka T, Sies H. Preferential relative porphyrin enrichment in solar keratoses upon topical application of delta-aminolevulinic acid methylester. *Photochem Photobiol.* 1998;68:218–221.
3. Wiegell S, Wulf H. Photodynamic therapy of acne vulgaris using 5-aminolevulinic acid versus methyl aminolevulinate. *J Am Acad Dermatol.* 2006;54: 647–651.
4. Morton CA, McKenna KE, Rhodes LE. Guidelines for topical photodynamic therapy: update. *Br J Dermatol.* 2008;159:1245–1266.
5. Padilla RS, Sebastian S, Jiang Z, Nindl I, Larson R. Gene expression patterns of normal human skin, actinic keratosis, and squamous cell carcinoma: a spectrum of disease progression. *Arch Dermatol.* 2010;146:288–293.
6. Marks R, Rennie R, Selwood TS. Malignant transformation of solar keratoses to squamous cell carcinoma. *Lancet.* 1988;1:795–797.
7. Dodson JM, DeSpain J, Hewett JE, Clark DP. Malignant potential of actinic keratoses and the controversy over treatment. A patient-oriented perspective. *Arch Dermatol.* 1991;127:1029–1031.
8. Mittelbronn MA, Mullins DL, Ramos Caro FA, Flowers FP. Frequency of pre-existing actinic keratosis in cutaneous squamous cell carcinoma. *Int J Dermatol.* 1998;37: 677–681.

9. Guenthner ST, Hurwitz RM, Buckel LJ, Gray HR. Cutaneous squamous cell carcinomas consistently show histologic evidence of in situ changes: a clinicopathologic correlation. *J Am Acad Dermatol*. 1999;41:443–448.

10. Lober B, Lober C. Actinic keratosis is squamous cell carcinoma. *South Med J*. 2000;93:650–655.

11. Takemiya M, Ohtsuka H, Miki Y. The relationship between solar keratoses and squamous cell carcinomas among Japanese. *J Dermatol*. 1990;17:342–346.

12. Anwar J, Wrone D, Kimyai Asadi A, Alam M. The development of actinic keratosis into invasive squamous cell carcinoma: evidence and evolving classification schemes. *Clin Dermatol*. 2004;22:189–196.

13. Marks R, Foley P, Goodman G, Hage BH, Selwood TS. Spontaneous remission of solar keratoses: the case for conservative management. *Br J Dermatol*. 1986;115:649–655.

14. Thai K-E, Fergin P, Freeman M, et al. A prospective study of the use of cryosurgery for the treatment of actinic keratoses. *Int J Dermatol*. 2004;43:687–692.

15. Lubritz RR, Smolewski SA. Cryosurgery cure rate of actinic keratoses. *J Am Acad Dermatol*. 1982;7:631–632.

16. Freeman R, Knox J, Heaton C. The treatment of skin cancer. A statistical study of 1,341 skin tumors comparing results obtained with irradiation, surgery, and curettage followed by electrodessication. *Cancer*. 1964;17:535–538.

17. Lawrence N, Cox SE, Cockerell CJ, Freeman RG, Cruz PD Jr. A comparison of the efficacy and safety of Jessner's solution and 35% trichloroacetic acid vs 5% fluorouracil in the treatment of widespread facial actinic keratoses. *Arch Dermatol*. 1995;131:176–181.

18. Simmonds W. Double-blind investigation comparing a 1%-vs-5% 5-fluorouracil topical cream in patients with multiple actinic keratoses. *Cutis*. 1973;12:615–617.

19. Lebwohl M, Dinehart S, Whiting D, et al. Imiquimod 5% cream for the treatment of actinic keratosis: results from two phase III, randomized, double-blind, parallel group, vehicle-controlled trials. *J Am Acad Dermatol*. 2004;50:714–721.

20. Szeimies R-M, Gerritsen M-JP, Gupta G, et al. Imiquimod 5% cream for the treatment of actinic keratosis: results from a phase III, randomized, double-blind, vehicle-controlled, clinical trial with histology. *J Am Acad Dermatol*. 2004;51:547–555.

21. Korman N, Moy R, Ling M, et al. Dosing with 5% imiquimod cream 3 times per week for the treatment of actinic keratosis: results of two phase 3, randomized, double-blind, parallel-group, vehicle-controlled trials. *Arch Dermatol*. 2005;141:467–473.

22. Wolf JJ, Taylor JR, Tschen E, Kang S. Topical 3.0% diclofenac in 2.5% hyaluronan gel in the treatment of actinic keratoses. *Int J Dermatol*. 2001;40:709–713.

23. Szeimies RM, Karrer S, Radakovic-Fijan S, et al. Photodynamic therapy using topical methyl 5-aminolevulinate compared with cryotherapy for actinic keratosis: a prospective, randomized study. *J Am Acad Dermatol*. 2002;47:258–262.

24. Tarstedt M, Rosdahl I, Berne B, Svanberg K, Wennberg A. A randomized multicenter study to compare two treatment regimens of topical methyl aminolevulinate (Metvix)-PDT in actinic keratosis of the face and scalp. *Acta Derm Venereol*. 2005;85:424–428.

25. Radakovic-Fijan S, Blecha-Thalhammer U, Kittler H, Hönigsmann H, Tanew A. Efficacy of 3 different light doses in the treatment of actinic keratosis with 5-aminolevulinic acid photodynamic therapy: a randomized, observer-blinded, intrapatient, comparison study. *J Am Acad Dermatol*. 2005;53:823–827.

26. Jeffes EW, McCullough JL, Weinstein GD, et al. Photodynamic therapy of actinic keratosis with topical 5-aminolevulinic acid. A pilot dose-ranging study. *Arch Dermatol*. 1997;133:727–732.

27. Jeffes EW, McCullough JL, Weinstein GD, Kaplan R, Glazer SD, Taylor JR. Photodynamic therapy of actinic keratoses with topical aminolevulinic acid hydrochloride and fluorescent blue light. *J Am Acad Dermatol*. 2001;45:96–104.

28. Piacquadio D, Chen D, Farber H, et al. Photodynamic therapy with aminolevulinic acid topical solution and visible blue light in the treatment of multiple actinic keratoses of the face and scalp: investigator-blinded, phase 3, multicenter trials. *Arch Dermatol*. 2004;140:41–46.

29. Kurwa HA, Yong Gee SA, Seed PT, Markey AC, Barlow RJ. A randomized paired comparison of photodynamic therapy and topical 5-fluorouracil in the treatment of actinic keratoses. *J Am Acad Dermatol*. 1999;41:414–418.

30. Alexiades Armenakas M, Geronemus R. Laser-mediated photodynamic therapy of actinic keratoses. *Arch Dermatol*. 2003;139:1313–1320.

31. Pariser D, Lowe N, Stewart D, et al. Photodynamic therapy with topical methyl aminolevulinate for actinic keratosis: results of a prospective randomized multicenter trial. *J Am Acad Dermatol*. 2003;48:227–232.

32. Pariser D, Loss R, Jarratt M, et al. Topical methyl-aminolevulinate photodynamic therapy using red light-emitting diode light for treatment of multiple actinic keratoses: a randomized, double-blind, placebo-controlled study. *J Am Acad Dermatol*. 2008;59:569–576.

33. Freeman M, Vinciullo C, Francis D, et al. A comparison of photodynamic therapy using topical methyl aminolevulinate (Metvix) with single cycle cryotherapy in patients with actinic keratosis: a prospective, randomized study. *J Dermatolog Treat*. 2003;14:99–106.

34. Kaufmann R, Spelman L, Weightman W, et al. Multicentre intraindividual randomized trial of topical methyl aminolaevulinate-photodynamic therapy vs. cryotherapy for multiple actinic keratoses on the extremities. *Br J Dermatol*. 2008;158:994–999.

35. Morton C, Campbell S, Gupta G, et al. Intraindividual, right-left comparison of topical methyl aminolaevulinate-photodynamic therapy and cryotherapy in subjects with actinic keratoses: a multicentre, randomized controlled study. *Br J Dermatol*. 2006;155:1029–1036.

36. Ruiz-Rodrguez R, Lpez L, Candelas D, Pedraz J. Photorejuvenation using topical 5-methyl aminolevulinate and red light. *J Drugs Dermatol*. 2008;7:633–637.

37. Alexiades Armenakas M, Geronemus R. Laser-mediated photodynamic therapy of actinic cheilitis. *J Drugs Dermatol*. 2004;3:548–551.

38. Cox NH, Eedy DJ, Morton CA. Guidelines for management of Bowen's disease: 2006 update. *Br J Dermatol*. 2007;156:11–21.

39. Lehmann P. Methyl aminolaevulinate-photodynamic therapy: a review of clinical trials in the treatment of actinic keratoses and nonmelanoma skin cancer. *Br J Dermatol.* 2007;156:793–801.

40. Morton CA, Whitehurst C, Moseley H, McColl JH, Moore JV, Mackie RM. Comparison of photodynamic therapy with cryotherapy in the treatment of Bowen's disease. *Br J Dermatol.* 1996;135:766–771.

41. Salim A, Leman JA, McColl JH, Chapman R, Morton CA. Randomized comparison of photodynamic therapy with topical 5-fluorouracil in Bowen's disease. *Br J Dermatol.* 2003;148:539–543.

42. Morton C, Horn M, Leman J, et al. Comparison of topical methyl aminolevulinate photodynamic therapy with cryotherapy or fluorouracil for treatment of squamous cell carcinoma in situ: results of a multicenter randomized trial. *Arch Dermatol.* 2006;142:729–735.

43. Morton CA, Whitehurst C, Moore JV, MacKie RM. Comparison of red and green light in the treatment of Bowen's disease by photodynamic therapy. *Br J Dermatol.* 2000;143:767–772.

44. Dijkstra AT, Majoie IM, van Dongen JW, van Weelden H, van Vloten WA. Photodynamic therapy with violet light and topical 6-aminolaevulinic acid in the treatment of actinic keratosis, Bowen's disease and basal cell carcinoma. *J Eur Acad Dermatol Venereol.* 2001;15:550–554.

45. Truchuelo M, Fernández-Guarino M, Fleta B, Alcántara J, Jaén P. Effectiveness of photodynamic therapy in Bowen's disease: an observational and descriptive study in 51 lesions. *J Eur Acad Dermatol Venereol.* 2012;26: 868–874.

46. Tan B, Sinclair R, Foley P. Photodynamic therapy for subungual Bowen's disease. *Australas J Dermatol.* 2004; 45:172–174.

47. Brookes PT, Jhawar S, Hinton CP, Murdoch S, Usman T. Bowen's disease of the nipple—a new method of treatment. *Breast.* 2005;14:65–67.

48. Usmani N, Stables G, Telfer N, Stringer M. Subungual Bowen's disease treated by topical aminolevulinic acid-photodynamic therapy. *J Am Acad Dermatol.* 2005;53: S273–S276.

49. Wong TW, Sheu HM, Lee JY, Fletcher RJ. Photodynamic therapy for Bowen's disease (squamous cell carcinoma in situ) of the digit. *Dermatol Surg.* 2001;27:452–456.

50. Ball SB, Dawber RP. Treatment of cutaneous Bowen's disease with particular emphasis on the problem of lower leg lesions. *Australas J Dermatol.* 1998;39:63–68.

51. Souza CS, Felício LBA, Bentley MV, et al. Topical photodynamic therapy for Bowen's disease of the digit in epidermolysis bullosa. *Br J Dermatol.* 2005;153:672–674.

52. Guillen C, Sanmartin O, Escudero A, Botella Estrada R, Sevila A, Castejon P. Photodynamic therapy for in situ squamous cell carcinoma on chronic radiation dermatitis after photosensitization with 5-aminolevulinic acid. *J Eur Acad Dermatol Venereol.* 2000;14:298–300.

53. Yang CH, Lee JC, Chen CH, Hui CY, Hong HS, Kuo HW. Photodynamic therapy for Bowenoid papulosis using a novel incoherent light-emitting diode device. *Br J Dermatol.* 2003;149:1297–1299.

54. Stables GI, Stringer MR, Robinson DJ, Ash DV. Erythroplasia of Queyrat treated by topical aminolaevulinic acid photodynamic therapy. *Br J Dermatol.* 1999; 140:514–517.

55. Lee M, Ryman W. Erythroplasia of Queyrat treated with topical methyl aminolevulinate photodynamic therapy. *Australas J Dermatol.* 2005;46:196–198.

56. Calzavara Pinton PG, Venturini M, Sala R, et al. Methylaminolaevulinate-based photodynamic therapy of Bowen's disease and squamous cell carcinoma. *Br J Dermatol.* 2008;159:137–144.

57. Sotiriou E, Apalla Z, Ioannides D. Complete resolution of a squamous cell carcinoma of the skin using intralesional 5-aminolevulinic acid photodynamic therapy intralesional PDT for SCC. *Photodermatol Photoimmunol Photomed.* 2010;26:269–271.

58. Fantini F, Greco A, Del Giovane C, et al. Photodynamic therapy for basal cell carcinoma: clinical and pathological determinants of response. *J Eur Acad Dermatol Venereol.* 2011;25:896–901.

59. Christensen E, Mork C, Skogvoll E. High and sustained efficacy after two sessions of topical 5-aminolaevulinic acid photodynamic therapy for basal cell carcinoma: a prospective, clinical and histological 10-year follow-up study. *Br J Dermatol.* 2012;166:1342–1348 [Epub ahead of print].

60. Wang I, Bendsoe N, Klinteberg CA, et al. Photodynamic therapy vs. cryosurgery of basal cell carcinomas: results of a phase III clinical trial. *Br J Dermatol.* 2001;144: 832–840.

61. Rhodes L, de Rie M, Leifsdottir R, et al. Five-year follow-up of a randomized, prospective trial of topical methyl aminolevulinate photodynamic therapy vs surgery for nodular basal cell carcinoma. *Arch Dermatol.* 2007;143:1131–1136.

62. Rhodes L, de Rie M, Enstrm Y, et al. Photodynamic therapy using topical methyl aminolevulinate vs surgery for nodular basal cell carcinoma: results of a multicenter randomized prospective trial. *Arch Dermatol.* 2004;140:17–23.

63. Calzavara Pinton PG. Repetitive photodynamic therapy with topical delta-aminolaevulinic acid as an appropriate approach to the routine treatment of superficial non-melanoma skin tumours. *J Photochem Photobiol B Biol.* 1995;29:53–57.

64. Foley P, Freeman M, Menter A, et al. Photodynamic therapy with methyl aminolevulinate for primary nodular basal cell carcinoma: results of two randomized studies. *Int J Dermatol.* 2009;48:1236–1245.

65. Basset-Seguin N, Ibbotson S, Emtestam L, et al. Topical methyl aminolaevulinate photodynamic therapy versus cryotherapy for superficial basal cell carcinoma: a 5 year randomized trial. *Eur J Dermatol.* 2008;18:547–553.

66. Soler AM, Warloe T, Berner A, Giercksky KE. A follow-up study of recurrence and cosmesis in completely responding superficial and nodular basal cell carcinomas treated with methyl 5-aminolaevulinate-based photodynamic therapy alone and with prior curettage. *Br J Dermatol.* 2001;145:467–471.

67. Peng Q, Warloe T, Berg K, et al. 5-Aminolevulinic acid-based photodynamic therapy. Clinical research and future challenges. *Cancer.* 1997;79:2282–2308.

68. Szeimies RM, Ibbotson S, Murrell DF, et al. A clinical study comparing methyl aminolevulinate photodynamic therapy and surgery in small superficial basal cell carcinoma (8–20 mm), with a 12-month follow-up. *J Eur Acad Dermatol Venereol.* 2008;22:1302–1311.

69. Mosterd K, Thissen MR, Nelemans P, et al. Fractionated 5-aminolaevulinic acid-photodynamic therapy vs. surgical excision in the treatment of nodular basal cell carcinoma: results of a randomized controlled trial. *Br J Dermatol.* 2008;159:864–870.

70. Anolik R, Weiss ET, Hunzeker C, et al. Investigation of the effectiveness of non-coherent blue light in intralesional photodynamic therapy of basal cell carcinoma. In: American Society for Laser Medicine and Surgery Annual Meeting; 2011; Grapevine, TX.

71. Itkin A, Gilchrest B. delta-Aminolevulinic acid and blue light photodynamic therapy for treatment of multiple basal cell carcinomas in two patients with nevoid basal cell carcinoma syndrome. *Dermatol Surg.* 2004;30: 1054–1061.

72. Kopera D, Cerroni L, Fink Puches R, Kerl H. Different treatment modalities for the management of a patient with the nevoid basal cell carcinoma syndrome. *J Am Acad Dermatol.* 1996;34:937–939.

73. Kwasniak L, Schweiger ES, Tonkovic-Capin V. A patient with nevoid basal cell carcinoma syndrome treated successfully with photodynamic therapy: case report and review of the literature. *J Drugs Dermatol.* 2010;9: 167–168.

74. Chapas A, Gilchrest B. Broad area photodynamic therapy for treatment of multiple basal cell carcinomas in a patient with nevoid basal cell carcinoma syndrome. *J Drugs Dermatol.* 2006;5:3–5.

75. Oseroff A, Shieh S, Frawley N, et al. Treatment of diffuse basal cell carcinomas and basaloid follicular hamartomas in nevoid basal cell carcinoma syndrome by wide-area 5-aminolevulinic acid photodynamic therapy. *Arch Dermatol.* 2005;141:60–67.

76. Winkelhorst JT, Brokelman WJ, Tiggeler RG, Wobbes T. Incidence and clinical course of de-novo malignancies in renal allograft recipients. *Eur J Surg Oncol.* 2001;27: 409–413.

77. Sanchez EQ, Marubashi S, Jung G, et al. De novo tumors after liver transplantation: a single-institution experience. *Liver Transpl.* 2002;8:285–291.

78. Hiesse C, Rieu P, Kriaa F, et al. Malignancy after renal transplantation: analysis of incidence and risk factors in 1700 patients followed during a 25-year period. *Transplant Proc.* 1997;29:831–833.

79. Webb MC, Compton F, Andrews PA, Koffman CG. Skin tumours posttransplantation: a retrospective analysis of 28 years' experience at a single centre. *Transplant Proc.* 1997;29:828–830.

80. Jensen P, Hansen S, Møller B, et al. Skin cancer in kidney and heart transplant recipients and different long-term immunosuppressive therapy regimens. *J Am Acad Dermatol.* 1999;40:177–186.

81. Hoxtell EO, Mandel JS, Murray SS, Schuman LM, Goltz RW. Incidence of skin carcinoma after renal transplantation. *Arch Dermatol.* 1977;113:436–438.

82. Lindelöf B, Sigurgeirsson B, Gäbel H, Stern RS. Incidence of skin cancer in 5356 patients following organ transplantation. *Br J Dermatol.* 2000;143: 513–519.

83. Hartevelt M, Bavinck J, Kootte A, Vermeer B, Vandenbroucke J. Incidence of skin cancer after renal transplantation in The Netherlands. *Transplant Proc.* 1990;49:506–509.

84. Dragieva G, Hafner J, Dummer R, et al. Topical photodynamic therapy in the treatment of actinic keratoses and Bowen's disease in transplant recipients. *Transplantation.* 2004;77:115–121.

85. de Graaf Y, Kennedy C, Wolterbeek R, Collen A, Willemze R, Bavinck JB. Photodynamic therapy does not prevent cutaneous squamous-cell carcinoma in organ-transplant recipients: results of a randomized-controlled trial. *J Invest Dermatol.* 2006;126: 569–574.

86. Willey A, Mehta S, Lee P. Reduction in the incidence of squamous cell carcinoma in solid organ transplant recipients treated with cyclic photodynamic therapy. *Dermatol Surg.* 2010;36:652–658.

87. Dragieva G, Prinz BM, Hafner J, et al. A randomized controlled clinical trial of topical photodynamic therapy with methyl aminolaevulinate in the treatment of actinic keratoses in transplant recipients. *Br J Dermatol.* 2004;151:196–200.

88. Piaserico S, Belloni Fortina A, Rigotti P, et al. Topical photodynamic therapy of actinic keratosis in renal transplant recipients. *Transplant Proc.* 2007;39:1847–1850.

89. Wulf HC, Pavel S, Stender I, Bakker-Wensveen CA. Topical photodynamic therapy for prevention of new skin lesions in renal transplant recipients. *Acta Derm Venereol.* 2006;86:25–28.

90. Rittenhouse Diakun K, Van Leengoed H, Morgan J, et al. The role of transferrin receptor (CD71) in photodynamic therapy of activated and malignant lymphocytes using the heme precursor delta-aminolevulinic acid (ALA). *Photochem Photobiol.* 1995; 61:523–528.

91. Lam M, Lee Y, Deng M, et al. Photodynamic therapy with the silicon phthalocyanine pc 4 induces apoptosis in mycosis fungoides and Sezary syndrome. *Adv Hematol.* 2010;2010:896161.

92. Edstrm DW, Porwit A, Ros AM. Photodynamic therapy with topical 5-aminolevulinic acid for mycosis fungoides: clinical and histological response. *Acta Derm Venereol.* 2001;81:184–188.

93. Edstrm D, Hedblad M-A. Long-term follow-up of photodynamic therapy for mycosis fungoides. *Acta Derm Venereol.* 2008;88:288–290.

94. Coors E, von den Driesch P. Topical photodynamic therapy for patients with therapy-resistant lesions of cutaneous T-cell lymphoma. *J Am Acad Dermatol.* 2004; 50:363–367.

95. Nardelli A, Stafinski T, Menon D. Effectiveness of photodynamic therapy for mammary and extra-mammary Paget's disease: a state of the science review. *BMC Dermatol.* 2011;11:13.

96. Schultz EW, Krueger AP. Inactivation of *Staphylococcus* bacteriophage by methylene blue. *Proc Soc Exp Biol Med.* 1928;26:100–101.

97. Iinuma S, Farshi SS, Ortel B, Hasan T. A mechanistic study of cellular photodestruction with 5-aminolaevulinic acid-induced porphyrin. *Br J Cancer.* 1994;70: 21–28.

98. Steinbach P, Weingandt H, Baumgartner R, Kriegmair M, Hofstdter F, Knchel R. Cellular fluorescence of the endogenous photosensitizer protoporphyrin IX following exposure to 5-aminolevulinic acid. *Photochem Photobiol.* 1995;62:887–895.

99. Ross EV, Romero R, Kollias N, Crum C, Anderson RR. Selectivity of protoporphyrin IX fluorescence for condylomata after topical application of 5-aminolaevulinic acid: implications for photodynamic treatment. *Br J Dermatol.* 1997;137:736–742.

100. Schroeter C, Pleunis J, van Nispen tot Pannerden C, Reineke T, Neumann HAM. Photodynamic therapy: new treatment for therapy-resistant plantar warts. *Dermatol Surg.* 2005;31:71–75.

101. Smucler R, Jatsov E. Comparative study of aminolevulic acid photodynamic therapy plus pulsed dye laser versus pulsed dye laser alone in treatment of viral warts. *Photomed Laser Surg.* 2005;23:202–205.

102. Stender IM, Na R, Fogh H, Gluud C, Wulf HC. Photodynamic therapy with 5-aminolevulinic acid or placebo for recalcitrant foot and hand warts: randomised double-blind trial. *Lancet.* 2000;355:963–966.

103. Schroeter CA, Kaas L, Waterval JJ, Bos PM, Neumann HAM. Successful treatment of periungual warts using photodynamic therapy: a pilot study. *J Eur Acad Dermatol Venereol.* 2007;21:1170–1174.

104. Chen K, Chang BZ, Ju M, Zhang XH, Gu H. Comparative study of photodynamic therapy vs CO₂ laser vaporization in treatment of condylomata acuminata: a randomized clinical trial. *Br J Dermatol.* 2007;156: 516–520.

105. Wang HW, Zhang LL, Miao F, Lv T, Wang XL, Huang Z. Treatment of HPV infection-associated cervical condylomata acuminata with 5-aminolevulinic acid-mediated photodynamic therapy. *Photochem Photobiol.* 2012;88: 565–569 [Epub ahead of print].

106. Mel TB. Uptake of protoporphyrin and violet light photodestruction of *Propionibacterium acnes.* *Z Naturforsch [C].* 1987;42:123–128.

107. Kjeldstad B, Johnsson A. An action spectrum for blue and near ultraviolet inactivation of *Propionibacterium acnes*; with emphasis on a possible porphyrin photosensitization. *Photochem Photobiol.* 1986;43:67–70.

108. Papageorgiou P, Katsambas A, Chu A. Phototherapy with blue (415 nm) and red (660 nm) light in the treatment of acne vulgaris. *Br J Dermatol.* 2000;142: 973–978.

109. Hamilton FL, Car J, Lyons C, Car M, Layton A, Majeed A. Laser and other light therapies for the treatment of acne vulgaris: systematic review. *Br J Dermatol.* 2009; 160:1273–1285.

110. Haedersdal M, Togsverd Bo K, Wulf HC. Evidence-based review of lasers, light sources and photodynamic therapy in the treatment of acne vulgaris. *J Eur Acad Dermatol Venereol.* 2008;22:267–278.

111. Genina EA, Bashkatov AN, Simonenko GV, Odoevskaya OD, Tuchin VV, Altshuler GB. Low-intensity indocyanine-green laser phototherapy of acne vulgaris: pilot study. *J Biomed Opt.* 2004;9:828–834.

112. Haedersdal M, Togsverd Bo K, Wiegell S, Wulf H. Long-pulsed dye laser versus long-pulsed dye laser-assisted photodynamic therapy for acne vulgaris: a randomized controlled trial. *J Am Acad Dermatol.* 2008;58: 387–394.

113. Hongcharu W, Taylor CR, Chang Y, Aghassi D, Suthamjariya K, Anderson RR. Topical ALA-photodynamic therapy for the treatment of acne vulgaris. *J Invest Dermatol.* 2000;115:183–192.

114. Hörfelt C, Funk J, Frohm Nilsson M, Wiegleb-Edstrm D, Wennberg AM. Topical methyl aminolevulinate photodynamic therapy for treatment of facial acne vulgaris: results of a randomized, controlled study. *Br J Dermatol.* 2006;155:608–613.

115. Pollock B, Turner D, Stringer MR, et al. Topical aminolaevulinic acid-photodynamic therapy for the treatment of acne vulgaris: a study of clinical efficacy and mechanism of action. *Br J Dermatol.* 2004;151:616–622.

116. Rojanamatin J, Choawawanich P. Treatment of inflammatory facial acne vulgaris with intense pulsed light and short contact of topical 5-aminolevulinic acid: a pilot study. *Dermatol Surg.* 2006;32:991–996.

117. Yeung C, Shek S, Bjerring P, Yu C, Kono T, Chan H. A comparative study of intense pulsed light alone and its combination with photodynamic therapy for the treatment of facial acne in Asian skin. *Lasers Surg Med.* 2007;39:1–6.

118. Tuchin V, Genina E, Bashkatov A, Simonenko G, Odoevskaya O, Altshuler G. A pilot study of ICG laser therapy of acne vulgaris: photodynamic and photothermolysis treatment. *Lasers Surg Med.* 2003;33:296–310.

119. Gold M, Bridges T, Bradshaw V, Boring M. ALA-PDT and blue light therapy for hidradenitis suppurativa. *J Drugs Dermatol.* 2004;3:S32–S35.

120. Schweiger E, Riddle C, Aires D. Treatment of hidradenitis suppurativa by photodynamic therapy with aminolevulinic acid: preliminary results. *J Drugs Dermatol.* 2011;10:381–386.

121. Sotiriou E, Apalla Z, Maliamani F, Ioannides D. Treatment of recalcitrant hidradenitis suppurativa with photodynamic therapy: report of five cases. *Clin Exp Dermatol.* 2009;34:e235–e236.

122. Passeron T, Khemis A, Ortonne J-P. Pulsed dye laser-mediated photodynamic therapy for acne inversa is not successful: a pilot study on four cases. *J Dermatolog Treat.* 2009;20:297–298.

123. Strauss RM, Pollock B, Stables GI, Goulden V, Cunliffe WJ. Photodynamic therapy using aminolaevulinic acid does not lead to clinical improvement in hidradenitis suppurativa. *Br J Dermatol.* 2005;152:803–804.

124. Neimann A, Porter S, Gelfand J. The epidemiology of psoriasis. *Expert Rev Dermatol.* 2006;1:63–75.

125. Schlaak JF, Buslau M, Jochum W, et al. T cells involved in psoriasis vulgaris belong to the Th1 subset. *J Invest Dermatol.* 1994;102:145–149.

126. Boehncke WH, Knig K, Kaufmann R, Scheffold W, Prmmer O, Sterry W. Photodynamic therapy in psoriasis: suppression of cytokine production in vitro and recording of fluorescence modification during treatment in vivo. *Arch Dermatol Res.* 1994;286:300–303.

127. Bissonnette R, Tremblay J-F, Juzenas P, Boushira M, Lui H. Systemic photodynamic therapy with aminolevulinic acid induces apoptosis in lesional T lymphocytes of psoriatic plaques. *J Invest Dermatol.* 2002;119: 77–83.

128. Smits T, Kleinpenning MM, van Erp PEJ, van de Kerkhof PCM, Gerritsen MJP. A placebo-controlled randomized study on the clinical effectiveness, immunohistochemical changes and protoporphyrin IX accumulation in fractionated 5-aminolevulinic acid-photodynamic therapy in patients with psoriasis. *Br J Dermatol.* 2006; 155:429–436.

129. Stringer MR, Collins P, Robinson DJ, Stables GI, Sheehan Dare RA. The accumulation of protoporphyrin IX in plaque psoriasis after topical application of 5-aminolevulinic acid indicates a potential for superficial photodynamic therapy. *J Invest Dermatol*. 1996;107: 76–81.

130. Silver H. Psoriasis vulgaris treated with hematoporphyrin. *Arch Dermatol Syphilol*. 1937;36:1118–1119.

131. Boehncke WH, Sterry W, Kaufmann R. Treatment of psoriasis by topical photodynamic therapy with polychromatic light. *Lancet*. 1994;343:801.

132. Robinson DJ, Collins P, Stringer MR, et al. Improved response of plaque psoriasis after multiple treatments with topical 5-aminolaevulinic acid photodynamic therapy. *Acta Derm Venereol*. 1999;79:451–455.

133. Beattie PE, Dawe RS, Ferguson J, Ibbotson SH. Lack of efficacy and tolerability of topical PDT for psoriasis in comparison with narrowband UVB phototherapy. *Clin Exp Dermatol*. 2004;29:560–562.

134. Radakovic Fijan S, Blecha Thalhammer U, Schleyer V, et al. Topical aminolaevulinic acid-based photodynamic therapy as a treatment option for psoriasis? Results of a randomized, observer-blinded study. *Br J Dermatol*. 2005;152:279–283.

135. Schleyer V, Radakovic Fijan S, Karrer S, et al. Disappointing results and low tolerability of photodynamic therapy with topical 5-aminolaevulinic acid in psoriasis. A randomized, double-blind phase I/II study. *J Eur Acad Dermatol Venereol*. 2006;20:823–828.

136. Collins P, Robinson DJ, Stringer MR, Stables GI, Sheehan Dare RA. The variable response of plaque psoriasis after a single treatment with topical 5-aminolaevulinic acid photodynamic therapy. *Br J Dermatol*. 1997;137:743–749.

137. Orringer J, Hammerberg C, Hamilton T, et al. Molecular effects of photodynamic therapy for photoaging. *Arch Dermatol*. 2008;144:1296–1302.

138. Issa MCA, Pieiro-Maceira J, Vieira MTC, et al. Photorejuvenation with topical methyl aminolevulinate and red light: a randomized, prospective, clinical, histopathologic, and morphometric study. *Dermatol Surg*. 2010;36:39–48.

139. Dover J, Bhatia A, Stewart B, Arndt K. Topical 5-aminolevulinic acid combined with intense pulsed light in the treatment of photoaging. *Arch Dermatol*. 2005;141:1247–1252.

140. Alster T, Tanzi E, Welsh E. Photorejuvenation of facial skin with topical 20% 5-aminolevulinic acid and intense pulsed light treatment: a split-face comparison study. *J Drugs Dermatol*. 2005;4:35–38.

141. Marmur E, Phelps R, Goldberg D. Ultrastructural changes seen after ALA-IPL photorejuvenation: a pilot study. *J Cosmet Laser Ther*. 2005;7:21–24.

142. Asilian A, Davami M. Comparison between the efficacy of photodynamic therapy and topical paromomycin in the treatment of Old World cutaneous leishmaniasis: a placebo-controlled, randomized clinical trial. *Clin Exp Dermatol*. 2006;31:634–637.

143. Halldin C, Gillstedt M, Paoli J, Wennberg A-M, Gonzalez H. Predictors of pain associated with photodynamic therapy: a retrospective study of 658 treatments. *Acta Derm Venereol*. 2011;91:545–551.

144. Grapengiesser S, Ericson M, Gudmundsson F, Lark O, Rosn A, Wennberg AM. Pain caused by photodynamic therapy of skin cancer. *Clin Exp Dermatol*. 2002;27: 493–497.

145. Sandberg C, Stenquist B, Rosdahl I, et al. Important factors for pain during photodynamic therapy for actinic keratosis. *Acta Derm Venereol*. 2006;86:404–408.

146. Steinbauer J, Schreml S, Babilas P, et al. Topical photodynamic therapy with porphyrin precursors—assessment of treatment-associated pain in a retrospective study. *Photochem Photobiol Sci*. 2009;8:1111–1116.

147. Moloney FJ, Collins P. Randomized, double-blind, prospective study to compare topical 5-aminolaevulinic acid methylester with topical 5-aminolaevulinic acid photodynamic therapy for extensive scalp actinic keratosis. *Br J Dermatol*. 2007;157:87–91.

148. Kasche A, Luderschmidt S, Ring J, Hein R. Photodynamic therapy induces less pain in patients treated with methyl aminolevulinate compared to aminolevulinic acid. *J Drugs Dermatol*. 2006;5:353–356.

149. Rud E, Gederaas O, Hgset A, Berg K. 5-Aminolevulinic acid, but not 5-aminolevulinic acid esters, is transported into adenocarcinoma cells by system BETA transporters. *Photochem Photobiol*. 2000;71:640–647.

150. Fritsch C, Stege H, Saalmann G, Goerz G, Ruzicka T, Krutmann J. Green light is effective and less painful than red light in photodynamic therapy of facial solar keratoses. *Photodermatol Photoimmunol Photomed*. 1997; 13:181–185.

151. Paoli J, Halldin C, Ericson MB, Wennberg AM. Nerve blocks provide effective pain relief during topical photodynamic therapy for extensive facial actinic keratoses. *Clin Exp Dermatol*. 2008;33:559–564.

152. Serra Guillen C, Hueso L, Nagore E, et al. Comparative study between cold air analgesia and supraorbital and supratrochlear nerve block for the management of pain during photodynamic therapy for actinic keratoses of the frontotemporal zone. *Br J Dermatol*. 2009;161: 353–356.

153. Halldin CB, Paoli J, Sandberg C, Gonzalez H, Wennberg AM. Nerve blocks enable adequate pain relief during topical photodynamic therapy of field cancerization on the forehead and scalp. *Br J Dermatol*. 2009;160:795–800.

CHAPTER 9

Laser Treatment of Cutaneous Scarring

Elliot T. Weiss and Jeremy A. Brauer

CUTANEOUS SCARRING

The ability to safely and effectively treat cutaneous scarring with laser therapy represents an invaluable skill for the practicing laser surgeon. Various types of scarring may result from traumatic injury, surgical procedures, inflammation, or infection. A basic understanding of the pathophysiology of scarring, the different types of scars, and the most appropriate laser therapy for each type is essential to successfully treating cutaneous scars. While a challenging task, successful treatment of scarring generates immense patient satisfaction and renewed patient self-confidence.

HYPERTROPHIC AND ERYTHEMATOUS SCARS

Hypertrophic scarring can occur after surgical procedures, inflammatory conditions, or traumatic injury to the skin. This aberrant scarring frequently occurs in predisposed individuals or in wounds under increased tension, pressure, or movement. Histologically, hypertrophic scars consist of compact, thickened collagen bundles and prominent microvasculature. Keloid scars have dense, proliferative nodules of collagen and a paucity of microvasculature compared with hypertrophic scars, and this difference in vessel density may explain, in part, the poor response of keloids to laser therapy. Affected individuals may frequently complain of discomfort or pruritus at the site of these scars, and patients frequently seek medical treatments for symptomatic or cosmetic improvement of hypertrophic scars. Persistent and excessive erythema, to some degree, often accompanies hypertrophic scarring.

The laser treatment of choice for hypertrophic and erythematous scars is the vessel-specific 585/595-nm pulsed dye laser (PDL) (Figure 9-1). Numerous studies have demonstrated efficacy in reducing scar erythema as well as scar volume, texture, and pruritus with PDL

treatments. The exact mechanism by which PDL improves hypertrophic scarring is not completely understood. PDL use for these scars is largely based on the concept of selective photothermolysis, in which oxyhemoglobin in scar vasculature selectively absorbs the laser energy resulting in thermal injury and coagulation of microvasculature.[1] This selective destruction of scar microvasculature is thought to result in reduced collagen density within the scar and perhaps decreased endothelial cell stimulation of scar fibroblasts. Histologically, the prominence of microvasculature in hypertrophic scars and the relative paucity of microvasculature in keloid scars are notable, and this difference in vessel density may explain, in part, the poor response of keloids to PDL. Other therapeutic effects of PDL correlated to scar improvement include suppression of fibroblast proliferation and activation of fibroblast apoptosis.[2] Additionally, suppression of TGF-beta1 expression and upregulation of matrix metalloproteinase have been correlated to scar regression following PDL treatment.[3] TGF-beta is known to enhance extracellular matrix, and collagen and fibronectin production by dermal fibroblasts,[4] and, based on animal models, overproduction of TGF-beta can produce excessive scar formation.[5,6] Inhibition of TGF-beta signaling may explain, in part, the histologic changes seen in scars treated with PDL.

Over many years of treating hypertrophic and keloidal scars, our experience has been that keloid scars, particularly established ones, respond very poorly to laser surgery and are more appropriately treated with non-laser interventions such as intralesional kenalog and 5-fluorouracil (5-FU) and/or excision and pressure bandaging. We frequently utilize the PDL with intralesional 5-FU for erythematous, hypertrophic scars and routinely observe symptomatic improvement as well as improved color and elevation after a series of treatments. For hypertrophic scarring due to surgery or trauma, the published literature and our extensive clinical experience over the past several years strongly support the use of

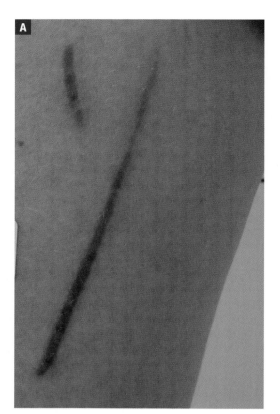 

▲ **FIGURE 9-1 A.** Erythematous scars resulting from trauma prior to treatment. **B.** Erythematous scars resulting from trauma 1 month after three treatments with a pulsed dye laser.

nonablative fractional resurfacing (NAFR) and ablative fractional resurfacing (AFR). Due to the prolonged healing and erythema typically seen after AFR of off-face scarring, we typically reserve AFR for facial scars and utilize NAFR for off-face scarring. Nonablative fractional treatment consistently leads to improved scar texture, pliability, and height in treated hypertrophic scars. The safety profile of nonablative fractional treatments and the lack of postprocedure pigmentary sequelae are important advantages over traditional ablative procedures. In order to manage the variable presentations of scarring, we at times combine PDL and nonablative fractional treatments, as appropriate, to treat scars with some degree of erythema and hypertrophy.

More recently, in an ongoing prospective clinical trial at our center using a novel picosecond alexandrite 755-nm laser, we have observed preliminary success in the treatment of hypertrophic and erythematous scars.

HYPOPIGMENTED SCARS

The final appearance of cutaneous scars depends on the etiology, depth of injury, wound tension, and variations in healing.[7] Immediately after healing, scars are usually red to pink in color, and over the course of months scars mature and their color approaches that of the surrounding skin.[8] Normal scars are hypopigmented, to some degree, compared with the surrounding skin. The exact cause of this hypopigmentation is debated, but hypomelanocytosis, hypomelanosis, and optical factors have been implicated. Depending on the surface area of the scar and the shape, the hypopigmentation may be the most striking feature noted by patients.

Laser treatment of hypopigmented scars remains a challenging task. The earliest, successful laser studies utilized the stimulating effects of ultraviolet light on melanocytes. The 308-nm excimer laser generates high-intensity coherent light in the UVB spectrum, and the excimer has demonstrated variable success in treating a variety of types of hypopigmented scars. Nonetheless, without periodic maintenance treatments, the beneficial effects of the excimer laser are short lived and typically diminish over a 6-month period. Our experience, in agreement with published series, supports the role of NAFR and AFR for hypopigmented scars. The exact mechanism of the repigmentation observed after fractional resurfacing is unknown, but suggested mechanisms include repopulation of normal melanocytes from adjacent healthy tissue and direct stimulation of scar melanocytes. Improvements in the degree of skin atrophy from fractional resurfacing may also alter the optical characteristics of the scar resulting in observed improvements in hypopigmentation. Extensive data from our clinic indicate that both NAFR and AFR of hypopigmented scars result in improvements in both pigmentation and skin texture that lasts greater than 6 months after the final treatment.[9] We routinely observe improvement after the first treatment, and additional treatments typically lead to incremental improvement.

As with hypertrophic and erythematous scars, improvement in hypopigmented scarring has also been recently noted in an ongoing prospective clinical trial at our center using a novel picosecond alexandrite 755-nm laser.

ATROPHIC ACNE SCARRING

Atrophic scarring resulting from inflammatory cystic acne is cosmetically concerning to patients and a frequent cause of social distress. For these reasons, patients often seek treatments to improve the appearance of these scars. Inflammation in and around cystic lesions may cause sufficient damage to dermal connective tissue to result in an atrophic depressed scar. Acne scars are frequently categorized as the narrow and deep ice-pick scars, the slightly wider depressed boxcar scars, or the smoother soft rolling scars.

The first successful attempts to improve acne scarring with laser devices utilized tissue ablating lasers. Traditional fully ablative lasers smooth the skin surface, and the thermal coagulation of dermis stimulates collagen and connective tissue production improving tissue atrophy within the scars. While efficacious in the improvement of the atrophy and appearance of acne scars, fully ablative laser treatments are associated with a relatively high risk of additional scarring and delayed hypopigmentation of treated skin. For these reasons, traditional ablative resurfacing fell out of favor, and laser surgeons began using safer, but less effective, nonablative laser devices. These nonablative lasers (1320-nm ND:YAG, 1450-nm diode, 1064-nm ND:YAG) selectively heat dermal tissue and stimulate neocollagenesis while avoiding the epidermal damage that necessitates prolonged healing.

The advent of fractional photothermolysis revolutionized the treatment of acne scarring by allowing physicians to once again safely use both ablative and nonablative wavelengths to generate deep coagulation or ablation of scar tissue and dermis without widespread epidermal damage. Fractional resurfacing shortens patient recovery and postoperative erythema, and it mitigates the risks of dyspigmentation and scarring associated with traditional laser resurfacing. Improvement in atrophic acne scarring with NAFR has been well reported in the literature,[10] (Figure 9-2) and NAFR

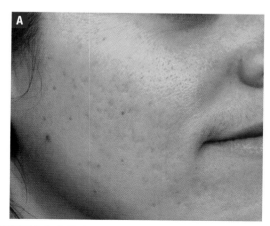
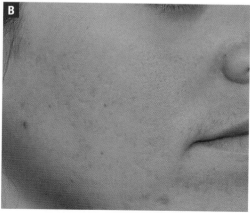

▲ **FIGURE 9-2 A.** Facial acne scarring prior to treatment. **B.** Facial acne scarring 1 month after five treatments with a nonablative fractional 1550-nm laser.

has been safely used to improve acne scars in darker skin types as well.[11] Depending on the severity of scarring, 3 to 5 treatments at monthly intervals are typically recommended, and patients generally notice gradual improvement with each successive treatment.

AFR combines the benefits of deep tissue ablation and coagulation with the more rapid healing and improved safety profile associated with fractional photothermolysis. For atrophic acne scarring, we believe AFR typically results in greater clinical benefit with fewer treatments. For severe acne scarring, AFR becomes our treatment of choice and NAFR becomes our second choice. In 1 study at our center, PRIMOS imaging technology was utilized to measure the depth of acne scars before and after 2 to 3 AFR treatments.[12] The overall average quantitative improvement in scar depth seen in that study was 66.8%.

SURGICAL SCARS

Although scarring from surgical procedures is inevitable, the appearance of the resulting scar often determines the overall satisfaction of the patient. Wound tension, surgical technique, defect size, and other wound healing variables determine the ultimate appearance of the scar. Postoperative scarring may therefore present in various forms, and laser therapy must be individually tailored to meet the needs of the patient. Uncomplicated surgical scarring typically results in a thin hypopigmented scar. Some degree of persistent erythema, atrophy, or hypertrophy may exist along the scar depending on the location, depth, and breadth of surgical defect.

Various laser devices have been used to attempt to improve the cosmetic appearance of postsurgical scars, and ablative resurfacing lasers were the first devices used for this purpose. The CO_2 laser uses the 10,600-nm wavelength, which targets water, to cause precise levels of tissue ablation and thermal damage. The 2940-nm erbium yttrium-aluminum-garnet (Er:YAG) laser is another tissue ablating laser frequently used for scar revision. This wavelength is highly absorbed by water, so penetration is shallower than for the CO_2 laser, and the Er:YAG has short-, variable-, or dual-pulsed modes of operation. These devices allow the user to ablate and smooth the skin to a precise tissue depth, and the large zone of thermal coagulation drives robust dermal remodeling and neocollagenesis. In general, fully ablative resurfacing of surgical scars improves the clinical appearance, but prolonged healing time, risk of further scarring,

prolonged erythema, and risk of pigment alteration significantly limit its application to certain clinical situations. We frequently use the erbium laser to flatten focal areas of hypertrophy on facial scars or to smooth the edges of surgical defects allowed to heal by secondary intention.

Clinical experience and published data support the use of the PDL for both erythematous and erythematous, hypertrophic surgical scars. The authors believe that optimal results are obtained with multiple monthly treatments performed with purpuric settings (7.5 J, 1.5 milliseconds, 10 mm). Purely macular erythema typically resolves in 1 to 2 treatments; however, greater degrees of hypertrophy necessitate increased numbers of treatment sessions. We frequently combine intralesional 5-FU with PDL treatment to flatten and soften elevated firm scars. For improving pigmentation, texture, and overall appearance of off-face scars, we utilize monthly NAFR treatments to minimize posttreatment erythema. The greater the degree of textural or pigmentary irregularity, the greater the number of NAFR treatment sessions needed. Typically, 3 to 5 treatment sessions are required to obtain optimal results. For facial scars, our treatment of choice for textural and pigmentary irregularity, atrophy, and mild hypertrophy is AFR[13] (Figure 9-3). While patients will notice incremental improvement with each treatment, moderate-to-severe scarring will necessitate 3 to 4 treatment sessions to reach an optimal end point.

CASE STUDIES

PDL: Erythematous and Hypertrophic Scarring

PATIENT SELECTION For all laser treatments, selecting the appropriate candidate is paramount to successful outcomes. Patients whose scars present with prominent blanching erythema with or without hypertrophy are candidates for treatment with the PDL. Patients should be fully educated on the need for multiple treatment sessions and the fact that treatment will not completely remove the scar. With the exception of very extensive burn scars, PDL treatments last only several minutes at most and do not generally require local or general anesthesia. If a patient is unable to tolerate treatment of his or her scar, an application of commercially available anesthetic creams is often sufficient to allow treatment to proceed.

TECHNIQUE The patient should be positioned comfortably on a well-lit examination table with opaque safety

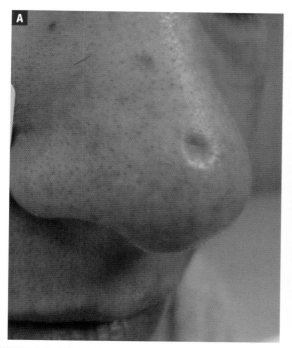
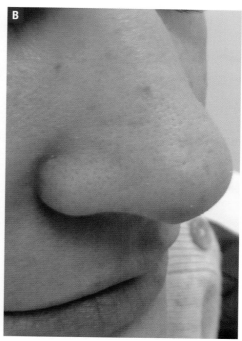

▲ **FIGURE 9-3** **A.** Surgical scar on nose prior to treatment. **B.** Surgical scar on nose 3 years after one treatment with an ablative fractional CO_2 laser.

goggles covering both eyes. All cosmetics and sunscreen should be removed from the treatment area. After confirming adequate eye protection for all individuals in the treatment room, the treating physician should then apply nonoverlapping pulses sufficient to completely treat the scar and the immediate surrounding skin.

EXPECTED RESULTS Beginning almost immediately after treatment, the treated area will develop purpura at the site of each laser pulse. Mild edema of the treatment area may occur transiently. Patients may also report a temporary stinging sensation lasting minutes. Treatment-induced purpura generally resolves gradually within 7 to 10 days. Improvement in scar erythema, softening of scar tissue, and scar flattening occur slowly over the month following treatment. Improvement is incremental, and symptomatic improvement in pruritus and discomfort typically occurs after multiple treatments (Figures 9-4 to 9-6).

POSTPROCEDURE INSTRUCTIONS Postprocedure care following PDL treatment is minimal. Patients are instructed to apply a petrolatum-based ointment in the rare event that crusting occurs. Patients are otherwise instructed to ice the area immediately following treatment, if they report discomfort. In order to minimize swelling when treating on the cheeks or near the eyes, patients are instructed to ice for 20 minutes after treatment. Makeup can be applied after treatment, and strict photoprotection of the treatment area is recommended.

PEARLS AND PITFALLS In general, the PDL has a wide margin of safety when the physician is aware of several important principles. In order to protect the epidermis of treated skin, epidermal cooling must be activated during treatment. Additionally, when treating darker skin types or tan skin, the treating physician should avoid utilizing very short pulse widths (0.45 millisecond) in order to minimize the risk of epidermal crusting and subsequent hypopigmentation. Epidermal whitening or graying should alert the treating physician to halt treatment and modify treatment parameters. Pulse stacking is not recommended when using short pulse durations and higher fluencies since the resulting bulk heating may lead to ulceration or further scarring.

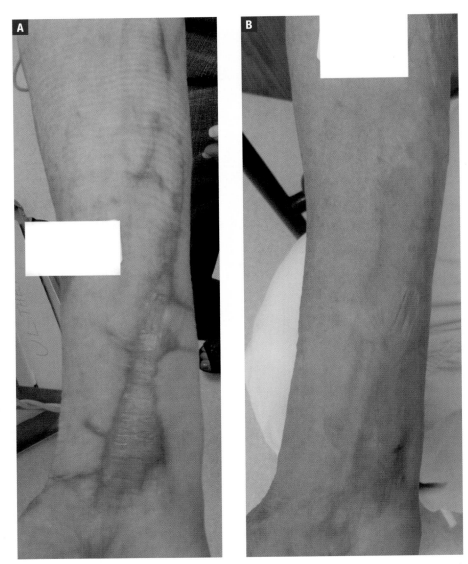

▲ **FIGURE 9-4 A.** Erythematous and hypertrophic scar prior to treatment. **B.** Erythematous and hypertrophic scar 1 month after six treatments with a pulsed dye laser and one treatment with a nonablative fractional 1927-nm laser.

AFR and NAFR: Atrophic Acne Scarring

PATIENT SELECTION Our general belief is that active acne should be tightly controlled before treatment to improve scarring is initiated. Patients who present with atrophic acne scarring of the face, neck, and chest are candidates for fractional resurfacing. In order to minimize the duration of posttreatment erythema, we generally prefer NAFR over AFR for diffuse acne

scarring of the back or chest. Individuals undergoing treatment with oral isotretinoin should wait approximately 6 months after discontinuation to begin laser treatment.

TECHNIQUE In general, for NAFR of acne scarring, adequate pain control is achieved with use of topical anesthetic and intramuscular ketorolac. When utilizing AFR for facial/neck acne scarring, premedication with

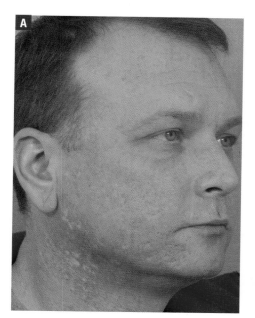
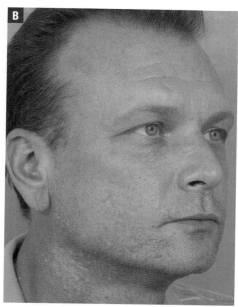

▲ **FIGURE 9-5** **A.** Facial acne scarring prior to treatment. **B.** Facial acne scarring 3 months after three treatments with an ablative fractional CO_2 laser.

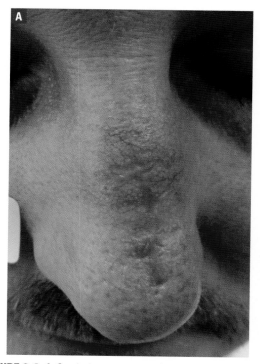
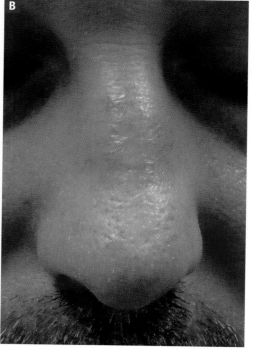

▲ **FIGURE 9-6** **A.** Surgical scar on nose prior to treatment. **B.** Surgical scar on nose 4 months after one treatment with an ablative fractional CO_2 laser.

an oral anxiolytic and an oral narcotic is preferred. In addition to topical anesthetic cream and intramuscular ketorolac, regional nerve blocks are performed 15 to 20 minutes before facial AFR treatment. Unless contraindicated, AFR and NAFR acne scarring patients receive oral corticosteroid for 3 days to minimize swelling.

The depth of treatment is guided by the degree of and depth of scarring, with more severe scarring best addressed with high pulse energy resurfacing. The treating physician should use caution and avoid overlapping pulses or passes during treatment. We additionally utilize forced air cooling to minimize discomfort and bulk heating of the treatment area. When utilizing AFR around the eyes, metal ocular shields are placed in the patient's eyes for the duration of treatment.

EXPECTED RESULTS For NAFR, acne scarring generally requires a series of 3 to 5 monthly treatments depending on the severity of scarring. Patients may begin to see improvement as early as the second or third treatment, and maximum improvement is seen 3 to 6 months after the final treatment. For AFR, acne scarring requires fewer treatments; a single treatment is often adequate for mild/moderate scarring and 2 to >3 treatments are required for moderate/severe scarring. Improvement is incremental with each treatment, and maximum improvement is observed 3 to 6 months after treatment.

POSTPROCEDURE INSTRUCTIONS Following treatment with NAFR, patients are instructed to expect swelling and erythema for several days followed by mild dryness and pink coloration that generally resolves several days later. For AFR, patients expect 3 to 4 days of weeping and crusting during which time they use distilled water soaks several times daily and apply liberal amounts of petrolatum-based ointment. AFR patients are seen 3 to 4 days after treatment for a wound check and the physician decides when the patient can switch to a non-petrolatum-based moisturizer. Patients are seen again approximately 1 week after treatment to ensure appropriate healing. Patients are prepared for swelling that can last up to a week and erythema that slowly fades over many weeks.

PEARLS AND PITFALLS The treating physician must set reasonable expectations for the patient before initiating treatment. Improvement in scarring rather than "removal" should be carefully stressed, and patients should understand that individual responses vary. No specific level of improvement should ever

be "guaranteed." Fractional resurfacing of active acne or acne scarring can lead to a temporary flare requiring oral antibiotics. Treating physicians should be aware of this potential complication and initiate therapy as soon as a flare is suspected.

Scarring as a result of bulk heating of treated tissue can occur from improper technique, excessive delivery of energy, or lack of tissue cooling. Meticulous technique and attention to energy delivery and tissue cooling avoids this pitfall altogether. The HSV status of all AFR and NAFR patients is obtained, and antiviral prophylaxis (3–5 days for NAFR, 7–10 days for AFR) is prescribed to all patients receiving facial treatments regardless of HSV status. For AFR patients, 1 week of oral antibiotic prophylaxis is prescribed, and patients return to clinic at 3 to 4 days and 1 week after treatment for an examination and wound check.

AFR and NAFR: Hypopigmented, Postsurgical, and Traumatic Scarring

PATIENT SELECTION Patients with hypopigmented, postsurgical, and traumatic scarring who seek improvement in the appearance of their scarring are candidates for laser treatment, unless obvious surgical revision is required. Individuals undergoing oral isotretinoin therapy should wait approximately 6 months after discontinuation to initiate laser therapy. For dark-skinned individuals and for off-face scarring, NAFR is preferred to minimize posttreatment erythema and PIH. For more severe scarring on the face, AFR is our treatment of choice.

TECHNIQUE For NAFR of discreet hypopigmented, traumatic, or postsurgical scars, adequate pain control is typically achieved with use of a topical anesthetic; however, use of injected local anesthesia eliminates the waiting time for topical anesthesia and universally results in a pain-free treatment. When utilizing AFR for discreet scars, we recommend infiltrating the scar and surrounding skin with local anesthesia to eliminate patient discomfort during treatment. The depth and percent coverage of treatment is guided by the degree of and depth of scarring, with more severe scarring best addressed with high pulse energy resurfacing. The entire scar and the immediate surrounding skin should be treated with nonoverlapping pulses to ensure uniform treatment. We additionally utilize forced air cooling to prevent bulk heating of the treatment area.

EXPECTED RESULTS When utilizing NAFR, improvement in scar pigmentation, texture, and appearance occurs gradually and requires multiple treatment sessions (3–6) for optimal results. More severe scarring requires a greater number of treatments. Patients generally begin to see improvement as early as the second or third treatment, and maximum improvement is seen several months after the final treatment. With AFR, fewer treatments are required; 1 to 2 treatments are often sufficient for mild/moderate scarring and 2 to >3 treatments are required for moderate/severe scarring. Improvement is incremental with each treatment, and maximum improvement is observed 3 to 6 months after treatment. Following AFR treatment on the face, posttreatment erythema typically resolves over 4 to 6 weeks.

POSTPROCEDURE INSTRUCTIONS Following treatment with NAFR, patients are instructed to expect mild swelling and erythema for several days followed by mild dryness and pink coloration that generally resolves within 7 to 10 days. For AFR, patients expect 3 to 4 days of weeping and crusting during which time they use distilled water soaks several times daily and apply liberal amounts of petrolatum-based ointment. AFR patients with focal scarring are instructed to continue applying petrolatum-based ointment until the treatment area is completely healed and reepithelialized. Patients usually switch to a non-petrolatum-based moisturizer approximately 5 to 7 days after treatment. Patients expect swelling that can last up to a week and erythema that slowly fades over many weeks.

PEARLS AND PITFALLS For both NAFR and AFR, the treatment depth and percentage coverage should be guided by the severity of scarring. Scars with deep atrophic depressions, severe textural irregularity, or extensive hypopigmentation are best treated with high pulse energy resurfacing. Milder textural irregularity or dyspigmentation is more appropriately treated with lower energy resurfacing. Treatment of off-face scarring with higher-energy AFR often leads to prolonged erythema, so patients must be prepared for this potential side effect. For this reason, we often utilize NAFR or occasionally low-energy AFR when treating off-face scarring to avoid prolonged treatment-induced erythema.

REFERENCES

1. Reiken SR, Wolfort SF, Berthiaume F, et al. Control of hypertrophic scar growth using selective photothermolysis. *Lasers Surg Med.* 1997;21(1):7–12.
2. Kuo YR, Wu WS, Jeng SF, et al. Activation of ERK and p38 kinase mediated keloid fibroblast apoptosis after flashlamp pulsed-dye laser treatment. *Lasers Surg Med.* 2005;36(1):31–37 [Erratum. *Lasers Surg Med.* 2005; 36(3):252].
3. Kuo YR, Wu WS, Jeng SF, et al. Suppressed TGF-beta1 expression is correlated with up-regulation of matrix metalloproteinase-13 in keloid regression after flashlamp pulsed dye laser treatment. *Lasers Surg Med.* 2005; 36(1):38–42.
4. Younai S, Nichter LS, Wellisz T, et al. Modulation of collagen synthesis by transforming growth factor-beta in keloid and hypertrophic scar fibroblasts. *Ann Plast Surg.* 1994;33(2):148–151.
5. Lin RY, Sullivan KM, Argenta PA, et al. Exogenous transforming growth factor-beta amplifies its own expression and induces scar formation in a model of human fetal skin repair. *Ann Surg.* 1995;222(2):146–154.
6. Lanning DA, Nwomeh BC, Montante SJ, et al. TGF-beta 1 alters the healing of cutaneous fetal excisional wounds. *J Pediatr Surg.* 1999;34(5):695–700.
7. Sahl WJ Jr, Clever H. Cutaneous scars: part I. *Int J Dermatol.* 1994;33(10):681–691.
8. Zitelli J. Wound healing for the clinician. *Adv Dermatol.* 1987;2:243–267.
9. Reddy KK, Brauer JA, Geronemus RG. Evidence for fractional laser treatment in the improvement of cutaneous scars. *J Am Acad Dermatol.* 2012;66(6):1005–1006.
10. Alster T, Tanzi E, Lazarus M. The use of fractional laser photothermolysis for the treatment of atrophic scars. *Dermatol Surg.* 2007;33:295–299.
11. Lee HS, Lee JH, Ahn GY, et al. Fractional photothermolysis for the treatment of acne scars: a report of 27 Korean patients. *J Dermatolog Treat.* 2008;19(1):45–49.
12. Chapas A, Brightman L, Sukal S, et al. Successful treatment of acneiform scarring with CO_2 ablative fractional resurfacing. *Lasers Surg Med.* 2008;40:381–386.
13. Weiss ET, Chapas A, Brightman L, et al. Successful treatment of atrophic postoperative and traumatic scarring with carbon dioxide ablative fractional resurfacing: quantitative volumetric scar improvement. *Arch Dermatol.* 2010;146(2):133–140.

CHAPTER 10

Home-use and Low-energy Laser and Light Devices

Kavitha K. Reddy and Roy G. Geronemus

 INTRODUCTION

Small devices designed for self-treatment in the home and out-of-office setting represent a major direction of medical technology. As the technological revolution has advanced, most medical devices, including laser and light devices, have continually become smaller, lighter, and increasingly user-friendly. This has led to rapid developments in the home-use and low-energy device category (Table 10-1), which is undergoing the early phases of a likely massive expansion in capabilities and market share.

HOME-USE DEVICE CHARACTERISTICS AND CONSIDERATIONS

The ideal home or out-of-office device should have several key characteristics. The optimal product provides treatment that adds to the value of or replicates in-office treatments. Many patients appreciate the principle of using a device as a replacement for drug treatment, to reduce drug dose or frequency, or to complement treatment by allowing synergistic effects or increased penetration of active ingredients. Ideally, the level of efficacy should be maximized and the treatments required for efficacy should be as short and few as possible. Ease of use and convenience, including potential for "hands-free" operation, are helpful benefits. Comfort is important, given anesthesia options are limited in the home setting. Side effects and "downtime" should be minimized. Safety is critical to protect individual patient and public health, and to promote patient and physician trust and confidence. The optimal product should be small and lightweight; wireless products increase convenience for the patient. Maintenance should be unnecessary or as simple as possible with technical support or warranties available. Cost is also a prominent factor in accessibility.

Patient and Operator Safety

Home-use devices are by nature designed for operation by nonphysicians, particularly by typical patients without any medical background or training in the use of such devices. "First, do no harm" is an important goal in medical treatment, whether in the home or in-office setting. Therefore, the threshold for safe operation must be set very low and instructions should be as simple and understandable as possible for persons of all education levels. Built-in safety mechanisms provide an additional level of protection. Risks of home laser and light devices are similar in nature to those of in-office devices, including risks of ocular damage, hyperpigmentation or hypopigmentation, and scarring. The intention is often for these risks to be significantly lower than if a nonphysician were to inappropriately use a more powerful in-office device. However, given patients may use these devices inappropriately due to unclear or inaccurate instructions, inadequate description of safety information and/or risks associated with use, and potential use of the device numerous times or for a significant cumulative amount of time, safety remains a large concern. Ocular risks remain the most serious. Ultraviolet (UV) light can cause corneal photokeratitis and lens cataracts, infrared radiation produces thermal hazards and opacities in the cornea and lens, and blue light can read to retinal damage and increase risks of age-related macular degeneration, a leading cause of blindness.[1] Unfortunately appropriate protective eyewear is not always provided or recommended by the manufacturer. Pigmentary changes are also a common risk, particularly in patients with skin of color, and are in many cases underestimated or omitted from product labeling.

The US Food and Drug Administration (FDA) has recognized the lack of a clear regulatory pathway for home-use device design, testing, and labeling and acknowledged public concern for the level of both safety and efficacy of these devices.[2] The FDA has

TABLE 10-1
Home Use and Low-energy Devices[a]

Type	Brand Name	Wavelength (nm)	FDA Approval	Indication	Skin Type	Dosing	Potential Risks	Safety Features	Cost (US$)[b]
Fractional nonablative	PaloVia	1410	Yes	Periorbital rhytids	Not described, caution advised in types III–VI	Daily for 4 weeks, and then twice weekly; high, medium, or low setting	Pigmentary changes; blistering; scabbing, scarring	Auto-shutoff Skin contact sensor	499
Fractional nonablative	Code name "Kovar"	1435	No	Not yet available	Not described, caution advised in types III–VI	Unclear; possibly twice weekly	Not available	Not available	Not available
Diode	HairMax LaserComb	655	Yes	Androgenetic alopecia	I–IV	8- to 15-min treatment, 3 times per week	Ocular risk, avoid directly looking at light	None specifically found	295
Diode	LaserCap	650	No	Androgenetic alopecia	I–IV	30 min every other day	Ocular risk, avoid directly looking at light	None specifically found	Request quote; currently available for sale only through authorized physicians
Diode	MEP-90 Hair Growth Stimulation System	650	Yes	Androgenetic alopecia in females	I–IV	20 min twice weekly for 6 months or more	Ocular hazard	None specifically found	Contact manufacturer for price
Diode	Tria Laser	810	Yes	Hair removal in brown and black hairs	I–III	Every 2 weeks up to 6 months or until hair does not regrow; 50% overlapping pulses recommended	Ocular hazard (class I)	White diffuser aperture reduces retinal hazard	395
Intense pulsed light (IPL)	Silk'n SensEpil	475–1200	Yes	Hair removal in brown and black hairs	I–III, caution with darker skin types	Every 2 weeks	Ocular hazard, pigmentary changes	Skin type sensor allows treatment on lighter skin types only; skin contact sensor	499
IPL	Claro	400–1100	Yes	Acne	Not described, caution with darker skin types	Daily 6-s treatment	Ocular hazard, pigmentary changes	None specifically found	195
IPL	No!no! Skin	480–2000	Yes	Acne (mild and moderate inflammatory only)	I–III; caution in darker skin types	Treat acne lesion with 2 pulses each 5 s apart; continue treating every 6–12 h until resolution	Ocular hazard, burn, scarring, pigmentary change	Recommend test on arm first for heat level	180

(continued)

133

TABLE 10-1
Home Use and Low-energy Devices[a] *(Continued)*

Type	Brand Name	Wavelength (nm)	FDA Approval	Indication	Skin Type	Dosing	Potential Risks	Safety Features	Cost (US$)[b]
Ultraviolet (NB-UVB)	Many; example Levia UVB	300–320	Yes	Psoriasis	I–VI	Two to 3 times weekly	Erythema, burn, pigment changes, ocular hazard	Protective eyewear provided	Contact manufacturer for price
Heat	Zeno Hot Spot	Heat; 118°F	Yes	Acne	I–VI, caution in darker skin types	Single 2.5-min treatment to acne lesion	Burn, pigmentary changes	Timer beeps ever 30 s; multitone sound at 2.5 min	40
Heat	ThermaClear	Heat; 222°F	Yes	Acne	I–VI, caution in darker skin types	2-s treatment twice daily	Burn, pigmentary changes	None specifically found	159
Heat	NoInoI Hair	Thermal heating	Yes	Hair removal in hair of all colors	I–VI; caution in darker skin types	Twice weekly for 6 weeks or more	Burn, pigmentary change	Safety switch activates power; heating filament activated only on rotation of skin roller; only lowest fluence is available for first 50 pulses; next 100 pulses allow any of the lowest 3 fluence levels	270
Light-emitting diode (LED)—blue	Tanda Clear	414	Yes	Acne	I–VI	Daily 6-min treatment	Ocular hazard	Goggles provided (level of protection unclear)	195
LED—blue	Tria Clarifying Blue Light	415	Yes	Acne	I–VI	Daily or several times weekly	Ocular hazard	Skin contact sensor	245
LED—red and blue	Omnilux Clear-U	415; 633	Yes	Acne (mild to moderate)	I–VI	20-min treatment twice weekly for 4 weeks	Ocular hazard	Goggles provided (level of protection unclear)	195
LED—red	Tanda Luxe	660	Yes	Periorbital rhytids	I–VI	Treat individual areas for 3 min or 12 min for full face; use twice weekly	Possible ocular hazard	Skin contact sensor Goggles provided (level of protection unclear)	195

[a]List does not include all products available to consumers.
[b]Cost and other data in this table were obtained from general Internet search and have not been verified by the manufacturers. Actual costs and device information should be determined by contacting the manufacturer or other authorized device seller.

announced the agency seeks to improve the safety, quality, and usability of home-use devices through the Medical Device Home Use Initiative, which has 5 goals: (1) to establish guidelines for manufacturers of home-use devices, (2) to develop a home-use device labeling repository, (3) to partner with home health accrediting bodies to support safe use, (4) to enhance postmarket oversight, and (5) to increase public awareness and education. An educational and interactive Web site has been developed for physicians and patients at www.fda.gov/homeusedevices. Caution should always be employed with home-use and low-energy devices, as with any medical or cosmetic device, recognizing each has potential risks associated with improper or even proper use. Fortunately, the balance of efficacy and safety appears to be improving with time. However, with rapid proliferation in new products, there will surely be difficulty in ensuring appropriate safety and efficacy for this large industry. Physician and patient vigilance and reporting will be crucial factors in protecting health, while also promoting optimal design and efficacy.

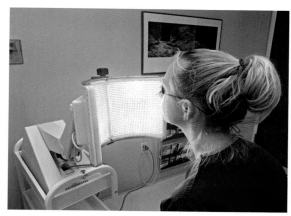

▲ **FIGURE 10-1** A patient receiving 590-nm yellow light LED low-level light therapy treatment after fractional nonablative laser treatment.

LOW-LEVEL LIGHT THERAPY

Low-level light therapy (LLLT) is a category of treatment utilizing low-energy laser or light energy to prevent or treat disease. LLLT has also been called low-level laser therapy, red light therapy, cold laser, soft laser, biostimulation, and/or photobiomodulation.[3,4] In particular, LLLT is defined by a power of 10^{-3} to 10^{-1} W, wavelength 300 to 10,600 nm, pulse rate 0 to 5000 Hz, pulse duration 1 to 500 milliseconds, total irradiation time of 10 to 3000 seconds, intensity (power/area) of 10^{-2} to 10^{0} W/cm², and dose (power × irradiation time/area) 10^{-2} to 10^{2} J/cm².[5,6] Currently, red and near-infrared (600–950 nm) wavelengths are the best studied with efficacy described for improvement in wound healing, pain reduction, anti-inflammatory, antiacne, anticancer, antibacterial, antiviral, antifungal, and antiaging rejuvenation purposes.[3,7,8] There are likely multiple mechanisms of action, most of which are poorly understood. Current proposed mechanisms of action include possible nitric oxide–induced disinhibition of cytochrome c oxidase, leading to an increase in adenosine triphosphate (ATP) production, with alterations in cellular metabolism, and/or production of singlet oxygen that may stimulate cell proliferation at low doses.[9]

The low-energy diode lasers (630–670 nm) have been shown to increase proliferation of follicular cells

and thickness of the resulting hairs.[10,11] Light-emitting diode (LED) devices in the 590 nm range (Figure 10-1) have been reported to produce improvement in signs of photoaging in 90% of patients after an 8-treatment series given over 4 weeks, along with 10% topographic improvement, increased collagen I staining, and reduction in matrix metalloproteinase-1 (MMP-1),[12–14] although further blinded, controlled, and/or larger studies are recommended to evaluate the efficacy of LED sources in reversal of aging-related skin changes.[15] Treatment with 590-nm LED array immediately after facial fractional nonablative laser treatment has been shown to reduce intensity and duration of post–fractional laser treatment erythema during the first 24 to 48 hours after treatment.[16]

Currently available LLLT LED devices designed for in-office treatment include 590 nm (GentleWaves, Light Bioscience, Virginia Beach, Virginia; Revitalight, Skin Care Systems, Chicago, Illinois), 630 nm (Omnilux, Photo Therapeutics, Montgomeryville, Pennsylvania), and 660 nm (LumiPhase-R, OpusMed, Montreal, Canada) devices. Home-use LLLT devices include low-level diode light devices for hair growth and LED devices intended primarily for skin rejuvenation discussed below.

Ultraviolet Light Devices

UV light represents the earliest form of light used to significantly affect human appearance and health. Several negative effects of UV irradiation exist, including photoaging and carcinogenesis.[17] UV light has been used for therapeutic treatment of selected inflammatory skin diseases for many years, including treatment of psoriasis, vitiligo, cutaneous T-cell lymphoma, and other dermatologic conditions. Home-use UV light devices for the treatment of dermatologic conditions were the first significant medical home light devices and have been available for many years. Broadband UV and narrowband UVB devices are produced by a number of manufacturers. Examples include the Levia UVB device (Lerner Medical Devices, Los Angeles, California) and the Derma-light-80 narrowband UVB device (National Biologic Corporation, Beachwood, Ohio). Some devices include available comb attachments that may be used for treatment of inflammatory scalp disorders.[18] Most of these devices require a prescription for shipment to a US address and many also require a physician-provided code for activation and settings selection to improve safety.

Antiacne Devices

Acne affects an estimated 80% of teenage and young adult patients, and for many continues through middle age as well. A number of over-the-counter and prescription products are currently used to prevent and treat acne, most commonly topical and oral products. Procedures for the prevention or treatment of acne have been increasing in popularity and availability. Facials, microdermabrasion, dermabrasion, chemical peels, and other methods of cleansing and exfoliation have been popular for many years. The more recent development of photodynamic and phototherapy protocols for the treatment of acne has provided alternative treatment options for acne and increased consumer interest in light- and laser-based acne treatments.

Proprionibacterium acnes bacteria residing in the pilosebaceous unit produce endogenous porphyrins (coproporphyrin III and protoporphyrin IX) that absorb blue and near-UV wavelengths, having an absorption peak at 415 nm.[19,20] The absorption of red light (660 nm) by *P. acnes* is lower than that for blue light (415 nm); however, red light penetrates more deeply. Absorption of visible light and/or heat by *P. acnes* with subsequent destruction by apoptosis, photothermal destruction, and effects on the surrounding pilosebaceous unit are the basis for treatment.[9] Several devices describe efficacy as a percentage of *P. acnes* bacteria killed; however, it is unclear that *P. acnes* levels themselves influence acne outcomes.[21] In addition, blue and red lights influence the inflammatory cytokine environment.[9,22] Red light activates macrophages, degranulates mast cells, activates neutrophils, and influences the growth factor balance.[9] Blue light decreases IL-1α in keratinocytes and intercellular adhesion molecule-1.[9] Blue and red lights appear to have efficacy in improving both comedonal and inflammatory acne, with the combination likely more effective than monotherapy.[23] Light treatments typically require 5 to 15 minutes of daily exposure to the face for improvement.

Several LED devices are marketed for the treatment of acne (Tanda Clear, Pharos Life Corporation, Cambridge, Ontario; Tria Clarifying Blue Light, Tria Beauty, Inc, Dublin, California; Omnilux Clear-U, Photo Therapeutics, Inc, Carlsbad, California). Blue and red wavelengths are the most popular, based on evidence of their efficacy in treating comedonal and inflammatory acne.[23] The Tanda Clear 414-nm blue light LED was studied using 21 subjects treated with a daily 6-minute treatment for 8 weeks. A statistically significant 30% to 50% decrease in open comedones and 35% reduction in papular acne was reported.[24] The Tria blue LED device (Figure 10-2) is recommended to be used daily for 5 minutes. A small study of 28 patients showed significant reductions in inflammatory and noninflammatory lesion count, although the device was used in combination with a 5% glycolic acid and 2% salicylic acid cleanser and a serum

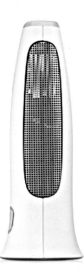

▲ **FIGURE 10-2** A blue light LED device for the treatment of facial acne. (*Source:* www.triabeauty.com.)

containing salicylic acid, niacinamide, and azelaic acid, which confounds the effect of the device alone.[25] A combination 415-nm blue (40 mW/cm[2]) and 633-nm red (70 mW/cm[2]) light LED device (Omnilux Clear-U) is available. A study of 21 subjects with inflammatory acne, each treated with self-administered 20-minute blue and 30-minute red light treatments, with several days between treatments over a period of 4 weeks, resulted in a lesion count reduction of 69% after 8 weeks of follow-up.[26]

A few heat-based (infrared) acne treatment devices (Zeno Hot Spot and Zeno Heat Treat, Tyrell, Inc, Houston, Texas; ThermaClear, Therative, Inc, Livermore, California) are available. The mechanism of action is activation of heat shock proteins in the *P. acnes* bacteria with resultant bacterial killing.[27] The Zeno manufacturer Web site reports 90% of treated acne lesions resolving or fading within 24 hours after a 2.5-minute treatment.[28] ThermaClear is applied for 2.5 seconds and reports 44% of treated lesions resolving at 5 days.[29]

A combination light and heat device (no!no! Skin, Radiancy, Inc, Orangeburg, New York) produces intense pulsed light (IPL) at 450 to 2000 nm (fluence 6 J/cm[2], treatment cycle 10 seconds). A double-blind placebo-controlled study of 63 subjects, each treated twice daily for 4 days, found 77% improvement based on visual analog scales in the treatment arm as compared with 16% in the placebo arm at 24 hours.[27] Another IPL device producing heat and light (CLARO, Solta Medical, Hayward, California) (400–1100 nm, fluence 6 J/cm[2], treatment cycle 6 seconds) has been developed for the treatment of acne. An unpublished study by the manufacturer reported 95% reduction in *P. acnes* bacteria after a single treatment exposure.[24]

Hair Growth Devices

A large portion of the population experiences reduced or absent hair growth as a result of varied medical causes, including androgenetic alopecia. Additionally, many patients seek to augment their natural level of hair density and/or hair growth rate to optimize their cosmetic appearance.

Two LLLT diode laser devices have been developed for the purpose of increasing hair growth. The wavelengths are believed to increase proliferative activity in the follicle, with conversion of vellus hairs to thicker and darker terminal hairs.[10,11] These devices may be used alone or in combination with currently popular topical and systemic medications such as minoxidil and finasteride.

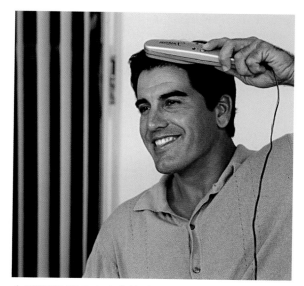

▲ **FIGURE 10-3** An individual uses a diode laser comb to promote hair growth. (*Source*: www.amazon.com/HairMax-HMFP-LaserComb/dp/B000C9M0UW.)

A 655-nm diode laser with 9 beams and total energy output of 45 mW (HairMax LaserComb, Lexington International LLC, Boca Raton, Florida) is FDA-approved for stimulation of hair growth (Figure 10-3). The device should be moved in sequential passes to cover the treatment area for a total of 10 to 15 minutes, and should be used at least 3 times per week on nonconsecutive days. A randomized double-blind sham-controlled study of 110 male patients with androgenetic alopecia demonstrated a statistically significant increase in mean terminal hair density in the treatment group (*P* < .0001).[30] The subjects also assessed themselves as having improved overall hair growth at 26 weeks of use.[30]

Also in the category of hair growth devices is a 650-nm diode laser device, fitted in a mesh hat framework, with 224 beams each emitting 5 mW with total energy output of 1120 mW (LaserCap, Transdermal Cap, Inc, Gates Mills, Ohio). The device may be worn under a hat and does not require combing or movement after placement, potentially increasing convenience for selected patients.

Another LLLT device for hair growth has been FDA-approved for treatment in women (MEP-90 Hair Growth Stimulation System, Midwest RF, Wisconsin). The treatment must be prescribed by a physician and consists of 82 low-level laser beams directed at the scalp while the patient is seated for 20 minutes, twice weekly for 6 months or longer. The company brochure reports a study of 36 subjects treated 20 minutes twice weekly for 18 weeks showed 97% of subjects with increased hair count of 20% or more, 89% of subjects with increased hair count of 30% or more, and 57% of subjects with increased hair count of 50% or more.[31]

Hair Removal Devices

Current laser hair removal technology uses selective photothermolysis targeting melanin in hair follicles and is effective for reduction in color, thickness, and growth rate of brown or black hairs. Other energy-based hair removal treatments include electrolysis and radio-frequency energy that heats and destroys the hair follicles. These are based on heat destruction as opposed to targeting of melanin and therefore may be effective for all colors of hair. Patients and physicians should be aware that laser-, light-, and heat energy–based hair removal as it currently stands does not always result in complete or "hair-free" results, but does typically result in improvement.

Laser hair removal results typically last 3 to 6 months after 1 treatment. "Permanent" or long-lasting results may be achieved after 5 to 6 sessions and typically require occasional maintenance or "touch-up" treatments. Home-use laser hair removal devices have a much lower fluence than in-office devices in order to reduce risks to the patient. Therefore, many more treatment sessions are required for efficacy. In addition, some patients may not ultimately achieve the same degree of hair removal as they would with in-office treatment. Home hair removal devices are used as an alternative to in-office treatment because of reduced costs and improved convenience for many patients, or many times as an adjunctive method to aid maintaining results after in-office laser hair removal.

A diode laser (Tria Laser, Tria Beauty, Inc) is among the most popular and effective current products for home laser hair removal (Figure 10-4). The Tria device produces an 810 nm wavelength, has 3 selectable fluences (high 22.0 J/cm^2, medium 17.5 J/cm^2, low 13.0 J/cm^2), 3 selectable pulse durations (600, 450, or 300 milliseconds), and 1.0 cm spot size. A single-center study was performed with 77 subjects with brown to black hair and skin types I to IV treated with 3 self-administered treatments performed every 3 weeks to evaluate safety and efficacy.[32] After the 3 treatments, mean hair reduction was 60% at 1 month, 41% at

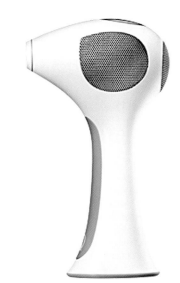

▲ **FIGURE 10-4** A popular diode laser home hair removal device. (*Source*: www.triabeauty.com.)

6 months, and 33% at 12 months. Transient erythema was the only observed side effect reported. Reasonable safety was demonstrated with 44 noncandidate subjects (having white, gray, red, or blonde hair, or skin type V or VI) who received a single staff-administered pulse at the non-hair-bearing site. The manufacturer advises the product should not be used on the face, neck, or genital areas, all of which are popular areas for hair removal. The spot size is smaller than that of most in-office lasers for hair removal. An average single axilla is estimated to take 10 to 15 minutes to treat and each upper and lower leg is estimated at 20 minutes.[33] The manufacturer instructions are for treatment every 2 weeks "up to 6 months or until the hair stops growing back."

An FDA-approved IPL device of 475 to 1200 nm for hair removal (Silk'n SensEpil, Home Skinovations, Yokneam, Israel) has settings of maximum fluence of 5 J/cm^2, pulse duration of <1 millisecond, pulse interval every 3.5 seconds, and 2.0 to 3.0 cm spot size. Treatment time is estimated at 2 to 3 minutes for an area the size of the axilla. The recent SensEpil model has a skin color sensor that prevents operation on types V and VI skin. A study of 34 subjects with 92 sites for hair removal was performed using self-treatment every 2 weeks for a total of 3 treatments.[34] After 3 months of follow-up, blinded assessment found reduced hair counts in 95% of patients, with a mean hair count reduction of 64%. A second study with 20 patients treated with the same treatment course showed a mean individual 40% to 61% hair count reduction after 3 months.[35] In 2 further studies also with treatments every 2 weeks, but with a higher total number of treatments (longer treatment course), widely differing results were found. One study of 20 patients showed efficacy increased after the longer treatment course to 72% hair reduction at 3 months,[36] and the other study of 10 patients showed only 10% hair reduction at 3 months.[37] Thinner hairs on the extremities responded better than thicker hairs on the axillary and inguinal regions. The most common side effect was transient perifollicular erythema, found in 25% to 50% of patients in these studies.

A heat-based hair removal device (no!no! Hair, Radiancy, Inc) uses thermal energy to target the hair follicle. Because the device does not target melanin, it can improve all types of hair. A study of 12 patients treated twice weekly for a total of 6 weeks reported results at 3-month follow-up of 44% hair loss on the legs and 15% hair loss in the inguinal (bikini) area.[38]

Rejuvenation Devices

FRACTIONAL NONABLATIVE DEVICES A fractional nonablative 1410-nm diode laser (Figure 10-5) with 15 mJ fluence and 10 milliseconds pulse duration has been FDA-approved for treatment of periorbital fine lines and wrinkles (PaloVia Skin Renewing Laser, Palomar Medical Technologies, Burlington, Massachusetts). Safety features of the device include a skin sensor

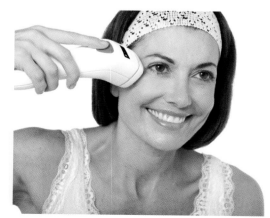

▲ **FIGURE 10-5** Use of a home nonablative fractional laser for the treatment of periorbital rhytids. (*Source*: www.palovia.com.)

requiring adequate contact for laser delivery, and an automatic shutoff after 25 scans for a period of 8 hours.[39] Histology has shown microthermal zones of injury extending to 250 μm.[24] The manufacturer-recommended treatment regimen is daily use for 1 month, followed by twice-weekly maintenance treatments.[39] Two prospective studies, 1 with 34 patients and 1 with 90 patients (total of 124 patients), each showed 90% of patients demonstrated 1 grade of improvement in periorbital rhytids as assessed by a blinded investigator after the initial 4-week treatment phase.[24] In both studies, 79% of patients maintained this grade of improvement after another 4 to 12 weeks of twice-weekly maintenance treatments. Patient self-assessment showed similar efficacy, with 87% of patients reporting reduction in periorbital rhytids.

Another fractional nonablative laser, a 1435-nm laser with high-speed scanner producing injury to 200 μm depth (temporarily code-named the "Kovar" device, Solta Medical; Philips, Einthoven, Holland), is under development and not yet FDA-approved.[40] The energy output is 1.2 W. The histology has shown transepidermal shuttle elimination and procollagen I formation similar in type to other fractionated devices. A study of 80 patients treated twice weekly on the face, neck, chest, and arms for 8 to 12 weeks has been reported to show statistically significant improvement in overall appearance, fine lines, pigmentation, age/sun spots, texture, firmness, and radiance at 1 and 4 weeks after the treatment course. At 8 weeks, 90% of patients were reported to have noticed improvement.[40]

LED devices are also widely marketed for the treatment of photoaging and rejuvenation of the skin. They utilize the principle of LLLT, and some wavelengths, particularly yellow and red lights, have been shown to increase collagen production and improve photoaging changes.[12] Several LED devices are available for home and portable use (Tanda Luxe, 660-nm red light LED device, Pharos Life Corporation; Baby Quasar, Quasar Biotech, Sarasota, Florida). As with many other home devices, further studies of these popular LED devices are needed to accurately evaluate efficacy for patients.

■ FUTURE DIRECTIONS

We are likely to witness an explosion in the variety of home-use laser and light devices available to consumers. Devices for prevention, diagnosis, and treatment of a wide variety of conditions will likely become commonplace in patient homes and other nonphysician-administered settings. Efficacy and safety will vary among these products, although with technological advancements theoretically the overall trend should result in continued improvements in both efficacy and safety. Appropriate monitoring and regulation for accuracy and transparency in safety and efficacy claims will be critical in safeguarding public health and confidence in home laser and light devices. Physician guidance provides a critical benefit in matching the appropriate device with the appropriate patient, evaluating and advocating for appropriate safety measures, and providing suggestions for individualizing and maximizing the potential benefits of use. Home-use and low-energy devices have the potential to significantly improve early, accessible, convenient, and effective prevention and treatment options for a wide variety of dermatologic conditions.

REFERENCES

1. Walker DP, Vollmer-Snarr HR, Eberting CL. Ocular hazards of blue-light therapy in dermatology. *J Am Acad Dermatol*. 2012;66(1):130–135.
2. U.S. Food and Drug Administration. *Medical Device Home Use Initiative*. <http://www.fda.gov/downloads/medicaldevices/productsandmedicalprocedures/home healthandconsumer/homeusedevices/UCM209056.pdf>; April 2010.
3. Sobanko JF, Alster TS. Efficacy of low-level laser therapy for chronic cutaneous ulceration in humans: a review and discussion. *Dermatol Surg*. 2008;34(8):991–1000.
4. Avram MR, Rogers NE. Hair transplantation for men. *J Cosmet Laser Ther*. 2008;10(3):154–160.
5. Posten W, Wrone DA, Dover JS, Arndt KA, Silapunt S, Alam M. Low-level laser therapy for wound healing: mechanism and efficacy. *Dermatol Surg*. 2005;31(3):334–340.
6. Schindl A, Schindl M, Pernerstorfer-Schon H, Schindl L. Low-intensity laser therapy: a review. *J Investig Med*. 2000;48(5):312–326.
7. Desmet KD, Paz DA, Corry JJ, et al. Clinical and experimental applications of NIR-LED photobiomodulation. *Photomed Laser Surg*. 2006;24(2):121–128.
8. Taub AF. Photodynamic therapy: other uses. *Dermatol Clin*. 2007;25(1):101–109.
9. Trelles MA, Mordon S, Calderhead RG. Facial rejuvenation and light: our personal experience. *Lasers Med Sci*. 2007;22(2):93–99.
10. Bouzari N, Firooz AR. Lasers may induce terminal hair growth. *Dermatol Surg*. 2006;32(3):460.
11. Bernstein EF. Hair growth induced by diode laser treatment. *Dermatol Surg*. 2005;31(5):584–586.
12. Weiss RA, McDaniel DH, Geronemus RG, et al. Clinical experience with light-emitting diode (LED) photomodulation. *Dermatol Surg*. 2005;31(9 pt 2):1199–1205.
13. Weiss RA, Weiss MA, Geronemus RG, McDaniel DH. A novel non-thermal non-ablative full panel LED photomodulation device for reversal of photoaging: digital

microscopic and clinical results in various skin types. *J Drugs Dermatol*. 2004;3(6):605–610.
14. Weiss RA, McDaniel DH, Geronemus RG, Weiss MA. Clinical trial of a novel non-thermal LED array for reversal of photoaging: clinical, histologic, and surface profilometric results. *Lasers Surg Med*. 2005;36(2):85–91.
15. Dierickx CC, Anderson RR. Visible light treatment of photoaging. *Dermatol Ther*. 2005;18(3):191–208.
16. Alster TS, Wanitphakdeedecha R. Improvement of post-fractional laser erythema with light-emitting diode photomodulation. *Dermatol Surg*. 2009;35(5):813–815.
17. Reddy KK, Gilchrest BA. Iatrogenic effects of photoprotection recommendations on skin cancer development, vitamin D levels, and general health. *Clin Dermatol*. 2011;29(6):644–651.
18. Stein KR, Pearce DJ, Feldman SR. Targeted UV therapy in the treatment of psoriasis. *J Dermatolog Treat*. 2008;19(3):141–145.
19. Charakida A, Seaton ED, Charakida M, Mouser P, Avgerinos A, Chu AC. Phototherapy in the treatment of acne vulgaris: what is its role? *Am J Clin Dermatol*. 2004;5(4):211–216.
20. Bhardwaj SS, Rohrer TE, Arndt K. Lasers and light therapy for acne vulgaris. *Semin Cutan Med Surg*. 2005;24(2):107–112.
21. Shaheen B, Gonzalez M. A microbial aetiology of acne: what is the evidence? *Br J Dermatol*. 2011;165(3):474–485.
22. Cunliffe WJ, Goulden V. Phototherapy and acne vulgaris. *Br J Dermatol*. 2000;142(5):855–856.
23. Papageorgiou P, Katsambas A, Chu A. Phototherapy with blue (415 nm) and red (660 nm) light in the treatment of acne vulgaris. *Br J Dermatol*. 2000;142(5):973–978.
24. Metelitsa AI, Green JB. Home-use laser and light devices for the skin: an update. *Semin Cutan Med Surg*. 2011;30(3):144–147.
25. Wheeland RG, Dhawan S. Evaluation of self-treatment of mild-to-moderate facial acne with a blue light treatment system. *J Drugs Dermatol*. 2011;10(6):596–602.
26. Sadick NS. Handheld LED array device in the treatment of acne vulgaris. *J Drugs Dermatol*. 2008;7(4):347–350.
27. Sadick NS, Laver Z, Laver L. Treatment of mild-to-moderate acne vulgaris using a combined light and heat energy device: home-use clinical study. *J Cosmet Laser Ther*. 2010;12(6):276–283.
28. Tyrell Inc. <http://www.myzeno.com/hotspot-the-science-behind-hotspot/>. Accessed 01.04.12.
29. ThermaClear for acne. *Med Lett Drugs Ther*. 2007;49(1263):51–52.
30. Leavitt M, Charles G, Heyman E, Michaels D. HairMax LaserComb laser phototherapy device in the treatment of male androgenetic alopecia: a randomized, double-blind, sham device-controlled, multicentre trial. *Clin Drug Investig*. 2009;29(5):283–292.
31. Midwest RF. *MEP-90 Brochure*. <http://www.midwestrf.com/mep90/literature/MEP-90%20Brochure.pdf>. Accessed 01.04.12.
32. Wheeland RG. Simulated consumer use of a battery-powered, hand-held, portable diode laser (810 nm) for hair removal: a safety, efficacy and ease-of-use study. *Lasers Surg Med*. 2007;39(6):476–493.
33. Tria Beauty. Manufacturer website. <http://www.triabeauty.com/home-laser-hair-removal>. Accessed 01.04.12.

34. Mulholland RS. Silk'n—a novel device using Home Pulsed Light for hair removal at home. *J Cosmet Laser Ther.* 2009;11(2):106–109.

35. Alster TS, Tanzi EL. Effect of a novel low-energy pulsed-light device for home-use hair removal. *Dermatol Surg.* 2009;35(3):483–489.

36. Gold MH, Foster A, Biron JA. Low-energy intense pulsed light for hair removal at home. *J Clin Aesthet Dermatol.* 2010;3(2):48–53.

37. Elm CM, Wallander ID, Walgrave SE, Zelickson BD. Clinical study to determine the safety and efficacy of a low-energy, pulsed light device for home use hair removal. *Lasers Surg Med.* 2010;42(4):287–291.

38. Spencer JM. Clinical evaluation of a handheld self-treatment device for hair removal. *J Drugs Dermatol.* 2007;6(8):788–792.

39. Palomar Medical Technologies. Manufacturer website. <http://www.palovia.com>. Accessed 01.04.12.

40. Zachary C. <http://www.drzachary.net/2011/04/03/home-use-skin-rejuvenating-devices-will-duke-it-out-in-2012/>. Accessed 01.04.12.

CHAPTER 11

Treatment of Leg Veins

Jeremy A. Brauer and Julie K. Karen

EPIDEMIOLOGY

Lower extremity venous disease is a common concern among dermatology patients. Leg veins are visibly present or symptomatic in greater than 50% of the adult population, with approximately 25% of the adult population suffering from varicose veins.[1,2] Among individuals with varicosities, more than one quarter suffer from superficial venous insufficiency (SVI).[1] There is a direct relationship between prevalence of varicosities and age as well as gender. Among those less than 25 years of age, less than 8% of women and 1% of men suffer from varicose veins, whereas more than half of women and more than one third of men aged 65 to 74 are affected.[3]

Studies have demonstrated that symptomatic varicose veins negatively impact quality of life.[4] Symptoms classically associated with SVI include fatigue, heaviness, aching, burning, pain, pruritus, edema, and cramping. Recent evidence points toward SVI as a cause of restless legs syndrome (RLS).[5] Prolonged standing, excessive warmth, menses, pregnancy, as well as oral contraceptives or other hormonal therapies often aggravate these symptoms. Patients often relate improvement in their symptoms with ambulation, compression therapy, leg elevation, and cooler ambient temperatures.

Early on, patients with SVI develop dilated, protuberant, and torturous veins, so-called varicose veins. With more advanced disease, patients may develop an eczematous or stasis dermatitis, pigmentary alteration of the skin, as well as lipodermatosclerosis, and atrophie blanche. Most severely, this condition can result in the formation of venous stasis erosions and ulcers, which are classically located over the medial malleolus. At this stage, patients may suffer from recurrent cellulitis, or, eventually, even malignant degeneration.

LEG VEIN ANATOMY AND PHYSIOLOGY

The lower extremity vascular system is comprised of both superficial and deep vessels, with interconnections throughout. The superficial venous system is one of primary collecting veins that are relatively distensible and thin-walled. The superficial vessels run within the skin and subcutaneous tissue and connect by epifascial perforating veins to the deeper vasculature within the muscular system.[6,7] Chief among the superficial vessels are the great saphenous vein (GSV) and the small saphenous vein (SSV).

The GSV drains the majority of the leg, with its origin at the medial aspect of the foot. It passes anteriorly to the medial malleolus before traveling upward along the anteromedial aspect of the calf and then the medial aspect of the thigh, terminating at the saphenofemoral junction near the groin. A normal GSV measures approximately 3 to 4 mm in diameter within the thigh. The SSV drains the posterior and lateral leg, and originates at the lateral foot, before traveling along the midline of the calf. Termination is variable, although most commonly, the SSV enters into the popliteal vein at or around the knee at the saphenopopliteal junction. The GSV and SSV are encased by superficial fascia, but tributaries to these veins lie superficial to this fascia. An intersaphenous connecting vein, the vein of Giacomini, is sometimes present. The lateral subdermic venous system drains the lateral thigh and leg.

The deep venous system of the thigh includes the common femoral vein with femoral vein and deep femoral vein branches, and the popliteal vein. The posterior and anterior tibial, peroneal, and gastrocnemius veins comprise the deep venous system of the calf. Major perforating veins connecting the 2 systems include the Hunterian, Dodd, Boyd, and Cockett.

In a properly functioning venous system, blood is first collected by superficial venous capillaries, followed by larger superficial veins, passing through 1-way valves directing blood flow upward and inward to the deep veins and eventually centrally to the heart and lungs. Failure of these valves produces a dysfunctional high-pressure system with improper flow between the deep and superficial systems, ultimately resulting in dilation of distensible superficial vessels. The precise etiology of SVI is unknown. Intrinsic factors, including genetics, advanced age, female gender, and obesity, are believed to combine with such extrinsic factors as prolonged standing, pregnancy, and, occasionally, trauma to contribute to its pathogenesis.

Most telangiectasias are visible as bright red or purple vessels. These superficial telangiectasias (0.03–0.3 mm in diameter) connect with larger red or blue postcapillary venulectasias (0.4–2.0 mm). Telangiectasias and venulectasias can collectively be referred to as "spider veins." These directly connect to still larger blue reticular veins (2–4 mm) situated deeper in the dermis. Varicose veins are typically blue, torturous, and palpable beneath the skin and typically measure 3 mm or more in diameter.

■ APPROACH TO THE PATIENT

The initial consultation should always include a thorough history and circumferential inspection of the lower extremities with photographic documentation. Clinical evaluation alone may be an unreliable indicator of underlying SVI, and, therefore, when indicated, noninvasive diagnostic evaluations may also be performed.[8] It is important to be able to identify which patients will require imaging. This group usually presents with 1 or more of the following findings on history or physical examination: complaints of symptoms previously discussed including aching, pain, burning, swelling, fatigue, or restless legs; signs such as bulging varicosities in the zones of influence of the saphenous venous systems, edema, induration, or stasis dermatitis; history of prior vein surgery; or a strong family history of varicose veins or venous disease. For these individuals, noninvasive imaging can help to delineate the nature and extent of underlying venous disease. The utility of handheld Doppler (HDD) is limited by its inability to discriminate between superficial and deep reflux in the popliteal fossa, as well as the fact that it does not provide specific anatomic information. Duplex imaging has become the gold standard for assessing the pattern and severity of lower extremity superficial venous disease and defining intervention protocols.[9]

■ TREATMENT

Algorithmic Approach to the Patient

The goal of treatment is to efficiently and reproducibly achieve pan-endothelial vascular obliteration, irrespective of the vessel size. The algorithm employed starts with addressing, when present, incompetence of the saphenous system and its branches, followed by treatment of reticular veins, and finally spider veins.

Compression

Compression treatment utilizing graduated compression stockings has a place in the management of superficial venous disease, and in some situations may serve as primary therapy. More often, compression serves as an adjunctive treatment after more invasive procedures. Compression has been shown to improve efficacy of vein treatments, reduce the risk of thromboembolism, and increase rate of recovery. However, optimum duration of compression after intervention remains unclear.[10–13]

In a study by Weiss et al, 30 female sclerotherapy patients were randomly assigned to wear compression stockings (20–30 mm Hg) during "all waking hours" for 3 days, 1 week, or 3 weeks.[11] Ten additional patients who received sclerotherapy did not apply stockings, and served as control subjects. Their varicose veins were evaluated at 1, 2, 6, 12, and 24 weeks for reduction in size and total number, as well as hyperpigmentation, matting, edema, and ulceration. All 3 compression groups showed statistically significant improvement in vessel size and number at 6 weeks when compared with the control group. However, by the end of the study, only the 1- and 3-week groups showed statistically significant improvement when compared with controls, with the latter group showing improved efficacy and reduced hyperpigmentation. After visual sclerotherapy, this chapter's authors encourage patients to wear compression stockings (typically 20–30 mm Hg) for 1 to 2 weeks. Patients may remove their stockings for brief showers and prior to bed. Higher strength compression is reserved for following treatment of larger vessels, including after ultrasound-guided foam sclerotherapy (UGFS) or endovenous ablation procedures. Immediate postinjection compression in the form of cotton balls secured with tape along treated vessels is thought by some to be beneficial, although this technique has not been rigorously studied. When this technique is employed, compression stockings are applied on top of the cotton balls at the conclusion of the treatment session.

Sclerotherapy

Sclerotherapy is the gold standard treatment for heterogeneous, nonvaricose leg veins and small varicosities. It became a widely accepted procedure after a publication in the early 1970s demonstrated successful

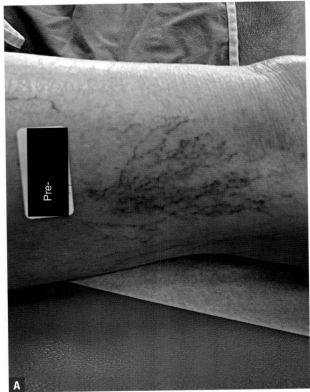
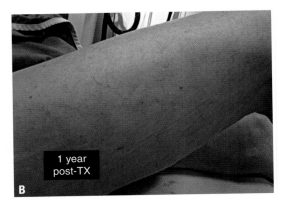
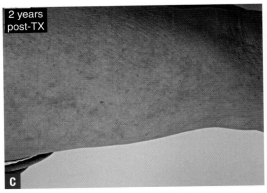

▲ **FIGURE 11-1** Pretreatment (**A**), at 1 year (**B**), and at 2 years (**C**) following 3 sessions of sclerotherapy of the lateral subdermal venous system using POL 0.5% and glycerin 72% mixed 2:1 with lidocaine with epinephrine.

treatment of venous ulcers.[14] More recent studies have shown approximately 60% to 70% improvement in cosmesis per treatment session, as well as marked improvement in subjective pain and discomfort[15,16] (Figure 11-1). This procedure involves the intravenous injection of a sclerosant, defined as any foreign substance known to induce endothelial damage. Although an "ideal" sclerosant does not yet exist, safe and effective sclerotherapy can be achieved when appropriate sclerosant concentrations and volumes are matched to vessel size.[16]

Sclerosants are divided into 3 categories: hyperosmolar or hypertonic, detergent or emulsifier, and toxins or chemical irritants (Table 11-1). Hyperosmolar or hypertonic solutions include hypertonic saline and hypertonic saline + dextrose (Sclerodex™). Chromated glycerin, which is commonly classified as a chemical irritant, may act in a similar fashion to these agents. The mechanism of action of these agents is thought to involve both dehydration and direct denaturation of

TABLE 11-1
Common Sclerosing Solutions

	Category	FDA-Approved
Hypertonic saline, 23.4%	Hyperosmolar	Not for sclerotherapy; yes for other uses
Hypertonic saline + dextrose (HSD)	Hyperosmolar	No
Polidocanol	Detergent	Yes
Sodium tetradecyl sulfate (STS)	Detergent	Yes
Ethanolamine oleate	Detergent	Yes[a]
Sodium morrhuate	Detergent	Yes[a]
Chromated glycerin	Chemical irritant	Not for sclerotherapy; yes for other uses
Polyiodide iodine	Chemical irritants	No
Sodium salicylate	Chemical irritants	No

[a]These agents were grandfathered in, but their use is rare.

cell surface proteins. These agents are slow-acting and require prolonged contact time (minutes) with the vessel wall. They are inexpensive, and are less likely than other agents to elicit allergy. However, because they have a very local effect due to rapid dilution, they are relatively ineffective at treating larger veins. Additionally, these agents may affect nerve endings present within the adventitia of vessels and thereby cause significant pain during treatment. Furthermore, extravasation of hypertonic saline may result in ulceration and consequent scarring.

Detergent solutions act by dissolution of endothelial cell membranes. Chief among this category are sodium tetradecyl sulfate (STS) and polidocanol (POL), both FDA-approved for the treatment of leg veins. Ethanolamine oleate and sodium morrhuate, 2 agents approved for the sclerosis of bleeding esophageal varices, are technically included in this category but are not recommended for the treatment of lower extremity veins due to a high risk of tissue necrosis and anaphylactic reactions. STS and POL are relatively fast acting, with distant spread of effect allowing for treatment of large networks and larger vessels. These are versatile agents that are generally painless when properly injected. Relative to hypertonic agents, there is a higher risk of allergy and greater associated expense.

Liquid detergent solutions can be combined with a gas and agitated in order to create foam. Room air is most commonly employed for foam preparation, although carbon dioxide (CO_2) or a 70% CO_2/30% oxygen (O_2) mixture may also be used.[17,18] In 2000, Tessari described a simple technique to achieve the creation of foam, whereby 1 part liquid detergent is

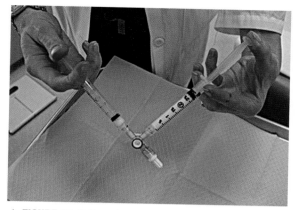

▲ **FIGURE 11-2** Foam is created via the Tessari technique. One part liquid detergent is combined with 4 parts air and agitated using a stopcock.

mixed with 3 or 4 parts room air and agitated via a 2- or 3-way stopcock[17,19] (Figure 11-2). Each microbubble of foam contains the full strength of solution, thus enabling use of lesser concentrations with enhanced effect (Figure 11-3). Foam more efficiently displaces blood and permits for prolonged contact with the vessel intima due to slow washout, further translating into greater efficacy at lower concentrations. Additionally, foam is echogenic and therefore useful as a contrast agent when performing UGFS.[20] Foam sclerotherapy is indicated in treating leg ulcer patients with superficial vein reflux, and patients with recurrent varicose veins.[21]

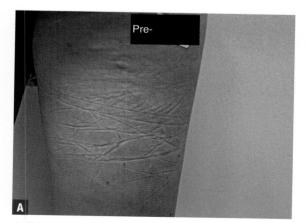

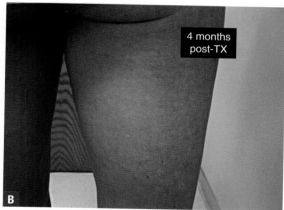

▲ **FIGURE 11-3** Pretreatment (**A**) and 4 months after (**B**) a single session of sclerotherapy utilizing POL 0.25% foam.

Foam sclerotherapy appears to carry an increased risk of pigmentary alteration relative to liquid sclerotherapy, especially when used to treat darker-skinned individuals or vessels that are larger or situated more superficially. Patients should be warned of this potential. Additionally, there is a risk of transient neurologic events, most commonly scotoma and migraine with aura. These neurologic symptoms have classically been considered transient ischemic attacks (TIAs) attributable to passage of air into the cerebral circulation through a patent foramen ovale or other septal defect.[22-24] However, recent evidence points toward a different pathogenesis, namely, a role for such vasoactive substances as endothelin, released in response to endothelial damage.[23] Further studies are needed to better define the nature of these events. Limiting injection volumes per session can help to reduce the risk for these dreaded events.

Chemical irritants and toxins include salts such as polyiodide iodine, sodium salicylate, alcohols, and heavy metals. Chromated glycerin is also typically included in this category. These agents act as cell surface protein poisons and result in full thickness injury at the site of injection within seconds, with a high risk of necrosis. With the exception of glycerin, these agents are rarely, if ever, used in the United States. Glycerin is FDA-approved for ophthalmologic use, although its use as a sclerosant is off-label. This chapter's authors commonly utilize a preparation of 72% glycerin mixed 2:1 with lidocaine (either with or without epinephrine) to treat spider veins. Many phlebologists consider glycerin to be the agent that is least likely to cause matting or pigmentary alteration. Additionally, glycerin has been used to successfully treat matting that occurs following sclerotherapy.

Contraindications to sclerotherapy include allergy to sclerosant(s), pregnancy, lactation, inability to ambulate, acute superficial thrombophlebitis or deep vein thrombosis (DVT), active local infections, advanced peripheral arterial disease, and severe systemic disease. For individuals with a history of DVT or known hypercoagulable state, caution should be exercised, and a hematologist consulted prior to proceeding with treatment.

Sclerotherapy complications can be classified as frequent but temporary, uncommon but self-limited, and rare but major.[24] Most adverse events are frequent but temporary, and include variable results with the need for multiple treatments, local tenderness or urticaria, pigmentary alteration, bruising, telangiectatic matting (TM), and intravascular microthrombus formation.[25,26] Less common, but self-limited problems

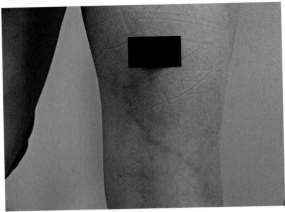

▲ **FIGURE 11-4** Golden brown pigmentation corresponding to dermal hemosiderin is evident along the posterior aspect of the thigh. The linear pattern is classic for post-sclerotherapy pigmentation induced by detergent sclerosants.

include superficial thrombophlebitis, nerve damage, and necrosis or ulceration with possible scarring. Major, but rare side effects include intra-arterial injection, anaphylaxis, thromboembolic events, or neurologic events. Many of these side effects can be minimized by careful patient screening, matching of sclerosant type, concentration, and volume to vessel size, minimizing injection pressure, eliminating sources of proximal reflux when present, maintaining adequate compression, and strictly avoiding sun.

Post-sclerotherapy pigmentation (PSP) typically manifests as a linear golden brown discoloration along the course of a treated vessel (Figure 11-4). Osmotic sclerosants that elicit maximal injury at the site of injection have been reported to cause a more punctate form. PSP is essentially a hemosiderin tattoo, due to ineffective digestion of extravasated hemosiderin.[24] It occurs independent of concurrent drug ingestion or underlying disease. Resolution within 1 year is the norm, with approximately 1% to 2% of cases persisting longer. Etiologic factors include sclerosant type and concentration, intraoperative technique, gravitational and/or other intravascular pressure, vessel diameter, innate tendency toward cutaneous pigmentation, and compliance with posttreatment compression. Concomitant ingestion of certain medications, such as minocycline, may contribute to a unique pigmentary pattern. Minocycline pigmentation is typically slate gray to blue and commonly persists for more than a year.

PSP is more common with use of higher sclerosant concentrations or foam, when treating vessels around the ankle, as well as after treatment of larger and/or superficial vessels. The highest rates of hyperpigmentation reported have been with STS, with which it occurs in approximately 10% to 30% of patients.[25] Use of glycerin and POL appears to be less likely to result in hyperpigmentation. However, rates of pigmentation are probably comparable for sclerosants when used in concentrations that represent an equivalent denaturing effect.

PSP can be minimized with meticulous technique including treatment of proximal sites of reflux, avoidance of excessive injection pressures, and use of a minimally effective sclerosant concentration. Proper patient counseling, including discontinuation of any oral minocycline, strict sun avoidance, and adequate posttreatment compression, may help to minimize this complication. Unfortunately, there is no perfectly effective way to treat post-sclerotherapy hyperpigmentation. Laser therapy may present a reasonable option, with favorable results being reported with Q-switched laser devices (532, 694, 755, and 1064 nm).[24]

TM presents as clusters of very fine pink and red vessels that give a blushed appearance to the skin (Figure 11-5). The precise etiology is not known;

however, some posit neoangiogenesis due to cytokine release in susceptible individuals.[26] Concurrent hormonal replacement therapy increases one's risk of developing matting.

Matting, which occurs following sclerotherapy, typically resolves spontaneously within several months, but occasionally may persist. Employing the minimal effective sclerosant concentration as well as the lowest possible infusion pressure to deliver the sclerosant can minimize this side effect. Re-treatment with a milder sclerosant such as glycerin, better visualization and treatment of any feeding vessels, and treatment of proximal reflux sources may minimize this complication overall.[24] Laser treatment (potassium titanyl phosphate [KTP], pulsed dye lasers [PDL]) can be employed to treat matting, but carries a risk of pigmentary alteration. If purple or violaceous matting results, duplex should be performed to interrogate for underlying reflux. For some individuals, it may be prudent to defer further treatment until cessation of hormone supplements.

Cutaneous necrosis is most often the result of extravasation or backflow of a strong sclerosant into smaller, more superficial vessels. This uncommon but dreaded side effect can be minimized by meticulous technique, including careful selection of the appropriate strength and volume of a sclerosant, massaging or injection of dilutant at the site of bleb formation, and application of topical nitroglycerin for prolonged blanching.[26] Ulceration may also result from inadvertent intra-arterial injection. If on injection, intra-arterial injection is suspected by patient report of pain or observation of profound blanching, injection should be stopped immediately. Massage and topical nitroglycerin should be applied. In severe cases, patients should be hospitalized for monitoring, anticoagulation, and supportive care. Superficial thrombophlebitis can develop days to weeks after treatment, usually after discontinuation of compression therapy. Compression, along with leg elevation and nonsteroidal anti-inflammatory agents, is the best way to treat this complication.

DVT is a rare adverse event, but may occur when larger vessels are injected, such as with UGFS.[27] When injection of larger vessels is performed, limb elevation and activation of the calf muscle pump immediately following injection can help to minimize passage of active sclerosant into deep system patients. Additionally, patients should ambulate following the procedure and compression stockings must be worn. Care should be taken to avoid injecting an individual prior to long travel or other planned immobility.

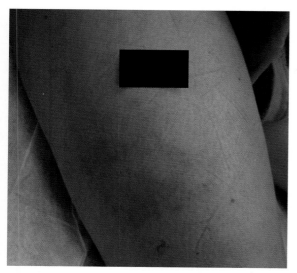

▲ **FIGURE 11-5** Telangiectatic matting. Three weeks following treatment with POL 0.5% liquid, a faint blush to the skin corresponding to new vessel formation is evident. The matting resolved without treatment in 4 months.

LASER AND LIGHT SOURCES

Lower extremity vessels are traditionally less responsive to lasers and light sources than facial vessels. Within an individual, leg vessels are heterogeneous with respect to size, depth, caliber, and flow characteristics precluding a singularly effective laser. Moreover, relative to their facial counterparts, leg vessels are larger in size, situated deeper in the dermis, and transport higher concentrations of deoxygenated blood. Finally, these vessels often have elevated hydrostatic pressure, even when underlying venous disease is not readily apparent.

Limitations aside, lasers and light sources are increasingly utilized in the management of cosmetic and medically significant lower extremity disease. Specifically, these devices may be advantageous when treating noncannulizable microtelangiectasia, persistent matting after sclerotherapy, or otherwise persistent vessels. Additionally, patients often express interest in laser treatments due to unsatisfactory experience with prior sclerotherapy, a fear of needles, or a desire for "newer and better" technologies. Additionally, individuals may be unwilling to comply with compression after sclerotherapy, or may falsely believe that laser treatment is less painful.[28]

Laser Fundamentals and Percutaneous Laser Treatment

Selective photothermolysis mandates 3 basic criteria: (1) a wavelength must be preferentially absorbed by the target chromophore (hemoglobin); (2) the pulse duration must not exceed the thermal relaxation time of the target to limit transference of thermal energy to perivascular tissue; and (3) the fluence or energy density must be sufficient to damage the target.[29]

The chromophore hemoglobin has 3 major absorption peaks in the visible spectrum (418, 542, and 577 nm), as well as a broad peak within the near-infrared region. Accordingly, a wide range of lasers should effectively treat leg vessels. The following lasers are employed in the treatment of leg veins: 532-nm KTP lasers, 585- to 595-nm PDL, 500- to 1200-nm intense pulsed light (IPL) devices, 755-nm alexandrite, 800- to 940-nm diodes, and 1064-nm pulsed neodymium:yttrium-aluminum-garnet (Nd:YAG) lasers.

Pulse duration selection should be based on target vessel size. Blood vessels are nonuniformly absorbing structures, with blood (hemoglobin) acting as a strong absorbing portion and the vessel wall as a weaker portion. Although hemoglobin is the target chromophore, effective vessel closure requires heating of the vessel wall via diffusion from blood. The term *thermal damage time* connotes the extended duration exposure time needed to effectively destroy nonuniformly absorbing structures such as blood vessels.[30]

Millisecond pulse durations are best suited for the treatment of leg telangiectasia. Mathematical modeling has demonstrated that comparable intravascular temperatures are achieved when employing pulse durations within the range of 3 to 100 milliseconds. Longer pulse durations result in more consistent vessel closure.[31] Additionally, purpura, thrombosis, and hyperpigmentation are more common when higher radiant exposures and shorter pulse durations are employed.[32]

Available spot sizes vary depending on the specific device. Larger spot sizes are associated with decreased scatter and increased depth of penetration. However, larger spot sizes are also associated with a narrower safety margin due to a risk of volumetric heating, especially at longer wavelengths. Selecting a spot size that is slightly larger than the target vessel diameter will optimize absorption by the vessel, while minimizing side effects.[30]

High radiant exposures are generally required to effectively treat leg veins with lasers, resulting in a significant risk of epidermal damage. Various means of selective epidermal cooling have been developed and are critical to safe and effective targeting of dermal blood vessel targets. Among the most commonly employed methods are contact cooling (ie, sapphire window or copper plate), cryogen spray cooling, convection air cooling, and aluminum rollers or cold gels. These methods extract heat from the epidermis while allowing necessary peak temperatures to be attained within underlying dermal vessels.[33]

Visible light devices in the range of 532 to 595 nm closely match the absorption peaks of hemoglobin within this portion of the spectrum. However, for vessels with diameters or depths of greater than 1 mm, the optical penetration depth of these devices is too shallow for effective treatment.[30] KTP and PDL are useful for patients with difficult-to-cannulate, pink or red, linear, fine-caliber (<1 mm) vessels. The KTP laser, with a wavelength of 532 nm, approximates the second absorption peak of oxyhemoglobin. However, at this wavelength there is significant competing absorption by melanin resulting in a significant risk of pigmentary alteration, especially in suntanned skin or individuals with greater constitutive pigmentation. Use of larger (3–5 mm) spot sizes, longer pulse widths (10–50 milliseconds), and higher fluences (14–20 J/cm^2) have resulted in superior results.[34]

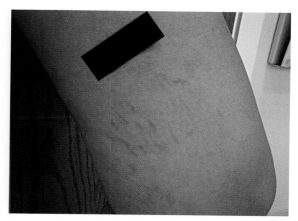

▲ **FIGURE 11-6** Diffuse hyperpigmented patches and persistent vessels are evident following use of pulsed dye laser in a dark-skinned individual.

The first-generation PDL was the first to be developed based on the principles of selective photothermolysis. Initially employed successfully in the treatment of vascular malformations and facial telangiectasias, this device did not have as much success when directed toward the treatment of leg telangiectasias due to limited depth of penetration and relatively short pulse duration.[35–38] Additionally, purpura and posttreatment pigmentary alteration was common.[39] The second-generation (595 nm) PDL offers longer and variable pulse durations and can effectively treat vessels up to 1 mm in diameter and depth,[40] although hyperpigmentation remains a concern, especially in patients with greater constitutive pigmentation (Figure 11-6).

IPL sources emit wavelengths from 500 to 1200 nm, but are commonly used with 550- and 570-nm filters to allow for delivery of yellow and red lights. Similar to the KTP and PDL, these devices can be effective in treatment of small (less than 1 mm), superficial (depth of less than 1 mm), pink to red telangiectasias. However, results are highly variable due to the range of adjusted parameters based on patient skin type, vessel diameter, and depth, as well as operator experience.[41]

Near-infrared devices penetrate more deeply and can achieve closure of deeper and larger, purple to blue veins that carry a higher proportion of deoxygenated blood. These devices take advantage of the broad 750 to 1100 nm absorption band of oxyhemoglobin, providing greater depth of penetration and treatment of larger (up to 3 mm) vessels. When comparing results of short (532 nm) wavelengths with those of long (1064 nm) wavelengths in the treatment of leg veins, it was found that both are capable of treating smaller (<0.3 mm deep and wide) vessels; however, at 532 nm only the circumference of the vessel is heated, compared with a complete and uniform heating with the deeper penetrating 1064 nm wavelength.[42]

Long-pulsed alexandrite lasers have a wavelength of 755 nm and pulse durations of 3 to 20 milliseconds, and can penetrate between 2 and 3 mm in depth. Ideal candidates are of skin types I to III in absence of suntan, with vessels between 0.4 and 2 mm in diameter. Higher fluences, greater than 50 J/cm^2, in combination with skin cooling are required for safe and effective treatment of leg telangiectasias. Posttreatment purpura and hyperpigmentation are commonly observed, the latter reportedly observed in up to 35% of treated patients and lasting 3 months or more. Kauvar and Lou reported greater than 75% improvement in 65% of patients treated with an 8 mm spot size, 3 milliseconds PW, and fluence of 60 to 80 J/cm^2.[43]

Various diode lasers have also been used to treat telangiectasia and reticular veins. With emission at 800, 810, and 940 nm, these lasers have relatively selective hemoglobin absorption with poor absorption by melanin. These lasers combine longer wavelengths with longer pulse durations to allow for successful use of these lasers in treatment of larger vessels in patients of skin types I to IV.[44–46]

Pulsed Nd:YAG lasers are millisecond-domain, 1064-nm lasers designed to treat larger telangiectasias, as well as reticular veins. At this wavelength hemoglobin has a lower absorption coefficient, requiring higher energies to achieve adequate penetration and vessel heating. This can result in increased pain secondary to volumetric heating, limiting its safety window and making adequate cooling and avoidance of pulse stacking essential in treatment with this specific wavelength. Unlike the previously discussed devices, these lasers have been safely used in the treatment of individuals of darker skin types. For the treatment of small vessels, employ a smaller spot size (about 2 mm), shorter pulse duration (15–30 milliseconds), and higher fluence (150–400 J/cm^2), whereas to treat larger vessels (1–3 mm), larger spot size (2–8 mm), longer pulse duration (30–50 milliseconds), and more moderate fluence (100–250 J/cm^2) are appropriate. The Nd:YAG lasers at 1064 nm presently provide the best results for percutaneous treatment of leg veins, permitting a monomodal therapy for treatment of small and larger vessels. However, trials comparing Nd:YAG laser treatment with sclerotherapy demonstrate equivalent results, with significant discomfort associated with laser therapy.

Recent studies suggest that more efficient treatment of leg veins may be achieved by employing a dual-wavelength device, Cynergy™ PDL (Cynosure), which couples a 585 nm and a 1064 nm pulse.[47] The rationale for using such a device is that the initial 585 nm pulse transforms hemoglobin into methemoglobin, which due to its higher absorption coefficient is more efficiently targeted by the subsequent 1064 nm pulse (enabling lower, and therefore safer, fluences).[48] Initial results are promising, although further study of this dual-wavelength device is warranted.

In summary, visible light lasers and IPL are reproducibly effective only for superficial, nonarborizing, pink and red telangiectasia not associated with proximal reflux. For vessels greater than 1 mm in depth and diameter, near-infrared lasers with millisecond pulse durations are required to achieve complete vessel thrombosis and transmural coagulation. Currently, of these devices, the 1064-nm Nd:YAG laser has shown the best results when employed properly with skin cooling and avoidance of pulse stacking.

Treatment of Truncal Varicose Veins

Historically, the treatment of truncal varicosities involved surgical methods including ligation and stripping. These procedures often require epidural or general anesthesia and have a significant risk of collateral damage to the arterial, nervous, and lymphatic systems. Postoperatively, there is a prolonged downtime that can be complicated by wound infections, permanent scarring, and unfortunate high rates of recurrent disease.

Minimally invasive treatments such as UGFS, endovenous laser ablation (EVLA), and radio-frequency ablation (RFA) are increasingly utilized in the management of truncal varicosities. While the medical indications of these procedures are similar, EVLA and RFA are generally preferred for vessels greater than 1.0 cm in diameter, whereas UGFS may be more appropriate for vessels smaller than 0.5 cm, previously treated or recurrent veins after surgery, markedly torturous veins, and incompetent perforator veins. UGFS has also proven helpful in treating venous ulceration.[49] These procedures have reduced serious side effects, cost, and pain with superior efficacy and patient satisfaction. The next section will focus on these minimally invasive procedures.

ULTRASOUND-GUIDED FOAM SCLEROTHERAPY UGFS entails intravenous injection of a foamed sclerosant under direct ultrasound visualization. Intravenous injection can be achieved directly or through a cannula or butterfly needle. Foam concentration and volume injected varies with diameter, depth, and length of targeted vessel. In accordance with the Second European Consensus Meeting report, volume of foam injected should generally not exceed 10 mL per session, although safe use of much higher volumes has been reported. Compression therapy should be applied posttreatment and maintained for approximately 2 weeks, although specific recommendations vary widely among practitioners.[50]

Saphenous closure rates are generally reported to be in the 80% to 90% range at 1 to 2 years of follow-up, although multiple treatments are necessary and occlusion rates appear to drop off with longer follow-up.[20,50,51] Prospective studies comparing UGFS with standard surgery are ongoing.

Side effects are similar to those observed with visual sclerotherapy and include bruising, pigmentary alteration, matting, and less commonly phlebitis or necrosis due to extravasation. Relative to liquid sclerotherapy postinflammatory pigmentary alteration is more commonly seen, but extravasation necrosis is less likely due to lesser concentrations employed with foaming technique. Limiting the volume and concentration of sclerosant injected, and enforcing posttreatment compression can help to limit these adverse events. Thrombotic and embolic events are exceedingly rare, although they have been reported. Limb elevation, engaging the calf muscular pump, and immediate manual compression of the relevant junction after foam injection have been hypothesized to reduce the risk of a DVT, although formal studies are lacking. For patients at elevated risk of thromboembolic complications, prophylactic low-molecular-weight heparin may be employed at the time of procedure, although routine prophylaxis is generally not recommended.

Migraine-like neurologic symptoms and scotomas have been reported following UGFS, although the precise incidence is not known.[22,23] These typically occur within minutes of injection and are self-limited. The pathophysiologic basis for such events is not fully understood. As noted previously, these events were generally considered transient neurologic events and thought attributable to air emboli due to passage of foam through a patent foramen ovale. Recent research purports to reclassify these events as migraine with aura and points toward an etiologic role for the vasoactive substance endothelin.[23]

ENDOVENOUS ABLATION PROCEDURES (EVLA, RFA) EVLA and RFA are gaining increasing popularity for the treatment of saphenous incompetence. They target deoxygenated hemoglobin and/or water (wavelengths

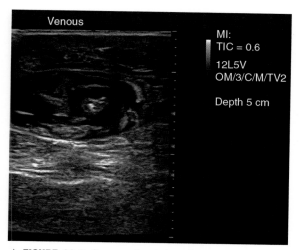

▲ **FIGURE 11-7** Cross-sectional view of great saphenous vein around which a cushion of tumescent anesthesia is visible.

810–1500 nm) and have shown reduction in serious side effects, cost, and pain with improvement in efficacy and patient satisfaction.[50] EVLA and RFA are effective in treating insufficiency of the GSV or SSV, and are the treatments of choice for veins greater than 1.0 cm in diameter. Both are performed in an outpatient setting under local tumescent anesthesia and ultrasound guidance[50] (Figure 11-7).

Preoperatively, duplex examination is performed to map out the incompetent vessel(s) and identify the access point. Topical nitropaste can be applied topically to the anticipated access point—typically at or above the knee for the GSV or mid-calf for the SSV—to facilitate needle access. Access to the diseased vessel is attained under ultrasound guidance with a hollow needle. A guidewire is then passed through the needle with caution, as risk for perforation and embolic events exists, especially in the setting of recurrent varicosities. Once the guidewire is in place, the needle is removed, and then an introducer sheath is passed over the guidewire. The guidewire is removed and the laser fiber is advanced and positioned a few centimeters distal to the junction. Tumescent anesthesia is then administered within the intrafacial plane above and below the vessel (Figure 11-8). This cushion of anesthesia compresses the vessel wall against the laser fiber, anesthetizes the entire course of the vessel, and achieves a thermal sink, thereby protecting surrounding vital structures from thermal injury. The laser is fired as it is withdrawn, typically in a continuous mode, along the course of the diseased vessel.

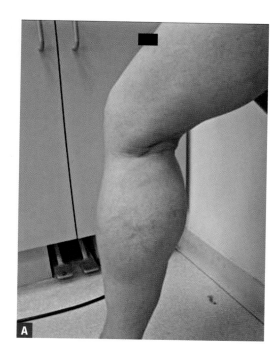

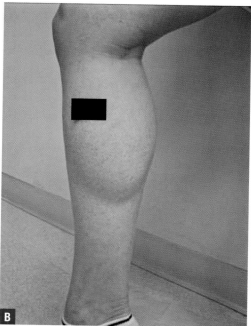

6 months s/p EVA + UGFS × 2

▲ **FIGURE 11-8** Patient with superficial venous insufficiency of the right GSV, pre-endovenous ablation (**A**) and post-endovenous ablation (**B**) with the CoolTouch CTEV (1320 nm) laser and 2 sessions of UGFS.

RFA is a similar technique to EVLA; however, electrodes at the end of the RFA catheter are in direct contact with the vessel wall and emit high radio-frequency energy as the catheter is withdrawn heating the tissue up to 85 to 120°C. This heat is conducted to deeper planes, resulting in destruction of the vessel wall, lumen obliteration, and contraction of perivascular collagen.[52] At higher temperatures (120°, VNUS ClosureFAST), faster pullback can be employed.

The majority of published series and systematic reviews of EVLA report occlusion rates exceeding 90%.[53] Several of the larger series, 1 involving 1000 patients, reported success rates ranging from 93% to 97% at least 2 years after therapy.[54–57] The first large case series examining RFA also demonstrated this technique to be effective in about 90% of treated limbs 2 years after intervention.[58] Both of these therapies have been met with greater patient satisfaction and fewer adverse events when compared with surgical vein stripping.[59–64] A recent meta-analysis demonstrated EVLA to be significantly more effective than RFA, stripping, and UGFS, with 3-year success rates of 95%, 84%, 78%, and 77%, respectively.[65]

The most common side effects of EVLA and RFA are ecchymosis and local phlebitic-type pain that generally abates within 1 to 2 weeks with compression and NSAIDs. Postprocedural bruising and discomfort may be reduced with longer-wavelength lasers that target water and are less likely to induce microperforations than hemoglobin-dependent devices. Less common side effects include skin burns, usually due to inadequate tumescence or careless technique. Neurologic injury is uncommonly seen, but may be more likely when the GSV is accessed below the knee or when treating the proximal SSV. The likelihood of DVT is less than 1% for both EVLA and RFA. This risk may be reduced with prophylactic anticoagulation for at-risk patients, proper positioning of the laser tip, ample tumescence, avoidance of prolonged inactivity or lengthy travel during the perioperative period, and encouraging patient ambulation in the days postprocedure. Scarring is limited to the access point and typically is minimal to nonexistent. Hyperpigmentation has been reported, although matting does not classically occur. Importantly, neovascularization at the SFJ, commonly seen after stripping, has not been reported. Partial or complete recanalization does occur in up to 10% of treated patients, although a smaller percentage manifest with recurrence of clinical symptoms.

In summary, since their introduction over a decade ago, these minimally invasive treatments are increasingly utilized in the management of medically significant lower extremity venous disease. Further comparative studies are ongoing and encouraged; however, relative to surgery, these procedures appear to be associated with less serious side effects, lesser cost, and improved patient outcomes.[55–57,66–69]

CONCLUSION

Endovenous technologies including UGFS, EVLA, and RFA have dramatically altered the way we manage symptomatic venous disease. For nonvaricose, heterogeneous lower extremity vessels, sclerotherapy remains the gold standard of therapy. Despite tremendous advances in cutaneous laser surgery, application of laser and light technology to leg veins remains an ongoing challenge. Near-infrared lasers equipped with novel cooling mechanisms, variable spot sizes and pulse durations, and higher fluences have vastly improved the safety and efficacy of percutaneous laser treatment of leg veins.

REFERENCES

1. Callam MJ. Epidemiology of varicose veins. *Br J Surg.* 1994;81(2):167–173.
2. Engel A, Johnson ML, Haynes SG. Health effects of sunlight exposure in the United States. Results from the first National Health and Nutrition Examination Survey, 1971–1974. *Arch Dermatol.* 1988;124(1):72–79.
3. Abramson JH, Hopp C, Epstein LM. The epidemiology of varicose veins. A survey in western Jerusalem. *J Epidemiol Community Health.* 1981;35(3):213–217.
4. Kurz X, Kahn SR, Abenhaim L, et al. Chronic venous disorders of the leg: epidemiology, outcomes, diagnosis and management. Summary of an evidence-based report of the VEINES task force. Venous Insufficiency Epidemiologic and Economic Studies. *Int Angiol.* 1999; 18(2):83–102.
5. Hayes CA, Kingsley JR, Hamby KR, et al. The effect of endovenous laser ablation on restless legs syndrome. *Phlebology.* 2008;23(3):112–117.
6. Marston WA. Evaluation of varicose veins: what do the clinical signs and symptoms reveal about the underlying disease and need for intervention? *Semin Vasc Surg.* 2010;23(2):78–84.
7. Tuchsen F, Hannerz H, Burr H, et al. Prolonged standing at work and hospitalisation due to varicose veins: a 12 year prospective study of the Danish population. *Occup Environ Med.* 2005;62(12):847–850.
8. Makris SA, Karkos CD, Awad S, et al. An "all-comers" venous duplex scan policy for patients with lower limb varicose veins attending a one-stop vascular clinic: is it justified? *Eur J Vasc Endovasc Surg.* 2006;32(6):718–724.
9. Cavezzi A, Labropoulos N, Partsch H, et al. Duplex ultrasound investigation of the veins in chronic venous disease of the lower limbs—UIP consensus document. Part II. Anatomy. *Vasa.* 2007;36(1):62–71.

10. Biswas S, Clark A, Shields DA. Randomised clinical trial of the duration of compression therapy after varicose vein surgery. *Eur J Vasc Endovasc Surg.* 2007;33(5):631–637.

11. Weiss RA, Sadick NS, Goldman MP, et al. Post-sclerotherapy compression: controlled comparative study of duration of compression and its effects on clinical outcome. *Dermatol Surg.* 1999;25(2):105–108.

12. Weiss RA, Duffy D. Clinical benefits of lightweight compression: reduction of venous-related symptoms by ready-to-wear lightweight gradient compression hosiery. *Dermatol Surg.* 1999;25(9):701–704.

13. Kern P, Ramelet AA, Wutschert R, et al. Compression after sclerotherapy for telangiectasias and reticular leg veins: a randomized controlled study. *J Vasc Surg.* 2007;45(6):1212–1216.

14. Henry ME, Fegan WG, Pegum JM. Five-year survey of the treatment of varicose ulcers. *Br Med J.* 1971;2(5760):493–494.

15. Goldman MP. Treatment of varicose and telangiectatic leg veins: double-blind prospective comparative trial between aethoxyskerol and sotradecol. *Dermatol Surg.* 2002;28(1):52–55.

16. Weiss RA, Weiss MA. Resolution of pain associated with varicose and telangiectatic leg veins after compression sclerotherapy. *J Dermatol Surg Oncol.* 1990;16(4):333–336.

17. Breu FX, Guggenbichler S, Wollmann JC. 2nd European Consensus Meeting on Foam Sclerotherapy 2006, Tegernsee, Germany. *Vasa.* 2008;37(suppl 71):1–29.

18. Wright D, Gobin JP, Bradbury AW, et al. Varisolve polidocanol microfoam compared with surgery or sclerotherapy in the management of varicose veins in the presence of trunk vein incompetence: European randomized controlled trial. *Phlebology.* 2006;21:180–190.

19. Tessari L. Nouvelle technique d'obtention de la sclero-mousse. *Phlebologie.* 2000;53:129–133.

20. Cabrera J, Redondo P, Becerra A, et al. Ultrasound-guided injection of polidocanol microfoam in the management of venous leg ulcers. *Arch Dermatol.* 2004;140(6):667–673.

21. Wright DD. What is the current role of foam sclerotherapy in treating reflux and varicosities? *Semin Vasc Surg.* 2010;23(2):123–126.

22. Ceulen RP, Sommer A, Vernooy K. Microembolism during foam sclerotherapy of varicose veins. *N Engl J Med.* 2008;358(14):1525–1526.

23. Gillet JL, Donnet A, Lausecker M, et al. Pathophysiology of visual disturbances occurring after foam sclerotherapy. *Phlebology.* 2010;25(5):261–266.

24. Munavalli GS, Weiss RA. Complications of sclerotherapy. *Semin Cutan Med Surg.* 2007;26(1):22–28.

25. Georgiev M. Postsclerotherapy hyperpigmentations: a one-year follow-up. *J Dermatol Surg Oncol.* 1990;16(7):608–610.

26. Davis LT, Duffy DM. Determination of incidence and risk factors for postsclerotherapy telangiectatic matting of the lower extremity: a retrospective analysis. *J Dermatol Surg Oncol.* 1990;16(4):327–330.

27. Gillet JL, Guedes JM, Guex JJ, et al. Side-effects and complications of foam sclerotherapy of the great and small saphenous veins: a controlled multicentre prospective study including 1,025 patients. *Phlebology.* 2009;24(3):131–138.

28. Coles CM, Werner RS, Zelickson BD. Comparative pilot study evaluating the treatment of leg veins with a long pulse ND:YAG laser and sclerotherapy. *Lasers Surg Med.* 2002;30(2):154–159.

29. Anderson RR, Parrish JA. Selective photothermolysis: precise microsurgery by selective absorption of pulsed radiation. *Science.* 1983;220(4596):524–527.

30. Kauvar AN, Khrom T. Laser treatment of leg veins. *Semin Cutan Med Surg.* 2005;24(4):184–192.

31. Ross EV, Domankevitz Y. Laser treatment of leg veins: physical mechanisms and theoretical considerations. *Lasers Surg Med.* 2005;36(2):105–116.

32. Parlette EC, Groff WF, Kinshella MJ, et al. Optimal pulse durations for the treatment of leg telangiectasias with a neodymium YAG laser. *Lasers Surg Med.* 2006;38(2):98–105.

33. Nelson JS, Milner TE, Anvari B, et al. Dynamic epidermal cooling during pulsed laser treatment of port-wine stain. A new methodology with preliminary clinical evaluation. *Arch Dermatol.* 1995;131(6):695–700.

34. Uebelhoer NS, Bogle MA, Stewart B, et al. A split-face comparison study of pulsed 532-nm KTP laser and 595-nm pulsed dye laser in the treatment of facial telangiectasias and diffuse telangiectatic facial erythema. *Dermatol Surg.* 2007;33(4):441–448.

35. Garden JM, Polla LL, Tan OT. The treatment of port-wine stains by the pulsed dye laser. Analysis of pulse duration and long-term therapy. *Arch Dermatol.* 1988;124(6):889–896.

36. Tan OT, Morrison P, Kurban AK. 585 nm for the treatment of port-wine stains. *Plast Reconstr Surg.* 1990;86(6):1112–1117.

37. Tan OT, Murray S, Kurban AK. Action spectrum of vascular specific injury using pulsed irradiation. *J Invest Dermatol.* 1989;92(6):868–871.

38. West TB, Alster TS. Comparison of the long-pulse dye (590–595 nm) and KTP (532 nm) lasers in the treatment of facial and leg telangiectasias. *Dermatol Surg.* 1998;24(2):221–226.

39. Goldman MP, Fitzpatrick RE. Pulsed-dye laser treatment of leg telangiectasia: with and without simultaneous sclerotherapy. *J Dermatol Surg Oncol.* 1990;16(4):338–344.

40. Hsia J, Lowery JA, Zelickson B. Treatment of leg telangiectasia using a long-pulse dye laser at 595 nm. *Lasers Surg Med.* 1997;20(1):1–5.

41. Schroeter CA, Neumann HA. An intense light source. The photoderm VL-flashlamp as a new treatment possibility for vascular skin lesions. *Dermatol Surg.* 1998;24(7):743–748.

42. Ross EV, Smirnov M, Pankratov M, et al. Intense pulsed light and laser treatment of facial telangiectasias and dyspigmentation: some theoretical and practical comparisons. *Dermatol Surg.* 2005;31(9 pt 2):1188–1198.

43. Kauvar AN, Lou WW. Pulsed alexandrite laser for the treatment of leg telangiectasia and reticular veins. *Arch Dermatol.* 2000;136(11):1371–1375.

44. Tierney E, Hanke CW. Randomized controlled trial: comparative efficacy for the treatment of facial telangiectasias with 532 nm versus 940 nm diode laser. *Lasers Surg Med.* 2009;41(8):555–562.

45. Trelles MA, Allones I, Alvarez J, et al. The 800-nm diode laser in the treatment of leg veins: assessment at 6 months. *J Am Acad Dermatol.* 2006;54(2):282–289.

46. Trelles MA, Martin-Vazquez M, Trelles OR, et al. Treatment effects of combined radio-frequency current and a 900 nm diode laser on leg blood vessels. *Lasers Surg Med.* 2006;38(3):185–195.

47. Trelles MA, Weiss R, Moreno-Moragas J, et al. Treatment of leg veins with combined pulsed dye and Nd:YAG lasers: 60 patients assessed at 6 months. *Lasers Surg Med.* 2010;42(9):609–614.

48. Mordon S, Brisot D, Fournier N. Using a "non uniform pulse sequence" can improve selective coagulation with a Nd:YAG laser (1.06 microm) thanks to Met-hemoglobin absorption: a clinical study on blue leg veins. *Lasers Surg Med.* 2003;32(2):160–170.

49. Pascarella L, Bergan JJ, Mekenas LV. Severe chronic venous insufficiency treated by foamed sclerosant. *Ann Vasc Surg.* 2006;20(1):83–91.

50. Nijsten T, van den Bos RR, Goldman MP, et al. Minimally invasive techniques in the treatment of saphenous varicose veins. *J Am Acad Dermatol.* 2009;60(1): 110–119.

51. Darke SG, Baker SJ. Ultrasound-guided foam sclerotherapy for the treatment of varicose veins. *Br J Surg.* 2006; 93(8):969–974.

52. Schmedt CG, Sroka R, Steckmeier S, et al. Investigation on radiofrequency and laser (980 nm) effects after endoluminal treatment of saphenous vein insufficiency in an ex-vivo model. *Eur J Vasc Endovasc Surg.* 2006;32(3): 318–325.

53. Navarro L, Min RJ, Bone C. Endovenous laser: a new minimally invasive method of treatment for varicose veins—preliminary observations using an 810 nm diode laser. *Dermatol Surg.* 2001;27(2):117–122.

54. Pannier F, Rabe E. Endovenous laser therapy and radiofrequency ablation of saphenous varicose veins. *J Cardiovasc Surg (Torino).* 2006;47(1):3–8.

55. Min RJ, Khilnani N, Zimmet SE. Endovenous laser treatment of saphenous vein reflux: long-term results. *J Vasc Interv Radiol.* 2003;14(8):991–996.

56. Agus GB, Mancini S, Magi G. The first 1000 cases of Italian Endovenous-laser Working Group (IEWG). Rationale, and long-term outcomes for the 1999–2003 period. *Int Angiol.* 2006;25(2):209–215.

57. Ravi R, Diethrich EB. Regarding "Diffuse phlegmonous phlebitis after endovenous laser treatment of the great saphenous vein". *J Vasc Surg.* 2006;44(4):912–913 [author reply 913].

58. Weiss RA. Comparison of endovenous radiofrequency versus 810 nm diode laser occlusion of large veins in an animal model. *Dermatol Surg.* 2002;28(1):56–61.

59. de Medeiros CA, Luccas GC. Comparison of endovenous treatment with an 810 nm laser versus conventional stripping of the great saphenous vein in patients with primary varicose veins. *Dermatol Surg.* 2005;31(12): 1685–1694.

60. Mekako AI, Hatfield J, Bryce J, et al. A nonrandomised controlled trial of endovenous laser therapy and surgery in the treatment of varicose veins. *Ann Vasc Surg.* 2006; 20(4):451–457.

61. Rasmussen LH, Bjoern L, Lawaetz M, et al. Randomized trial comparing endovenous laser ablation of the great saphenous vein with high ligation and stripping in patients with varicose veins: short-term results. *J Vasc Surg.* 2007;46(2):308–315.

62. Rautio TT, Perala JM, Wiik HT, et al. Endovenous obliteration with radiofrequency-resistive heating for greater saphenous vein insufficiency: a feasibility study. *J Vasc Interv Radiol.* 2002;13(6):569–575.

63. Puggioni A, Lurie F, Kistner RL, et al. How often is deep venous reflux eliminated after saphenous vein ablation? *J Vasc Surg.* 2003;38(3):517–521.

64. Perala J, Rautio T, Biancari F, et al. Radiofrequency endovenous obliteration versus stripping of the long saphenous vein in the management of primary varicose veins: 3-year outcome of a randomized study. *Ann Vasc Surg.* 2005;19(5):669–672.

65. van den Bos R, Arends L, Kockaert M, et al. Endovenous therapies of lower extremity varicosities: a meta-analysis. *J Vasc Surg.* 2009;49(1):230–239.

66. Puggioni A, Kalra M, Carmo M, et al. Endovenous laser therapy and radiofrequency ablation of the great saphenous vein: analysis of early efficacy and complications. *J Vasc Surg.* 2005;42(3):488–493.

67. Almeida JI, Raines JK. Radiofrequency ablation and laser ablation in the treatment of varicose veins. *Ann Vasc Surg.* 2006;20(4):547–552.

68. Merchant RF, DePalma RG, Kabnick LS. Endovascular obliteration of saphenous reflux: a multicenter study. *J Vasc Surg.* 2002;35(6):1190–1196.

69. Gale SS, Dosick SM, Seiwert AJ, et al. Regarding "Deep venous thrombosis after radiofrequency ablation of greater saphenous vein". *J Vasc Surg.* 2005;41(2):374 [author reply 374].

Index